The COVID-19 Pandemic: Epidemiology, Molecular Biology and Therapy

Edited by

Shama Parveen

Centre for Interdisciplinary Research in Basic Sciences
Jamia Millia Islamia
New Delhi
India

The COVID-19 Pandemic: Epidemiology, Molecular Biology and Therapy

Editor: Shama Parveen

ISBN (Online): 978-981-14-8187-1

ISBN (Print): 978-981-14-8185-7

ISBN (Paperback): 978-981-14-8186-4

need for a court order if at any point you breach any terms of this License Agreement. In no event will any delay or failure by Bentham Science Publishers in enforcing your compliance with this License Agreement constitute a waiver of any of its rights.

3. You acknowledge that you have read this License Agreement, and agree to be bound by its terms and conditions. To the extent that any other terms and conditions presented on any website of Bentham Science Publishers conflict with, or are inconsistent with, the terms and conditions set out in this License Agreement, you acknowledge that the terms and conditions set out in this License Agreement shall prevail.

Bentham Science Publishers Pte. Ltd.
80 Robinson Road #02-00
Singapore 068898
Singapore
Email: subscriptions@benthamscience.net

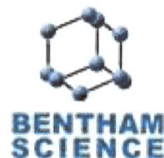

BENTHAM SCIENCE

CONTENTS

Irshad H. Naqvi, Md. Imam Faizan, Mohammad Islamuddin, Mohd Abdullah
Arpita Rai and Shama Parveen

Anwar Ahmed, Fahad N. Almajhdi, Md. Imam Faizan, Tanveer Ahmad and
Shama Parveen

FOREWORD

Zoonotic viruses are becoming a threat for mankind since they keep on jumping the species. The emergence of some of these viral infections that were seen in the 21st century include Avian Influenza, Ebola, Nipah, Sever Acute Respiratory Syndrome (SARS) and Middle East Respiratory Syndrome (MERS). But none of these epidemics reached this magnitude as Coronavirus Disease 2019 (COVID-19). This infection was first reported in December 2019 in Huanan seafood market, in the capital of China's Hubei province, Wuhan. Later, the infection spread to different parts of the globe leading to the pandemic. It has affected millions of people across the globe and has led to death of more than a million affected individuals. It reminds us of the Swine Flu pandemic of 1918-19 when millions of people died, and the morbidity was quite high. COVID-19 is caused by a beta coronavirus that is named as severe acute respiratory syndrome coronavirus-2 (SARS-CoV-2) because of its similarity with SARS CoV and other bat coronaviruses.

In these unprecedented times of the Coronavirus pandemic which is gripping the whole world, the idea of writing a book on **"The COVID-19 Pandemic: Epidemiology, Molecular Biology and Therapy"** by Dr. Shama Parveen is a very timely effort and is going to provide a comprehensive account for the readers about this topic. The first chapter of the book gives a general introduction to COVID-19 and the topics that are discussed in the book. This book has all the relevant and important topics covered. The next 3 chapters deal with the biology of the SARS-CoV-2 *i.e.,* morphology, genomic organization, proteins and viral replication; molecular characterization of major structural proteins of the pathogen and codon based characterization of S2 subunit of severe acute respiratory syndrome-related coronaviruses. This knowledge about the structure of the virus and its genomics is needed to develop the tools for diagnosis, prevention and treatment. The next chapters are on global epidemiology and transmission of COVID-19; risk factors for severe disease; clinical manifestations, management, pathogenesis and host immune response to COVID-19 and current diagnostic approaches to detect the infection. These chapters are of practical importance and are useful for the public health workers as well as for clinicians and laboratory personnel. The last few chapters are focussed on treatment and prevention and they cover some important topics like natural compounds and drug repurposing candidates as potential therapeutic agents against this infection. Finally, the last chapter focusses on COVID-19 vaccine development: challenges and current scenario.

The efforts put in by Dr. Shama Parveen and her team in compiling all the knowledge in a such a short time is highly commendable. Although there has been an explosion of knowledge on SARS-CoV-2 and COVID-19 and the WHO has named it as 'Infodemic', however a concise and accurate information which covers all the relevant fields in a single platform is lacking. This book will thus be extremely useful for scientists, researchers, doctors, epidemiologists and public health personnel as well students of Science and Virology.

Science and Medicine has made so much progress in the last 100 years and though this pandemic has brought the whole world on its knees, we must also appreciate the efforts of the scientific community in providing diagnostic assays for COVID-19 within 15 days and hopefully a vaccine within a year. With COVID-19, I believe it's God's way of telling us: **"Only Humans can Save Humans with Humanity and Knowledge".**

Dr. Shobha Broor
Ex Professor, Microbiology
AIIMS, New Delhi
Professor Emeritus
SGT University, Gurgaon
India

PREFACE

COVID-19 pandemic has affected almost every part of the globe with millions of infections and more than a million deaths. According to WHO, the infection has spread to almost all the countries and territories with USA, India, Brazil and Russia being the most affected ones. The infection is caused by a novel severe acute respiratory syndrome coronavirus 2 (SARS-CoV-2) that causes Coronavirus Disease 2019 (COVID-19). This pandemic originated as an outbreak in Wuhan, Hubei province in China at the end of 2019. Small animals like pangolin or bat are speculated to be the initial source of human infection in China leading to a local outbreak in Wuhan. Later, the infection spread its tentacles across the world through travellers and it was declared a pandemic by WHO on 11th March 2020. The longer incubation period, aerosol-mediated as well as air-borne spread and pre-symptomatic spread resulted in high transmission rates thereby infecting the humans at an unprecedented scale. The pandemic was fuelled further by the undiagnosed asymptomatic cases. Therefore, WHO recommended "isolation" of the infected patients and quarantining of the individuals who encountered the patients. Most of the countries implemented "lockdown" to take care of the ever-increasing cases and recommended "social distancing" to minimize human interactions. The pandemic has devastated all walks of life but the only saving grace is healing of the nature and nurturing of the environment. Thus, we have less polluted environment, more pristine forest and cleaner water bodies. The pandemic has impacted the social life and global economy as well.

SARS-CoV-2 is a Betacoronavirus like the two other human viruses which includes SARS and MERS of the same group. SARS-CoV-2 is spherical in shape having crown like surface structure formed by the spike (S) protein. Its genome is negative sense single stranded RNA of 30Kb that codes for 4 structural and 16 non-structural proteins. The S, M (membrane), E (envelope) and N (nucleocapsid) forms the structure of the virion. The non-structural proteins play a pivotal role in viral replication within the host cell cytoplasm following the entry of the virus.

The COVID-19 shows diverse clinical manifestations and results in asymptomatic, mild, severe and critical illness. The intense host immune response due to infection of the lower respiratory tract leads to generation of "cytokine storm". Further, complications like respiratory and multi-organ failure and septic shock in many cases cause death. Certain individuals (elderly, males, and type A blood group) and people with co-morbidities (diabetes, hypertension, existing respiratory disease, *etc*) are vulnerable to the severe infection. The most reliable diagnosis is based on the real time PCR assays and antigen detection during first few days of infection. At a later stage, the infection is detected by rapid tests or ELISA that are based on the detection of IgM/IgG serology. The treatment of the patients is symptomatic in the absence of antiviral drugs and prophylactic vaccine. Antipyretics, antivirals and supplements are used for the treatment of the COVID-19 patients. However, clinical trials of several antivirals and other drugs are going on at war footing to contain this infection. Interestingly, several vaccine candidates are also under clinical trials across the globe.

The present book "The COVID-19 Pandemic: Epidemiology, Molecular Biology and Therapy" deals with all the significant aspects of the ongoing COVID-19 pandemic including the pathogen (morphology, genome, proteins, structural protein genes, replication), global epidemiology, transmission, risk factors, clinical manifestation, management, host immune response, pathogenesis, diagnosis, therapeutic agents (antiviral and other drugs, natural compounds) and vaccines.

We hope that this book will provide basic but relevant information about the different aspects of COVID-19 to scientists, academicians and common citizens alike. Eventually, if this book inspires any one in any manner to become more civic and responsible citizen of the globe, we will achieve our goal.

Shama Parveen
Centre for Interdisciplinary Research in Basic Sciences
Jamia Millia Islamia
New Delhi
India

List of Contributors

Abu Hamza Centre for Interdisciplinary Research in Basic Sciences, Jamia Millia Islamia, New Delhi, India

Anwar Ahmed Center of Excellence in Biotechnology Research, College of Science, King Saud University, Riyadh, Saudi Arabia
Department of Biochemistry, College of Science King Saud University, Riyadh, Saudi Arabia

Arpita Rai Department of Oral Medicine and Radiology, Dental Institute Rajendra Institute of Medical Sciences Ranchi, Jharkhand, India

Arshi Islam Centre for Interdisciplinary Research in Basic Sciences, Jamia Millia Islamia, New Delhi, India

Asimul Islam Centre for Interdisciplinary Research in Basic Sciences, Jamia Millia Islamia, New Delhi, India

Ayesha Tazeen Centre for Interdisciplinary Research in Basic Sciences, Jamia Millia Islamia, New Delhi, India

Fahad N. Almajhdi Center of Excellence in Biotechnology Research, College of Science, King Saud University, Riyadh, Saudi Arabia
Department of Botany & Microbiology, College of Science, King Saud University, Riyadh, Saudi Arabia

Farah Deeba Centre for Interdisciplinary Research in Basic Sciences, Jamia Millia Islamia, New Delhi, India

Irshad H. Naqvi Dr. M. A. Ansari Health Centre, Jamia Millia Islamia, New Delhi, India

Maryam Sarwat Department of Pharmacology, Amity University, Noida, Uttar Pradesh, India

Md. Wasim Khan Centre for Interdisciplinary Research in Basic Sciences, Jamia Millia Islamia, New Delhi, India

Md. Imam Faizan Multidisciplinary Centre for Advanced Research and Studies, Jamia Millia Islamia, New Delhi, India
Centre for Interdisciplinary Research in Basic Sciences, Jamia Millia Islamia, New Delhi, India

Md. Shakir H. Haider Centre for Interdisciplinary Research in Basic Sciences, Jamia Millia Islamia, New Delhi, India

Mohammad Islamuddin Centre for Interdisciplinary Research in Basic Sciences, Jamia Millia Islamia, New Delhi, India

Mohammed Misbah Urrehmaan Department of Biotechnology, School of Chemical and Life Sciences Jamia Hamdard, New Delhi, India

Mohammed Khalid Parvez Department of Pharmacognosy, College of Pharmacy, King Saud University, Riyadh, Saudi Arabia

Mohd Abdullah Dr. M. A. Ansari Health Centre, Jamia Millia Islamia, New Delhi, India

Nasir Salam Department of Microbiology, Central University of Punjab, Bathinda, Panjab, India

Nazim Khan	Centre for Interdisciplinary Research in Basic Sciences, Jamia Millia Islamia, New Delhi, India
Nazish Parveen	Centre for Interdisciplinary Research in Basic Sciences, Jamia Millia Islamia, New Delhi, India
Priyanka Sinha	Centre for Interdisciplinary Research in Basic Sciences, Jamia Millia Islamia, New Delhi, India
Ravins Dohare	Centre for Interdisciplinary Research in Basic Sciences, Jamia Millia Islamia, New Delhi, India
Saba Parveen	Centre for Interdisciplinary Research in Basic Sciences, Jamia Millia Islamia, New Delhi, India
Saima Wajid	Department of Biotechnology, School of Chemical and Life Sciences Jamia Hamdard, New Delhi, India
Sajda Ara	Centre for Interdisciplinary Research in Basic Sciences, Jamia Millia Islamia, New Delhi, India
Shama Parveen	Centre for Interdisciplinary Research in Basic Sciences, Jamia Millia Islamia, New Delhi, India
Sher Ali	School of Basic Sciences and Research, Department of Life Sciences, Sharda University, Greater Noida, India
Syed Abuzar Raza Rizvi	Department of Biotechnology, School of Chemical and Life Sciences Jamia Hamdard, New Delhi, India
Syed Naqui Kazim	Centre for Interdisciplinary Research in Basic Sciences, Jamia Millia Islamia, New Delhi, India
Tanveer Ahmad	Multidisciplinary Centre for Advanced Research and Studies, Jamia Millia Islamia, New Delhi, India
Zoya Shafat	Centre for Interdisciplinary Research in Basic Sciences, Jamia Millia Islamia, New Delhi, India

CHAPTER 1

An Introduction to Coronavirus Disease 2019 (COVID-19)

Shama Parveen[1,*] and **Sher Ali**[2]

[1] Centre for Interdisciplinary Research in Basic Sciences, Jamia Millia Islamia, New Delhi, India

[2] School of Basic Sciences and Research, Department of Life Sciences, Sharda University, Greater Noida, India

Abstract: Severe acute respiratory syndrome coronavirus 2 (SARS-CoV-2) is the causative agent of the global pandemic of Coronavirus Disease 2019 (COVID-19). More than 24.8 million global cases and 0.84 million deaths have been reported until the 31st August 2020. SARS-CoV-2 is like other human coronaviruses *i.e.* SARS and Middle East respiratory syndrome (MERS) but its transmission rate is much higher, biology is more complicated, and mechanism of action is still elusive. Certain individuals like elderly, males, people with type A blood group and persons with co-morbidities (diabetes, hypertension, obesity, *etc.*) are susceptible to severe infection. One of the major concerns is that the asymptomatic individuals and persons in incubation period may also transmit the pathogen. Treatment of the affected individuals is symptomatic in the absence of antiviral drugs or vaccines. Collaborative clinical, epidemiological, molecular and immunological investigations are needed at war-footing across the globe to identify the evolutionary trajectories, mutational load, host immune response, therapeutics and vaccines against this pathogen. Pandemic has drastically affected the social life, economy, travel and transportation, educational systems, aviation, to name a few. However, it has a positive impact on the environment, wildlife, water bodies and forests. This warrants us to get ready to face aftermath scenario of this pandemic and rebuild the system. This by no means would be a simple task as it involves large scale resource mobilization, unprecedented development of sagging economy and infrastructures, rebooting the society, nations and the world after the default control-alt –delete mode of the pandemic.

Keywords: Clinical symptoms, COVID-19, Diagnosis, Epidemiology, Genome, Management, Natural compounds, Risk factors, SARS-CoV-2, Socio-economic-environmental effects, Therapeutics, Vaccines.

INTRODUCTION

The pandemic of COVID-19 has caused more than 24 million infections in diffe-

---

* **Corresponding author Shama Parveen:** Centre for Interdisciplinary Research in Basic Sciences, Jamia Millia Islamia, New Delhi, India; E-mails: sparveen2@jmi.ac.in and shamp25@yahoo.com

rent parts of the globe till 31st August 2020. The causative agent is known as severe acute respiratory syndrome coronavirus 2 (SARS-CoV-2). The infection started as a pneumonia outbreak in Wuhan, China at the end of 2019 and within a few months the infection spread its tentacles around the globe leading to an unprecedented pandemic. The present chapter illustrates the key features of the pathogen like morphology, genome organization, proteins and replication pattern. The S (spike), M (membrane), E (envelope) and N (nucleocapsid) are the structural proteins that are part of mature virion. We have carried out molecular characterization of these proteins employing phylogenetic, entropy and selection pressure analyses.

In addition, we have also focussed on some crucial aspects of the viral infection such as global epidemiology, transmission, risk factors, clinical manifestations, management of patients, pathogenesis and host immune response. In addition, we have also discussed the current diagnostic approaches for detection of viral infection. The existing and newer therapeutics against COVID-19, including antiviral drugs and natural compounds are highlighted. Finally, the candidates being evaluated for a prophylactic vaccine are shown. All these crucial attributes of the COVID-19 pandemic are discussed in the present book and are shown here diagrammatically (Fig. **1**).

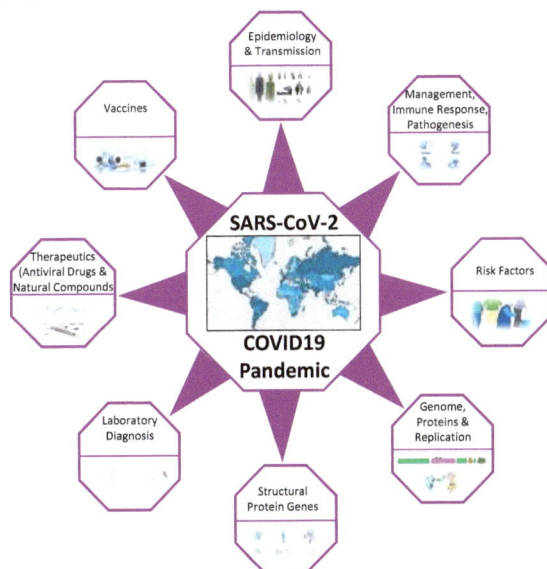

Fig. (1). The Pandemic of COVID-19. Different aspects of SARS-CoV-2 like genome, proteins (including structural proteins) and viral replication are studied. The world map was taken from the WHO website. In addition, the clinical manifestations and their management, pathogenesis and host immune response are taken into consideration for better management of the patients. Different aspects of the pandemic like epidemiology, transmission, risk factors, laboratory diagnosis, therapeutics and vaccine approaches are analysed for containment of the COVID-19 pandemic.

MORPHOLOGY, GENOME, PROTEINS AND VIRAL REPLICATION

SARS-CoV-2 is a spherical pathogen with S protein forming a crown like structure on its surface [1]. SARS-CoV-2 belongs to the family *Coronaviridae*, subfamily *Coronavirinae* and genera Betacoranviruses [2]. Other human pathogens of Betacoronaviruses include SARS and Middle East respiratory syndrome (MERS) that have caused outbreaks in China during 2002-03 and in Saudi Arabia during 2012-13, respectively [3]. The pathogen has showed much higher transmission rate but lower mortality rate as compared to its other two counterparts. SARS-CoV-2 genome shares genetic similarity with bat coronaviruses (88%), SARS (79%) and MERS (50%) [4]. The single stranded negative sense RNA genome of the virus is 30kb in length that codes for 4 structural and 16 non-structural proteins [5]. The structural proteins encompassing S, M, E and N are part of the mature virion. The non-structural proteins (nsp1-16) are present in infected cells and are involved in viral genome replication [5, 6]. The S protein is composed of S1 (binds to receptor) and S2 (host cell membrane fusion) subunits [7]. The receptor binding domain (RBD) of S protein binds to angiotensin converting enzyme 2 (ACE2) receptor on the host cell and determines the host cell tropism for successful infection [1]. The number of pathogen particles (viral load) coming in contact with the host cells is equally important. After the infection, the immune system of the host takes over whereas sometimes, the pathogen succeeds but, in many times, the viral onslaught can be eliminated. Thus, a robust immune system of the host acts as a natural life insurance.

STRUCTURAL PROTEINS

Structural proteins of SARS-CoV-2 have a crucial role in the pathogenicity as it facilitates the assembly and release of the virion [8]. The S, E and M proteins together form an envelope of the virus. The S glycoprotein of SARS-CoV-2 comprises two subunits; S1 which determines the virus host range and cellular tropism and S2 is involved in the virus-cell membrane fusion activity by HR1 [9] and HR2 [10]. The S2 subunit is highly conserved and thus, forms a target for antiviral compounds [10]. The E protein is the smallest structural protein. The M protein is the most abundant and is responsible for the shape of the envelope. The N protein together with the RNA forms the nucleocapsid inside the envelope. The proteins E and N interfere with the host immune response [8]. We have carried out the detailed molecular and genetic characterization of SARS-CoV-2 major structural protein genes using nucleotide composition, codon usage patterns, phylogenetic, entropy and selection pressure analyses. This data is likely to augment the information about the evolution, biology and adaptation of SARS-CoV-2 in the human host.

The S glycoprotein of the coronavirus is class I viral fusion protein. This outermost glycoprotein is initially synthesized as a single chain precursor which is approximately 1,300 amino acid residues in length [11, 12]. The protein undergoes trimerization upon folding [12]. It is the key target of neutralizing antibodies upon infection [12]. The S1 subunit consists of a signal peptide, the N-terminal domain (NTD) and the receptor-binding domain (RBD), whereas the S2 subunit contains fusion peptide (FP), the heptad repeats: HR 1 and HR2, transmembrane domain, (TM), and the cytoplasmic domain (CP) [2]. A study has reported 99% similarity of the S2 subunit of SARS-CoV-2 to the sequences of Bat-SL-CoVs [2], suggesting its conserved nature. Analysis of S2 subunit of Bat-SL-CoV, SARS-CoV and SARS-CoV-2 may help us to understand the evolutionary phenomena of these viruses. Therefore, we attempted phylogenetic and codon-based characterization of S2 subunit of the species *Severe acute respiratory syndrome-related coronavirus* (SARSr-CoV) that include Bat-S--CoV, SARS-CoV and SARS-CoV-2 employing selection pressure and Shannon entropy analyses. The N- and O-linked glycosylation pattern was also studied using the S2 subunit sequences. The information obtained from this data may help in the prediction of codon-based model of molecular evolution of the coronaviruses (CoVs), which may further assist in designing antiviral peptides against the S2 subunit of spike glycoprotein of CoVs.

GLOBAL EPIDEMIOLOGY AND TRANSMISSION

A cluster of cases of pneumonia of unknown aetiology was reported by China on 31st December 2019. Novel Coronavirus (2019-nCoV) was the newly identified causative pathogen in these cases. The initial cases were linked to a zoonotic transmission of the virus from small animals like pangolin, bats, *etc* to humans in a Seafood Market in Wuhan, Hubei province, China. Wuhan thus became the epicentre of this pneumonia outbreak in Mainland China. However, the exact source of the initial human infection is still not established. The pathogen was later named as severe acute respiratory syndrome coronavirus 2 (SARS-CoV-2) by the International Committee on Taxonomy of Viruses (ICTV) due to its similarity to SARS. The disease was named as Coronavirus Disease 2019 (COVID-19) by the World Health Organization (WHO) [13]. Subsequently, the viral infection showed significant human to human transmission in China fuelling a larger outbreak in the region. Later, the viral infection reached other parts of the world by the travellers leading to an unprecedented pandemic. WHO declared this outbreak a "Public Health Emergency of International Concern (PHEIC)" on 30th January 2020. The epidemic gradually spread its tentacles to almost every part of the globe leading to an unprecedented contagion. Consequently, it was declared a pandemic by WHO on 11th March 2020. Till 31st August 2020, more than 24 million global infections and 0.8 million deaths were reported. More than 216 countries/regions were affected though the most severely affected nations are the USA, Brazil, India, Russia, Peru and South Africa [14].

The mean R_0 value for SARS-CoV-2 is 3 (range is 2.2 to 5.7) suggesting high transmission capability of this pathogen [15]. It is also postulated that the transmission will decrease after attaining the threshold of the herd immunity that is expected to range between 60-68% for this pathogen [15]. This threshold can be reached after mass vaccination using prophylactic vaccine though that might take some time. Alternatively, this threshold can be reached by natural infection of the population. However, the second approach may have devastating consequences since a large part of the global population will be infected including the high-risk individuals. The most vulnerable people with co-morbidities would contribute to millions of deaths. Therefore, we should take appropriate precautions maintaining social distancing and overall hygiene to protect ourselves from this deadly infection. This will help us to develop immunity against COVID-19 gradually which in turn will assist in better management of the clinical cases.

The conventional modes of transmission of SARS-CoV-2 are the droplets from the infected persons which are aerosol mediated or air borne. In addition, fecal and fomites could also contribute. Nosocomial and familial mediated modes have contributed significantly propelling human to human transmission of this virus. However, the asymptomatic patients in incubation period are the most dangerous ones because they remain unpredictable to the extent of damage they can cause [16, 17]. In this context, the only possible way to contain this aspect is to undertake large scale swift testing across the spectra of society. However, the enhancement of testing facility poses another kind of challenge because that must be done by the Government. Management of any pandemic would be lot less challenging if epidemiological base is strong. However, this base cannot be developed overnight. This must be part of the overall policy decision in the context of human health care system. Similarly, scientific surveillance of the diseases would also provide correct picture of the pandemic. Overall, this needs cooperation, collaboration, sharing of the data and real time-based communication besides professional care of the patients.

RISK FACTORS

Several known and unknown risk factors have been described that contribute towards severity of the disease. It has been reported that certain category of individuals like elderly people [18, 19], males [20, 21], persons with type A blood group are more susceptible to severe COVID-19 disease [22]. Females are less susceptible to the infection as compared to males probably due to the difference in immune system, hormonal changes and specific habits like smoking/drinking

[23]. In addition, certain co-morbid conditions like diabetes, hypertension, cardiovascular, endocrine/ chronic respiratory diseases and obesity have been associated with an enhanced risk to severe SARS-CoV-2 infection [24]. Pregnant women are at a risk for developing different viral infections including SARS-CoV-2 [25]. There might be a risk of vertical transmission of the infection from mother to fetus. However, data on this line is scanty and needs larger number of such cases for the analysis before a definitive conclusion may be drawn.

CLINICAL SYMPTOMS AND MANAGEMENT

The disease may range from asymptomatic to mild to severe respiratory illness. The clinical manifestations comprise of high-grade fever, extreme weakness, body ache, cough, runny nose, congestion, difficulty in breathing, nausea or vomiting, diarrhoea, change in taste and smell [26]. Some patients may develop severe disease with respiratory syndrome that may lead to multi-organ failure and death [27]. The incubation period ranges from 2-14 days with median of 5-6 days. The human to human transmission of the infection occurs via aerosol/ droplet mediated methods and direct contact. The respiratory droplets containing virus particles are transferred among individuals during coughing, sneezing and talking [28]. Highly infected surfaces in the hospital set up, may also lead to substantial transmission. Maintenance of general good health particularly hand hygiene is the need of the hour. Household liquid soaps can be used for washing of hands for at least 20 seconds. Around 60-70% ethanol or 70% isopropanol solution can be used for disinfection of hands and surfaces in the absence of soap. A 10% solution of hypochlorite is generally used to disinfect surfaces at hospitals, laboratories, *etc*. WHO recommends physical distancing to avoid transmission of the virus [29]. Therefore, many countries promulgated a mandatory lockdown in 2020 to prevent the human to human transmission of COVID-19.

The infected patients are isolated in specified COVID Care Centres to prevent the transmission. The suspected patients are also quarantined to avoid the spread. Mild cases and the persons in contact with the positive patients are recommended to follow self-isolation at their homes to prevent infection of healthy individuals. Patients are given symptomatic treatment since specific drug against SARS-CoV-2 is not available. Patients with mild disease are treated with antipyretics drugs for fever and pain, antibiotics to prevent secondary bacterial infection, rehydration and nutritional supplements to boost the sagging immune system. Patients with severe disease are admitted to hospitals and are monitored regularly for oxygen saturation and other parameters to avoid the respiratory failure. The severe patients are given appropriate antiviral and other drugs that have shown efficacy against SARS-CoV-2 [30].

HOST IMMUNE RESPONSE AND PATHOGENESIS

Initially, the virus causes upper respiratory tract infection that subsequently moves to lower respiratory tract. The binding of the virus with ACE2 receptors present on the epithelial cells in alveoli in lungs leads to intense host immune response [31]. Numerous immune cells accumulate at the site of infection that releases an influx of chemicals known as "cytokine storm" to over-power the viral assault [32]. The damaged and dead immune cells along with a sticky fluid accumulate in the alveolar region is called exudate. This causes difficulty in breathing that sometimes lead to acute respiratory syndrome (ARSD) followed by multi-organ failure and death. Unfortunately, no part of the body is secure, and infection may reach to any part of the body including brain and heart, two most vital organs [27, 33].

DIAGNOSTICS

Diagnosis of COVID-19 is continuously evolving since researchers are trying to use the newer technologies for detection of SARS-CoV-2. Samples collected from upper respiratory tract (nasopharyngeal swabs, oropharyngeal swabs) or lower respiratory tract (bronchoalveolar lavage, endotracheal aspirates) or saliva are used to test for COVID-19. In addition, stool and urine samples can also be tested in severe hospitalized patients [34]. The recommended molecular tests are Real Time PCR assays that are specific and sensitive and can be done on suspected patients within first few days of symptoms. However, these tests are conducted in laboratories using sophisticated equipment and trained staff. In addition, the reagents required for these tests are costly thereby making them expensive that are not within the reach of many patients [35]. The serological approach involving testing for IgM and IgG antibodies by rapid tests and ELISA are much cheaper alternatives. These tests can be carried out in suspected patients after 6-7 days of the appearance of symptoms. Serology also has the advantage of giving the information of the past infection in a community. The rapid tests can be performed in a few minutes even at remote areas without specific training and can be used to screen a large population in case of a pandemic. Another, non-nucleic acid based antigen detection test detects viral antigen in nasal/pharyngeal specimens of the patient [36]. It is rapid, specific and implies current infection. However, the ideal diagnostic strategy for COVID-19 can be initial testing the viral genome by RT-PCR or antigen detection followed by IgM/IgG serology in the next week [37].

The assessment of viral load is simple to conduct but most difficult to confirm. This is because, the actual load would be the sum of the virus particles present in all the parts of the body. The assessment cannot be done for all the organs. Thus, the selective tissues or blood would reflect an estimate but not the real viral load when subjected to RT-PCR analysis [38]. This viral load business can be scaled up using samples from the dead bodies. However, this would have its own perils and problems and one must negotiate with logistic constraints to meet the challenges. We need well trained scientists whose knowledge about the viruses is deep and who desire to indulge in innovation. The availability of many well-trained scientists and innovators would be an asset to the country in general and the society in particular during such pandemic as we are witnessing.

THERAPEUTICS (ANTIVIRALS AND NATURAL COMPOUNDS)

No specific drug is available against SARS-CoV-2 since it is a comparatively newer pathogen as mentioned earlier. In addition, its biology is far from being understood. What we know however is based on the information from the other family members like SARS and MERS [39]. Thus, the need for drugs to treat the patients in view of the ongoing COVID-19 pandemic is warranted. However, drug development, like vaccine, is a long process involving manpower, money, materials and management besides several years of time. In the present scenario, several existing antiviral and other drugs are being tested on COVID-19 patients [40]. Drug repurposing is an attractive and economical option in the absence of specific treatment. Remdesivir, chloroquine/hydroxychloroquine, lopinavir/ritonavir, favipiravir, arbidol and several other drugs in different permutation and combinations are being tested and are under trials in different parts of the world [40]. World Health Organization has classified the type of drug treatment available for the COVID-19. The classification includes specific and broad spectrum antivirals (interferons, Interleukin-2, favipiravir, Umifenovir, Remdesivir, LPV/RTV), antimalarial (CQ/HCQ), antiparasitic (Niclosamide, Nitazoxanide), antibiotic (Carrimycin, Teicoplanin, Azithromycin), antifungal (Itraconazole), anti-inflammatory (Dexamethasone), immunosuppressants (thalidomide), inhibitors of kinase and protease (Imatinib mesylate, Camostat Mesilate), monoclonal antibodies (Eculizumab), immunomodulators (CD24), ACE inhibitors (Losartan), antiarrhythmic (Amiodarone), vasodilator (angiotensin 1-7), anticoagulant (Rivaroxaban), NSAID (Ibuprofen), mucolytic, antidepressant and others [41]. The classification also includes many non-drug candidates. Many of these combinations have shown to be effective in treatment of the COVID-19 patients. However, elaborate clinical trials on these drugs involving different population sets, dosage determination and side effects, if any will ultimately determine the exact therapeutic potential of these medications against SARS-CoV-2. Further, plasma derived from the recovered patients is also being used for therapy [40]. In addition, different curative tactics such as corticosteroids, vitamins, trace elements, immune enhancers are also being used to rejuvenate the feeble immune system of humans [42].

Further, many natural compounds derived from medicinal plants have been reported to be antiviral along with healing properties [43]. These can be used to augment the human immune system. Both computational and experimental approaches seem to be promising with respect to these compounds as they target SARS-CoV-2 at the molecular level. These compounds have shown to affect different structural (spike, envelope, and membrane) and non-structural (protease, RdRp, endonuclease) proteins of SARS-CoV-2 [44 - 46]. These include naturally occurring bioactive compounds (flavonoids, terpenes, and polyphenols, *etc.*) of plant origin that can acts as potential inhibitors of COVID-19 [47, 48]. We have reviewed different compounds encompassing Myricitrin, Baicalin, Hesperidin, Theaflavin, Apigenin, Isothymol, Curcumin, Tanin, *etc.* In addition, we have also examined several medicinal plants (*Curcuma longa, Vitis vinifera, Glycyrrhiza glabra, Malus domestica, Azadirachta indica, Camellia Sinensis, Nigella sativa, etc.*) that can be considered as pro-immune herbs for the humans. However, elaborate toxicity studies and clinical trials of these natural compounds will determine their doses and the overall therapeutic potential against SARS-CoV-2. Further, synergistic effect of the antiviral drugs and natural compounds on treatment of COVID-19 may be explored in clinical studies.

VACCINE DEVELOPMENT

There are several obstacles in vaccine development against SARS CoV2. One of the major hindrances is the risk of immune potentiation (increased infectivity) after immunization with whole virus or complete spike protein as described with previous SARS and MERS vaccine candidates [49]. The next hurdle is to identify the key target population. The primary high-risk population includes frontline health care workers, elderly individuals and persons with pre-existing chronic diseases [26]. Still another crucial impediment is availability of the vaccine at the earliest in the context of the on-going pandemic. Further, it should also be produced in large quantities for global distribution in addition to being economical so that it may reach the developing countries as well.

Vaccine development against this respiratory pathogen has been accelerated across the globe using different platforms encompassing nucleic acid, viral vector, recombinant protein, live attenuated viruses, inactivated viruses and virus like particles. Experience from the existing SARS and MERS vaccine contenders has assisted in speeding up the vaccine formulation efforts of SARS-CoV-2. Interestingly as of now (till 31st August 2020), we have about 190 vaccine candidates in the pre-clinical and clinical pipelines. Remarkably 39 different vaccine candidates are in various stages of clinical trials [50, 51]. Three of these candidates have received approval for emergency use. Further, the current tuberculosis vaccines are also being tested against SARS-CoV-2 [52, 53]. Thus, scientific community is leaving no stone unturned in search and formulation of a prophylactic vaccine.

CORONA WARRIORS

The Corona warriors encompassing doctors, nurses, paramedical staff, ambulance drivers and police forces are working day/ night to assist the mankind to fight this battle. Other Corona warriors include school, college, and university teachers who are taking continuous online classes and scientists busy with their experiments for the development of vaccine and therapeutic agents against this infection. Yet another lot of scientists are pursuing computational approaches to map the evolutionary trajectories of this virus to identify the possible drug targets. We must also acknowledge the support of delivery boys/agents who are supplying goods, essential commodities, groceries, *etc.* at our doorstep. Last but not the least, the lady of the house who not only has to ensure the availability of food on the table, on time, all the time but also has to adjust with the angularities of the spouse on the real time basis in addition to gracefully accommodating the tantrums and ever growing prank of the children. The poor lady starts the day as a tired soul and call off the day as the retired one. This pandemic has taught us many things of which one is to become a good citizen and develop high level of civic sense to have positive socio-economic impact on the society and environment.

SOCIO-ECONOMIC-ENVIRONMENTAL IMPACT

The on-going pandemic of COVID-19 has impacted the global economy, social life, travel and transportation, education and entertainment industries, small- and large-scale businesses, and environment and interpersonal relations [54 - 56]. However, the impact may vary from country to country and person to person depending upon its local dynamics, availability of sources and resources and involvement of government policies and implementing agencies. The long-term effects of the pandemic are envisaged to be an increased unemployment and rampant poverty. The national and international travel restrictions were enforced to limit the viral transmission but have also crippled the aviation industry. Many countries have implemented the lockdown between February to August, 2020 to prevent community transmission of the infection. Gatherings, parties and meetings were cancelled across the globe that affected the social life. Most of the companies and offices suggested that the employees should work from home and the virtual meetings were organized to minimize human interactions. Only the essential services were operative during the lockdown including hospitals, diagnostic centres, pharmacists, grocery stores, milk depots and law enforcement agencies. Closure of the markets, shopping malls, factories and trade of goods led to an increase in the unemployment and a rise in the prices of almost all the commodities. It may be noted that the domestic violence against women and children including physical and emotional abuse increased considerably during the lockdown period. Tourism, aviation and real estate sectors were hard-hit by the pandemic since the social distancing was implemented across the world. In addition, sports and entertainment industries were also paralyzed due to the pandemic. The Sensex and crude oil prices crashed at a remarkably low level. The loss of global economy due to this pandemic in 2020 is estimated more than 20 trillion US dollars according to a report published on 5th July 2020 [57].

The healthcare sector consisting of hospitals, diagnostic centres and pharmaceutical industries, drugs, supplements and diagnostic kits were in high demand due to ever increasing infection. In addition, the requirement for sanitizers, disinfectants and liquid/solid soaps increased dramatically since most of the people wish to maintain good hygiene. Fabrication of general medical supplies for hospitals and PPE kits for the health care workers was accelerated. There was an increased demand in the food sector due to panic buying and stock piling by many people in several countries of the world. Educational institutions like universities, schools were closed across the globe but most of these organizations started online classes to impart education ensuring the future prospects of the students.

However, the pandemic had a positive impact on the environment especially during the lockdown. Nature had heeled itself in the absence of human interference during the lockdown. Air pollution decreased dramatically due to the absence of aviation and vehicular transportation during the lockdown. The water bodies showed a massive decrease in pollution levels since factories were no longer discharging pollutants and toxic chemicals. However, random disposal of used face masks and medical waste is now polluting the environment, which will have severe consequences in the future. Therefore, all of us should act in an intelligent manner to take care of our well-being, our social life and the environment during this pandemic.

CONCLUDING REMARKS

The pandemic of COVID-19 has impacted the entire globe allowing only minimal social interactions in many countries. The number of cases is nonetheless increasing consistently. Maintenance of good hygiene and social distancing is the key to prevent community transmission of the infection. The rapid release of the SARS-CoV-2 genome resulted in the development of diagnostic kits on a fast track basis. Investigations on evolutionary trajectories and genomic variations will provide insight into the details on the global spread of the infection. Drug repurposing approaches have shown promising results, but trials are still underway to identify specific therapeutic agents against SARS-CoV-2. In addition, several candidate vaccines are undergoing trials at a pandemic speed across the globe.

The social life and global economy are also affected drastically by the pandemic. However, post pandemic, we should expect more hell due to rampant job loss, skewed health care system, stalled economy, burden of feeding the millions of people, finding a way to engage the daily wagers and numerous other unforeseen problems. Those who have recovered will have emotional, psychosomatic and rehabilitation issues. Such people would require medical counseling. There are far too many things that are at stake. The only way society can defeat this unseen enemy is to join head, hand and heart to mount a collective battle. It is envisaged that this book would prove to be a much-needed wakeup call for the society, system and the world in the larger interest of mankind.

CONSENT FOR PUBLICATION

Not Applicable.

CONFLICT OF INTEREST

The author declares no conflict of interest, financial or otherwise.

ACKNOWLEDGEMENTS

The research in our laboratory is funded by Council of Scientific and Industrial Research (CSIR), India (37(1697)17/EMR-II) and Central Council for Research in Unani Medicine (CCRUM), Ministry of Ayurveda, Yoga and Naturopathy, Unani, Siddha and Homeopathy (AYUSH), India (F.No.3-63/2019-CCRUM/Tech), India. Sher Ali is grateful for the financial support from DBT (BT/PR12828/AAQ/1/622/2015), New Delhi and JC Bose award (SR/S2/JCB-49/2011) from SERB-DST, New Delhi, India.

REFERENCES

[1]   Ashour HM, Elkhatib WF, Rahman MM, Elshabrawy HA. Insights into the recent 2019 novel coronavirus (SARS-CoV-2) in light of past human coronavirus outbreaks. Pathogens 2020; 9(3): 186.
[http://dx.doi.org/10.3390/pathogens9030186] [PMID: 32143502]

[2]   Chan JF, Kok KH, Zhu Z, *et al.* Genomic characterization of the 2019 novel human-pathogenic coronavirus isolated from a patient with atypical pneumonia after visiting Wuhan. Emerg Microbes Infect 2020; 9(1): 221-36.
[http://dx.doi.org/10.1080/22221751.2020.1719902] [PMID: 31987001]

[3]   Shanmugaraj B, Siriwattananon K, Wangkanont K, Phoolcharoen W. Perspectives on monoclonal antibody therapy as potential therapeutic intervention for Coronavirus disease-19 (COVID-19). Asian Pac J Allergy Immunol 2020; 38(1): 10-8.

[PMID: 32134278]

[4]   Lu R, Zhao X, Li J, *et al.* Genomic characterisation and epidemiology of 2019 novel coronavirus:
        implications for virus origins and receptor binding. Lancet 2020; 395(10224): 565-74.
        [http://dx.doi.org/10.1016/S0140-6736(20)30251-8] [PMID: 32007145]

[5]   Chen Y, Liu Q, Guo D. Emerging coronaviruses: Genome structure, replication, and pathogenesis. J
        Med Virol 2020; 92(4): 418-23.
        [http://dx.doi.org/10.1002/jmv.25681] [PMID: 31967327]

[6]   Romano M, Ruggiero A, Squeglia F, Maga G, Berisio R. A Structural View of SARS-CoV-2 RNA
        Replication Machinery: RNA Synthesis, Proofreading and Final Capping. Cells 2020; 9(5): 1267.
        [http://dx.doi.org/10.3390/cells9051267] [PMID: 32443810]

[7]   He Y, Zhou Y, Liu S, *et al.* Receptor-binding domain of SARS-CoV spike protein induces highly
        potent neutralizing antibodies: implication for developing subunit vaccine. Biochem Biophys Res
        Commun 2004; 324(2): 773-81.
        [http://dx.doi.org/10.1016/j.bbrc.2004.09.106] [PMID: 15474494]

[8]   Guo YR, Cao QD, Hong ZS, Tan YY, Chen SD, Jin HJ, *et al.* The origin, transmission and clinical
        therapies on coronavirus disease 2019 (COVID-19) outbreak–an update on the status. Mil Med Res
        2020; 7(11): 1-10.
        [http://dx.doi.org/10.1186/s40779-020-00240-0] [PMID: 31928528]

[9]   Yu F, Du L, Ojcius DM, Pan C, Jiang S. Measures for diagnosing and treating infections by a novel
        coronavirus responsible for a pneumonia outbreak originating in Wuhan. China: Microb Infect 2020
        Mar; 22(2): 74-9.
        [http://dx.doi.org/10.1016/j.micinf.2020.01.003]

[10]   Cascella M, Rajnik M, Cuomo A, Dulebohn SC, Di Napoli R. Features, evaluation and treatment
        coronavirus (COVID-19). StatPearls [Internet]. Treasure Island (FL): StatPearls Publishing; 2020 Jan.

[11]   Fehr AR, Perlman S. Coronaviruses: an overview of their replication and pathogenesis. Methods Mol
        Biol 2015; 1282: 1-23.
        [http://dx.doi.org/10.1007/978-1-4939-2438-7_1] [PMID: 25720466]

[12]   Walls AC, Tortorici MA, Snijder J, *et al.* Tectonic conformational changes of a coronavirus spike
        glycoprotein promote membrane fusion. Proc Natl Acad Sci USA 2017; 114(42): 11157-62.
        [http://dx.doi.org/10.1073/pnas.1708727114] [PMID: 29073020]

[13]   Zhou P, Yang XL, Wang XG, *et al.* A pneumonia outbreak associated with a new coronavirus of
        probable bat origin. Nature 2020; 579(7798): 270-3.
        [http://dx.doi.org/10.1038/s41586-020-2012-7] [PMID: 32015507]

[14]   Coronavirus disease (COVID-19) pandemic. World Health Organization (WHO). Available at:
        https://www.who.int/emergencies/diseases/novel-coronavirus-2019

[15]   Randolph HE, Barreiro LB. Herd Immunity: Understanding COVID-19. Immunity 2020; 52(5): 737-
        41.
        [http://dx.doi.org/10.1016/j.immuni.2020.04.012] [PMID: 32433946]

[16]   Guo ZD, Wang ZY, Zhang SF, *et al.* Aerosol and surface distribution of severe acute respiratory
        syndrome coronavirus 2 in hospital wards, Wuhan, China, 2020. Emerg Infect Dis 2020; 26(7): 1583-
        91.
        [http://dx.doi.org/10.3201/eid2607.200885] [PMID: 32275497]

[17]   Modes of transmission of virus causing COVID-19: World Health Organisation. Modes of
        transmission of virus causing COVID-19: implications for IPC precaution recommendations. 2020.
        Available from: https://www.who.int/news-room/commentaries/detail/modes-of-transmission-of--
        irus-causing-COVID-19-implications-for-ipc-precaution-recommendations

[18]   Blagosklonny MV. From causes of aging to death from COVID-19. Aging (Albany NY) 2020; 12(11):
        10004-21.

[http://dx.doi.org/10.18632/aging.103493] [PMID: 32534452]

[19]   Covid CD, Team R. Severe outcomes among patients with coronavirus disease 2019 (COVID-19)—United States, February 12–March 16, 2020. MMWR Morb Mortal Wkly Rep 2020; 69(12): 343-6.
[http://dx.doi.org/10.15585/mmwr.mm6912e2] [PMID: 32214079]

[20]   Surveillances V. The epidemiological characteristics of an outbreak of 2019 novel coronavirus diseases (COVID-19)—China, 2020. China CDC Weekly 2020; 2(8): 113-22.
[http://dx.doi.org/10.46234/ccdcw2020.032]

[21]   COVID-19 sex-disaggregated data tracker – Global Health 50/50 [Internet]. Globalhealth5050.org. 2020. Available from: https://globalhealth5050.org/covid19/sex-disaggregated-data-tracker/

[22]   Zhao J, Yang Y, Huang HP, *et al.* Relationship between the ABO Blood Group and the COVID-19 Susceptibility. medRxiv. 2020.
[http://dx.doi.org/10.1101/2020.03.11.20031096]

[23]   Klein SL, Flanagan KL. Sex differences in immune responses. Nat Rev Immunol 2016; 16(10): 626-38.
[http://dx.doi.org/10.1038/nri.2016.90] [PMID: 27546235]

[24]   Williamson EJ, Walker AJ, Bhaskaran K, *et al.* OpenSAFELY: factors associated with COVID-19 death in 17 million patients. Nature 2020; 584: 430-6.

[25]   Schwartz DA, Graham AL. Potential maternal and infant outcomes from (Wuhan) coronavirus 2019-nCoV infecting pregnant women: lessons from SARS, MERS, and other human coronavirus infections. Viruses 2020; 12(2): 194.
[http://dx.doi.org/10.3390/v12020194] [PMID: 32050635]

[26]   Huang C, Wang Y, Li X, *et al.* Clinical features of patients infected with 2019 novel coronavirus in Wuhan, China. Lancet 2020; 395(10223): 497-506.
[http://dx.doi.org/10.1016/S0140-6736(20)30183-5] [PMID: 31986264]

[27]   Wang T, Du Z, Zhu F, *et al.* Comorbidities and multi-organ injuries in the treatment of COVID-19. Lancet 2020; 395(10228): e52.
[http://dx.doi.org/10.1016/S0140-6736(20)30558-4] [PMID: 32171074]

[28]   Bourouiba L. Turbulent gas clouds and respiratory pathogen emissions: potential implications for reducing transmission of COVID-19. JAMA 2020; 323(18): 1837-8.
[http://dx.doi.org/10.1001/jama.2020.4756] [PMID: 32215590]

[29]   Chughtai AA, Seale H, Islam MS, Owais M, Macintyre CR. Policies on the use of respiratory protection for hospital health workers to protect from coronavirus disease (COVID-19). Int J Nurs Stud 2020; 105: 103567.
[http://dx.doi.org/10.1016/j.ijnurstu.2020.103567] [PMID: 32203757]

[30]   Arons MM, Hatfield KM, Reddy SC, *et al.* Presymptomatic SARS-CoV-2 infections and transmission in a skilled nursing facility. N Engl J Med 2020; 382(22): 2081-90.
[http://dx.doi.org/10.1056/NEJMoa2008457] [PMID: 32329971]

[31]   Zhang H, Penninger JM, Li Y, Zhong N, Slutsky AS. Angiotensin-converting enzyme 2 (ACE2) as a SARS-CoV-2 receptor: molecular mechanisms and potential therapeutic target. Intensive Care Med 2020; 46(4): 586-90.
[http://dx.doi.org/10.1007/s00134-020-05985-9] [PMID: 32125455]

[32]   Moore JB, June CH. Cytokine release syndrome in severe COVID-19. Science 2020; 368(6490): 473-4.
[http://dx.doi.org/10.1126/science.abb8925] [PMID: 32303591]

[33]   Xu Z, Shi L, Wang Y, *et al.* Pathological findings of COVID-19 associated with acute respiratory distress syndrome. Lancet Respir Med 2020; 8(4): 420-2.
[http://dx.doi.org/10.1016/S2213-2600(20)30076-X] [PMID: 32085846]

[34]   Wang W, Xu Y, Gao R, *et al.* Detection of SARS-CoV-2 in different types of clinical specimens. JAMA 2020; 323(18): 1843-4.
[http://dx.doi.org/10.1001/jama.2020.3786] [PMID: 32159775]

[35]   Wölfel R, Corman VM, Guggemos W, *et al.* Virological assessment of hospitalized patients with COVID-2019. Nature 2020; 581(7809): 465-9.
[http://dx.doi.org/10.1038/s41586-020-2196-x] [PMID: 32235945]

[36]   La Marca A, Capuzzo M, Paglia T, Roli L, Trenti T, Nelson SM. Testing for SARS-CoV-2 (COVID-19): a systematic review and clinical guide to molecular and serological in-vitro diagnostic assays. Reprod Biomed Online 2020; 41(3): 483-99.
[http://dx.doi.org/10.1016/j.rbmo.2020.06.001] [PMID: 32651106]

[37]   Xiang F, Wang X, He X, *et al.* Antibody detection and dynamic characteristics in patients with COVID-19. Clin Infect Dis 2020; 71(8): 1930-4.
[http://dx.doi.org/10.1093/cid/ciaa461] [PMID: 32306047]

[38]   Corman VM, Drosten C. Authors' response: SARS-CoV-2 detection by real-time RT-PCR. Euro Surveill 2020; 25(21): 2001035.
[http://dx.doi.org/10.2807/1560-7917.ES.2020.25.21.2001035] [PMID: 32489177]

[39]   Lu H. Drug treatment options for the 2019-new coronavirus (2019-nCoV). Biosci Trends 2020; 14(1): 69-71.
[http://dx.doi.org/10.5582/bst.2020.01020] [PMID: 31996494]

[40]   Lythgoe MP, Middleton P. Ongoing Clinical Trials for the Management of the COVID-19 Pandemic. Trends Pharmacol Sci 2020; 41(6): 363-82.
[http://dx.doi.org/10.1016/j.tips.2020.03.006] [PMID: 32291112]

[41]   World Health Organization. COVID 19 candidate treatments https://www.who.int/publications/m/item/covid-19-candidate-treatments

[42]   Zhang L, Liu Y. Potential interventions for novel coronavirus in China: A systematic review. J Med Virol 2020; 92(5): 479-90.
[http://dx.doi.org/10.1002/jmv.25707] [PMID: 32052466]

[43]   Hussain W, Haleem KS, Khan I, *et al.* Medicinal plants: a repository of antiviral metabolites. Future Virol 2017; 12(6): 299-308.
[http://dx.doi.org/10.2217/fvl-2016-0110]

[44]   Joshi RS, Jagdale SS, Bansode SB, *et al.* Discovery of potential multi-target-directed ligands by targeting host-specific SARS-CoV-2 structurally conserved main protease. J Biomol Struct Dyn 2020; May 5: 1-16.
[http://dx.doi.org/10.1080/07391102.2020.1760137] [PMID: 32329408]

[45]   Sinha SK, Shakya A, Prasad SK, *et al.* An *in-silico* evaluation of different Saikosaponins for their potency against SARS-CoV-2 using NSP15 and fusion spike glycoprotein as targets. J Biomol Struct Dyn 2020; 1-12.
[PMID: 32345124]

[46]   Borkotoky S, Banerjee M. A computational prediction of SARS-CoV-2 structural protein inhibitors from *Azadirachta indica* (Neem). J Biomol Struct Dyn 2020; 1-17.
[http://dx.doi.org/10.1080/07391102.2020.1774419] [PMID: 32462988]

[47]   Silva JKRD, Figueiredo PLB, Byler KG, Setzer WN. Essential Oils as Antiviral Agents. Potential of Essential Oils to Treat SARS-CoV-2 Infection: An *In-Silico* Investigation. Int J Mol Sci 2020; 21(10): 3426.
[http://dx.doi.org/10.3390/ijms21103426] [PMID: 32408699]

[48]   Sayed AM, Khattab AR. AboulMagd AM, Hassan HM, Rateb ME, Zaid H, Abdelmohsen UR. Nature as a treasure trove of potential anti-SARS-CoV drug leads: a structural/mechanistic rationale. RSC Advances 2020; 10(34): 19790-802.

[http://dx.doi.org/10.1039/D0RA04199H]

[49]   Jiang S, Bottazzi ME, Du L, *et al.* Roadmap to developing a recombinant coronavirus S protein receptor-binding domain vaccine for severe acute respiratory syndrome. Expert Rev Vaccines 2012; 11(12): 1405-13.
[http://dx.doi.org/10.1586/erv.12.126] [PMID: 23252385]

[50]   Draft landscape of COVID-19 candidate vaccines .WHO 2020 [Accessed 24 Jun 2020]. Available from: https://www.who.int/publications/m/item/draft-landscape-of-covid-19-candidate-vaccines

[51]   Praveen D. Coronavirus treatment: vaccines/drugs in the pipeline for COVID-19. 2020. https://www.clinicaltrialsarena.com/analysis/coronavirus-mers-cov-drugs/

[52]   BCG Vaccination to Protect Healthcare Workers Against COVID-19 (BRACE). 2020. https://clinicaltrials.gov/ct2/show/NCT04327206

[53]   Study to Assess VPM1002 in Reducing Healthcare Professionals' Absenteeism in COVID-19 Pandemic. 2020. https://clinicaltrials.gov/ct2/show/NCT04387409

[54]   Nicola M, Alsafi Z, Sohrabi C, *et al.* The socio-economic implications of the coronavirus pandemic (COVID-19): A review. Int J Surg 2020; 78: 185-93.
[http://dx.doi.org/10.1016/j.ijsu.2020.04.018]

[55]   Malik YS, Kumar N, Sircar S, *et al.* Coronavirus disease pandemic (COVID-19): challenges and a global perspective. Pathogens 2020; 9(7): 519.
[http://dx.doi.org/10.3390/pathogens9070519] [PMID: 32605194]

[56]   Noor S, Parveen S, Ali S. Impact of COVID-19 Pandemic on environment and socioeconomic dynamics. Cover Story, TerraGreen, Teri Press. 6th August 2020: 22-28.

[57]   SciTechDaily. https://scitechdaily.com/economic-pain-covid-19-pandemic-will-cost-global-economy-21-trillion/

CHAPTER 2

Morphology, Genomic Organization, Proteins and Replication of SARS-CoV-2

Nazim Khan[1], Arshi Islam[1], Abu Hamza[1], Zoya Shafat[1], Asimul Islam[1], Anwar Ahmed[2,3] and Shama Parveen[1,*]

[1] *Centre for Interdisciplinary Research in Basic Sciences, Jamia Millia Islamia, New Delhi, India*

[2] *Center of Excellence in Biotechnology Research, College of Science, King Saud University, Riyadh, Saudi Arabia*

[3] *Department of Biochemistry, College of Science, King Saud University, Riyadh, Saudi Arabia*

Abstract: The current pandemic disease (COVID-19) is caused by a highly infectious coronavirus known as severe acute respiratory syndrome coronavirus 2 (SARS-Co--2). It belongs to the family of *Coronaviridae,* subfamily *Orthocoronaa-virinae,* order *Nidovirales*. Coronaviruses (CoVs) are enveloped and spherical shaped pathogens with crown-like protrusions formed by S protein on the surface. The CoVs contain single-stranded positive-sense RNA with genome of 27-32 kb that encodes both structural and non-structural proteins. The Coronavirus genome encodes for at least 6 ORFs, among which two third parts include ORF 1a/1b, which encodes 16 non-structural proteins (nsp 1-16) that play a pivotal role in viral genome replication. The structural proteins are part of mature virion and include spike (S), envelope (E), membrane (M) and nucleocapsid (N) proteins. The S protein binds to the receptor (ACE2 or others) on the host cell and determines host tropism. Replication of CoVs is extremely complicated process and includes regulation at various stages including dependency on both the viral and host factors. The present chapter provides updated information about the morphology, genomic structure, properties and function of different proteins and their role in replication mechanism of SARS-CoV-2. The information about the proteins and their role in viral life cycle is likely to assist in the formulation of targeted therapeutic interventions and vaccines against this emerging respiratory pathogen.

Keywords: COVID-19, Genome, Morphology, Proteins, Replication, SARS-CoV-2.

INTRODUCTION

In December 2019, Coronavirus disease 2019 (COVID-19) began in Wuhan city of China and within a span of few months it has spread its tentacles across the

---
[*] **Corresponding author Shama Parveen:** Centre for Interdisciplinary Research in Basic Sciences, Jamia Millia Islamia, New Delhi, India; E-mails: sparveen2@jmi.ac.in and shamp25@yahoo.com

globe. WHO declared COVID-19 a pandemic on 11[th]March 2020. The disease is caused by newly identified coronavirus, severe acute respiratory syndrome coronavirus 2 (SARS-CoV-2). In the last two decades, two highly infectious zoonotic pathogenic coronaviruses of the same family *i.e.* SARS-CoV and Middle East respiratory syndrome coronavirus (MERS-CoV) have caused widespread epidemics with significant fatality rate in China and Saudi Arabia respectively [1]. Coronaviruses (CoVs) are enveloped pathogens containing single-stranded positive-sense RNA genome of 26-32 kb that encodes both structural and non-structural proteins [2, 3]. The four structural proteins spike (S), envelope (E), membrane (M) and nucleocapsid (N) play a major role in virus entry and replication in the host cell [1]. The spike protein is known to play a major role in viral transmission as it is known to have affinity for angiotensin converting enzyme 2 (ACE-2) receptors on the human host cell [4].

SARS-CoV-2 infection in humans leads to both symptomatic and asymptomatic cases. The incubation period of SARS-CoV-2 is about 14 days [5]. The infected persons usually show symptoms like fever, dry cough, shortness of breath, weakness, body ache and in severe cases, pneumonia [6, 7]. An infected person can transmit COVID-19 to humans through direct contact *via* respiratory droplets [8]. In severe cases, respiratory, hepatic, gastrointestinal and neurological complications are reported which may lead to multi-organ failure and mortality in some cases [6]. Millions of cases and deaths have been reported due to COVID-19 across the globe. Till 31st August 2020, more than 24 million cases and 0.83 million deaths were reported from different parts of the globe. The countries showing maximum infections include USA, Brazil and India [9]. The current situation thus warrants an urgent need of vaccines and therapeutic agents against SARS-CoV-2.

A deep insight into the mechanism of the viral genome replication, role of different proteins in the process and their interaction with host cell system is the need of the hour. These cellular events will provide data on the importance of different proteins in viral replication. These proteins can act as potential target of antiviral drugs and vaccines that will be a step towards management of the current COVID-19 pandemic. In the same context, we have provided a comprehensive overview about the morphology, genomic organization, structural and non-structural proteins of SARS-CoV-2 along with their role in viral life cycle.

VIRAL MORPHOLOGY

The structure of SARS-CoV-2 is quite like SARS-CoV [10]. The characteristic morphology of SARS-CoV-2 was revealed under the electron microscope with the size of the particles ranging between 70-90nm [11]. They are spherical in shape having the bulb like projections on the surface [12]. These projections on the viral surface is formed by the homotrimer of spike protein [13]. The spike protein is responsible for the initiation of viral infection by binding to the receptor in the host cell membrane [1]. The viral envelope is made up of host derived lipid bilayer [14]. This envelope consists of the major viral structural proteins viz. spike protein, membrane (M) protein and envelope (E) protein. Inside the envelope, a viral nucleocapsid is located. This nucleocapsid is formed by the nucleocapsid (N) protein which binds to RNA genome of the virus in a continuous bead on string type conformation [15, 16].

GENOMIC ORGANIZATION

SARS-CoV-2 belongs to the family of *Coronaviridae,* subfamily *Orthocoronaavirinae,* order *Nidovirales* which includes four CoV genera that are known as Alpha, Beta, Gamma and Delta-coronavirus. SARS-CoV-2 clusters into the genus Betacoronavirus and subgenus *Sarbecovirus,* which also include the other zoonotic coronaviruses *i.e.* SARS-CoV and MERS-CoV [17]. The phylogenetic analysis showed the similarity of SARS-CoV-2 with two bat derived coronavirus strains bat-SL-CoVZC45 and bat-SL-CoVZXC21 and SARS strain of 2002-2004 epidemic [18, 19]. Further, the studies have shown that SARS-CoV-2 has 54% identity at whole genomic level, 58% identity at non-structural proteins (nsps) coding region and 43% at structural protein coding region among other CoVs [19]. It was also concluded that the receptor binding domain of SARS-CoV and SARS-CoV-2 binds with the same receptor *i.e.*, ACE-2 in the host cell [20].

The 30kb single stranded positive sense RNA viral genome encodes both structural and non-structural proteins consisting of a total of 9860 amino acids [19, 21]. The non-structural proteins are encoded by polyprotein 1a/1ab, which is directly translated by genomic RNA and are responsible for the formation of replication-transcription complex in double membrane vesicles [22]. This complex synthesizes sub-genomic RNA through discontinuous transcription [23]. These sub-genomic RNAs are further responsible for the synthesis of sub-genomic mRNAs [24]. The Coronavirus genome encodes for at least 6 ORFs, among which two third parts include ORF 1a/1b that encodes 16 non-structural proteins (Fig. **1**). The gamma coronaviruses lack the nsp1 protein. The production of two polypeptides 1a and 1ab occurs through -1 frameshift between ORF 1a and 1b [25]. The other ORF's near 3'-terminus of the genome encodes at least four structural proteins spike (S), membrane (M), envelope (E) and nucleocapsid (N) protein. The sub genomic RNA also encodes HE protein, 3a/b protein and 4a/b protein [3]. RNA replication and translation are regulated by a highly structured un-translated regions (UTR) located at the 5' and 3' end of the genomic RNA.

Structurally, seven stem loop structures and a stem loop and a pseudoknot is present at the 5' and 3' end, respectively [26].

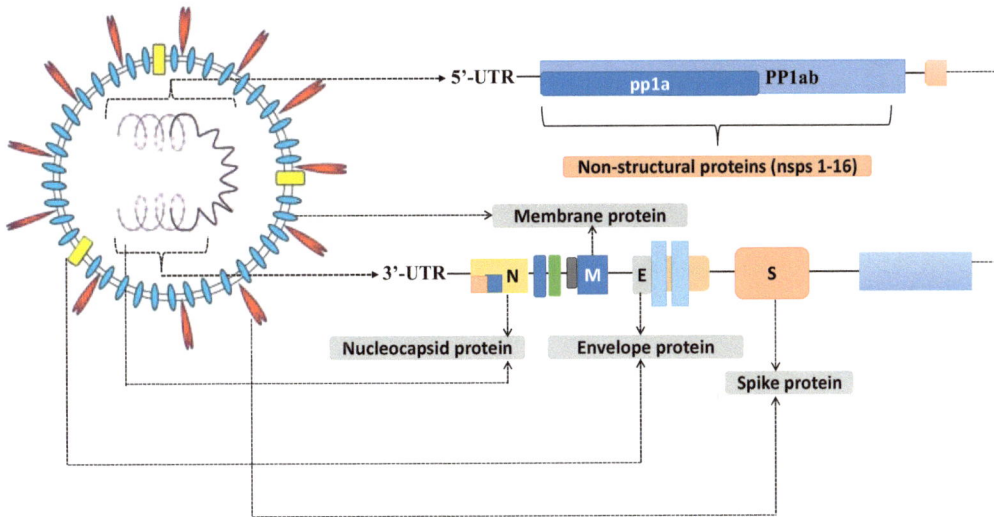

Fig. (1). The genomic organization of SARS-CoV-2. The structure of SARS-CoV-2 virus, the structural proteins and the corresponding open reading frames (ORFs). The viral envelope consists of major structural proteins including S (red protrusions), M (blue colour) and E (yellow colour) that surround the nucleocapsid. Nucleocapsid (N) protein is shown by the purple coloured dots around the helical viral genome. Both the structural and non-structural proteins (nsp 1-16) are also encoded by the viral genome. The genomic sequence is described as 5'-UTR-PP1ab-S-E-M-N-UTR-3'.

STRUCTURAL PROTEINS

Spike Protein (S-protein)

The club like protrusions of the SARS-CoV-2 under the electron microscope is due to the spike protein which appears as the homotrimer spikes on the viral surface [13, 27]. The S-protein is heavily glycosylated with a size of about 150kDa (Fig. **2**) [15]. The homology of S-protein of SARS-CoV-2 with SARS-CoV and MERS-CoV is about 76% and 34% respectively [27]. But the S protein of SARS-CoV-2 is slightly larger in size than the corresponding CoV counterpart [28]. The S-protein initiates the viral infection by the interaction of its receptor binding domain (RBD) with the host cell surface receptor like ACE-2 [1]. The CD209L was also reported to be as an alternative receptor [29]. The RBD in SARS-CoV and MERS-CoV is located at the C-terminus [30]. The clinically proven inhibitor of serine protease (TMPRSS2), *i.e.* camostat mesylate has shown reduced lung cell line infection with SARS-CoV-2 suggesting that the host cell serine protease TMPRSS2 along with ACE-2 is important for viral cell entry and can be considered for COVID-19 treatment [31]. The SARS-CoV-2 spike protein can be proteolytically activated by a variety of cellular proteases such as endosomal cysteine proteases (cathepsin B and L) other than TMPRSS2 [32].

Structurally, each monomer of S-protein is composed of two subunit S1 and S2. S1 is the globular form and helps in receptor binding whereas the S2 is the stem form and is important for the membrane fusion [27, 33]. The interaction of the S1 subunit with the receptor brings the conformational change in S2 subunit which leads to the fusion of cell membrane with the viral envelope that releases the nucleocapsid into the cytoplasm [34]. The S2 protein of SARS-CoV-2 has close sequence identity (93%) whereas S1 has only 68% identity with bat-SL-CoVZC45 and bat-SL-CoVZXC21 strains [18]. Further, in another study, it was found that the S2 subunit has 99% identity and S1 has 70% identity with these two bat strains [21]. The previous studies suggested that the expression of S protein near the cell membrane is responsible for the cell-cell fusion between the infected and adjacent uninfected cell in some Coronaviruses [35].

The S1 subunit consists of a signal peptide, an N-terminal Domain (NTD) and Receptor Binding Domain (RBD) while the S2 is composed of Fusion Peptide (FP), Heptad Repeat (HR1 and HR2), Transmembrane Domain (TM), and Cytoplasmic Domain (CD) [21]. The NTD is heavily N-glycosylated and is responsible for the entry of viruses in ER (endoplasmic reticulum) [36]. The RBD of S1 subunit has receptor binding motifs that interact with the host cell receptor and facilitate the virus attachment [37]. Recent investigations have suggested that SARS-CoV-2 have stronger interaction with the ACE-2 than the SARS-CoV and poses a substantial public health risk for human transmission *via* S-protein ACE-2 binding pathway [34].

The S1 and S2 domains get cleaved inside the endolytic vesicles by host cell protease during viral entry [15]. The cleavage occurs at S1/S2 site as well as S2' site in two steps, first is "priming cleavage" and then "activation cleavage" [38, 39]. The proteases responsible for the 'priming' proteolysis are furin, elastase, factor X and trypsin initiate the viral entry [39, 40].

This cleavage occurs at different sites in different Coronaviruses. According to amino acids, sequences of different CoVs diverse proteases are required for this cleavage [41]. SARS-CoV and SARS-CoV-2 have same S1/S2 site (AYT↓M). In both SARS-CoV-2 and SARS-CoV, this site is cleaved by Cathepsin L. The significance of this cathepsin L site is that the potent inhibitors can be designed against this that will help to prevent viral infection. SARS-CoV-2 has another furin-like protease site (RRAR↓SV) that is located towards the N-terminus to the Cathepsin L site, which is cleaved by furin. This site is absent in SARS-CoV [12, 42]. The significance of this furin site is that, the newly synthesized virions can be secreted in a 'preactivated 'state. Now these preactivated viruses can fuse and infect other cells without using cellular receptors such as ACE-2 [32].

Envelope Protein (E-protein)

The E protein of coronavirus is short integral membrane, multifunctional protein with a size about 8.4 to 12kDa with 76-109 amino acids [43 - 45]. It is smallest among all the structural proteins [46]. It is involved in the envelope formation, assembly, budding and virus maturation [15]. Thus, the E protein plays an important role in pathogenesis during the viral infection [47, 48]. This protein is the neutralizing antigen and thus a potential vaccine candidate [46]. Previous studies on this protein revealed that it interacts with other CoV protein and host cell receptor and functions as ion-channeling viroporin [48, 49]. It was also reported that the expression of this protein is very high inside the infected cell and majority of this protein is localized near the endo-membrane system (ERGIC) [50]. The protein at this location helps in viral assembly as well as budding and minor portion of it is incorporated into the virus envelope [51].

Membrane Protein (M-protein)

The M-protein is the most abundant structural protein and has size about 25-30kDa [15]. The M-protein gives the virion its shape and curvature. Previous studies have proposed that the two different conformations of M-protein allow it to bind with nucleocapsid and it may exist as dimers [52]. The M-protein of CoV has a small N-terminal glycosylated ectodomain, three transmembrane domains and comparatively much larger C-terminal endo-domain. This endo-domain extends the virion particle about 6-8nm and most of them does not contain signal sequences [53]. It plays a central role in virus assembly by interacting with all other structural proteins *via* significant protein-protein interaction [15].

The virus like particles (VLPs) cannot be formed from M-protein alone. Envelope of the virus is formed by interaction of the M-protein with the E-protein. This interaction also stimulates the envelope maturation [54]. The assembly of virion particle is completed by the binding of M-protein with nucleocapsid. This binding also promotes the stabilization of N-protein-RNA complex and internal core of the virion [15, 55]. The virus assembly is not dependent upon the glycosylation of this protein, but this state has important role in virus-host interaction [56, 57]. The interaction of M-protein with S-protein is also important for presence of S in the endoplasmic reticulum Golgi-intermediate compartment and its integration into virions, but it is not essential for the assembly process [58, 59].

Nucleocapsid (N-protein)

The N-protein is well conserved, and SARS-CoV-2 has 90% amino acid identity with the SARS-CoV counterpart [8, 60]. It is the one of the most abundant proteins in Coronaviruses [8] and is heavily phosphorylated [61]. This protein binds with CoV RNA genome and forms the ribonucleoprotein core [62]. The antibodies bind with the N-protein of SARS-CoV and works as antagonist to IFN-γ. But for SARS-CoV-2 it is still not completely known [19, 28]. The protein forms the helically symmetric nucleocapsid of the CoV and has two domains NTD (N-Terminal Domain) and CTD (C-Terminal Domain). The C-terminal domain is responsible for dimerization [63]. Both the domains use different mechanisms to bind RNA molecules in the form of beads [15, 64, 65]. It was also found that it binds with the replicase complex (nsp3) as well as the M-protein. This interaction is essential to bind the RTC (Replicase-Transcriptase Complex) with the viral genome and to package the genome into viral particles [65 - 67].

What we know about **structural** proteins

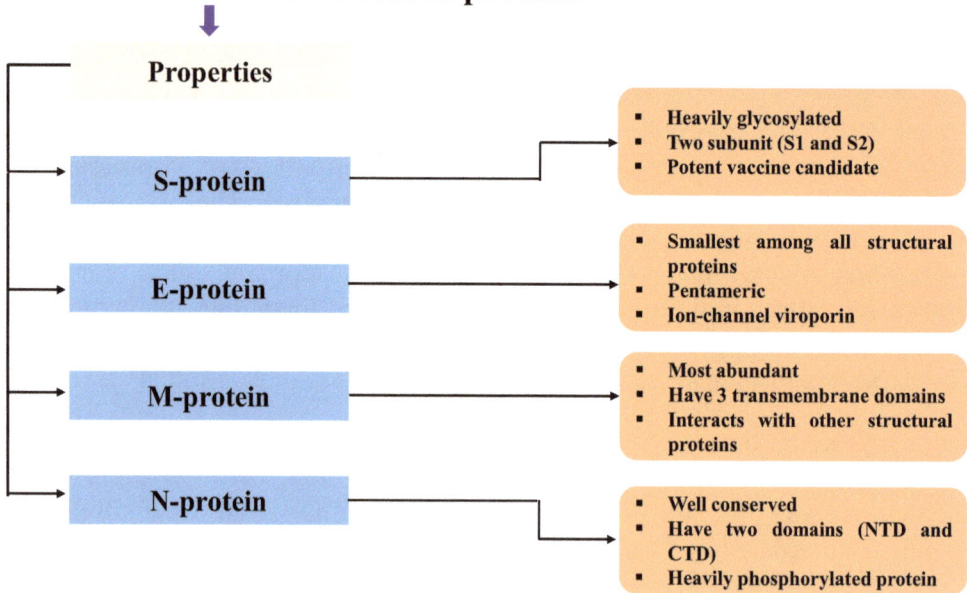

Fig. (2). Properties of structural proteins of SARS-CoV-2.

NON-STRUCTURAL PROTEINS

It has been reported that there is no significant difference between Orfs and non-structural proteins of SARS-CoV-2 and SARS-CoV [27]. The Orf1a and Orf1ab produces two polyproteins *i.e.* pp1a (that forms nsps 1-11) and pp1ab (that forms nsps 1-16), respectively. The nsp-11 in pp1a forms nsp-12 in pp1ab [15]. The replicase proteins cleaved by two or three proteases viz. papain like protease (PL-pro), a 3C-like proteases or main proteases (3CL-pro or M-pro) and a serine like proteases [68, 69]. The PL-proteases encoded by the nsp-3 cleaves nsp1/2, nsp2/3 and nsp3/4 and other is cleaved by M-pro (Table 1) [15].

The nsp-1 is the leader protein which functions as host mRNA inhibitor by binding with 40S subunit of ribosome that uses internal ribosome entry site (Fig. 3) [70]. It also inhibits interferon signaling [27, 71, 72]. The nsp-2 is the homolog of p65 protein [27]. The nsp-2 interacts with the host protein prohibition-1 and prohibition-2 that inhibits the host survival pathway [73]. The nsp-3 is known as PL-pro (papain like protease) which is important for the human infection. It has the protein hydrolase activity and property of de-Ubiquitinase (DUB). These properties of nsp-3 help the virus to block the host antiviral-immune response by inhibiting the expression of interferons [67, 74]. This also acts as antagonist to IFN pathway [75]. This protein is also responsible for the blocking the NF-κβ [75]. It was reported that the PLP of SARS-CoV-2 has 86% homology with the corresponding protein of SARS-CoV [27]. The nsp-4 helps in the double membrane vesicle formation (DMV) formation by interaction with nsp-3 and nsp-4 [76 - 78]. The nsp-4 protein has membrane spanning helices [76]. The nsp-5 has the 3C-like proteinase or M-protease activity that helps in polyprotein cleavage and inhibit the interferon signaling [27, 69, 77]. Antiviral drugs like Lopinavir and Ritonavir target this main 3C- proteinase [78]. The nsp-6 works with nsp-3 and nsp-4 for the DMV formation and can restrict autophagosome expansion. This activates omegasome pathway which induces autophagy [79, 80]. The nsp-6 protein also has membrane spanning helices [80]. The nsp-7 and nsp-8 works as the co-factor of nsp-12 and accelerate its polymerase activity [81]. Nsp-7 along with the nsp-8 forms a hexadecameric ring like structure by contributing 8 molecules from each [82]. Nsp-8 also acts as a primase [81]. The nsp-9 is the single-stranded RNA binding protein that provides the protection against the nucleases [83]. The nsp-10 is the growth factor like peptide (GFL-peptide) and make complexes with the nsp-14 and nsp-16 and stimulates their activities. It activates and stimulates the exonuclease activity and methyltransferase activity of nsp-14 respectively. Both these processes are required during the RNA cap formation [27, 84 - 87]. The nsp-12 is known as the RNA-dependent RNA polymerase (RdRp) [88]. The nsp-12 uses Mn^{2+} as metallic cofactor and nsp-7 and nsp-8 as protein cofactor [89]. It was reported that the antiviral drug Remdesivir (an adenosine analog) acts on the RdRp and can causes inhibition of RNA synthesis [90]. The nsp-13 is known as the helicase and it unwinds nucleic acid during viral replication [91]. The nsp-14 is the exoribonuclease (ExoN) which has the N7-methyltransferase activity and has role in the replication fidelity [86, 92]. The nsp-15 and nsp16 proteins exhibit the endoribonuclease and 2'-O- methyltransferase (2'-O-MTase) activities, respectively [84, 85, 93]. The endonuclease activity of nsp-15 uses Mn^{2+} as cofactor. This nsp-15 is conserved in Nidoviruses which acts as genetic marker as it is absent in other RNA viruses [94].

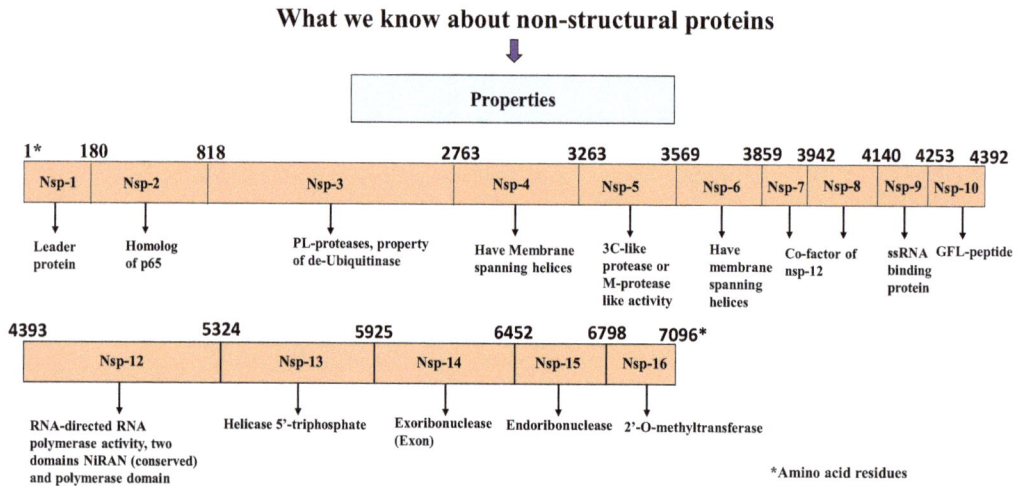

Fig. (3). Properties of non-structural proteins of SARS-CoV-2.

Table 1. Properties and functions of structural and non-structural proteins of SARS-CoV-2.

Proteins	Length (No. of Residues)	Functions
S	1273 residues [45]	Initiate infection by binding with the host's cell surface receptor [1], acts as vaccine candidate
E	75 residues [45]	Involved in the viral envelope formation, assembly [15], budding and pathogenesis [47, 48], acts as vaccine candidate [46]
M	222 residues [45]	Maintains shape and curvature [52], involved in viral assembly process [15]
N	419 residues [45]	Interacts with the M-protein and replicase complex to package the genome in viral particle [65 - 67]
nsp-1	180 residues [45]	Host mRNA inhibitor [71], inhibits interferon signaling [72]
nsp-2	638 residues [45]	Essential for viral replication, inhibits host survival pathway [73]
nsp-3	1945 residues [45]	Protein hydrolase activity (cleaves nsp1/2 and nsp 2/3), inhibit the expression of interferons, promoting cytokine expression [68, 74]
nsp-4	500 residues [45]	Helps in double membrane vesicle formation [76], interacts with nsp3 and nsp6 [79, 80]
nsp-5	306 residues [45]	Cleaves nsp3/4 [95], inhibits the interferon signaling [77]

(Table 1) cont.....

Proteins	Length (No. of Residues)	Functions
nsp-6	290 residues [45]	Interacts with nsp3 and nsp4 for DMV formation [79], restrict autophagosome expansion [80]
nsp-7	83 residues [45]	Accelerate polymerase activity [81]
nsp-8	198 residues [45]	Accelerate polymerase activity, primase [83]
nsp-9	113 residues [45]	Provides protection against nucleases, dimerization [82]
nsp-10	139 residues [45]	Stimulate the activity of nsp14 and nsp16, acts as allosteric activator [84 - 86]
nsp-12	932 residues [45]	Genome replication, viral proliferation through NiRAN [96]
nsp-13	601 residues [45]	Helps in genome replication, part of RNA capping machinery [95]
nsp-14	527 residues [45]	Function of N7-methyltransferase activity [86], role in the replication fidelity [92]
nsp-15	346 residues [45]	Cleaves at uridine residue required for viral infection [93]
nsp-16	298 residues [45]	Involved in mRNA capping (cap-1 (m7GpppNm-RNA) [84]

VIRAL GENOME REPLICATION

The droplets containing the virions are released into the environment by the infected person during sneezing or coughing. The virus then enters the healthy individuals *via* nose, eyes or mouth and enters the respiratory system. The virus is more likely to infect alveolar epithelial cells in lungs [97]. SARS-CoV-2 initiates infection by binding of its RBD in the S1 region of the S-protein with the ACE-2 receptor (Fig. **4**) [1]. The virus can also possibly gain entry through CD147 receptor into the host cell [98]. The coronavirus entry, *i.e.*, clathrin mediated endocytosis is regulated by host AP-2 associated protein kinase-I (AAKI), which activates the spike protein [78, 99]. This is further followed by the acid dependent proteolytic cleavage of S1 and S2 domain by the Cathepsin-L inside the endolytic vesicles during viral entry. The fusion domain of S-protein fuses the viral and host cell membranes and makes the entry of viral genome into the cytosol of the host cell [15].

After gaining the entry, the translation of viral genomic RNA takes place. Two large ORFs rep1a and rep1b produces two polyproteins pp1a and pp1ab, respectively. The ribosomal frame shifting plays a major role in expression of rep1a reading frame to rep1b with the utilization of slippery sequences (5'-UUUAAAC-3') and RNA pseudoknot. In most cases, the ribosome can melt the pseudoknot and continues elongation until the stop codon of rep1a leads to the production of pp1a. In the other case the pseudoknot blocks the ribosomal elongation on slippery sequence causing -1 frame shifting back to one nucleotide and continues elongation on rep1b leading to the translation of pp1ab [100, 101].The Orf1a and Orf1ab produces two polyproteins pp1a (that codes for nsps 1-11) and pp1ab (that codes for nsps 1-16), respectively. The nsp11 in pp1a forms nsp12 in pp1ab [15]. These polyproteins are further cleaved by proteases [papain like protease (PL-pro), 3C-like proteases or main proteases (3CL-pro or M-pro), serine like protease] [68, 69]. Subsequently, the replication complex forms and the production of genomic and sub-genomic RNA synthesis takes place during the process of viral RNA translation. The structural and accessory genes are located at the downstream of the replicase polyproteins. The sub-genomic RNA acts as mRNA for these genes. These sub-genomic and genomic RNA forms negative sense intermediate which contains both poly-uridylate and anti-leader sequences [102]. In the next event, the translation of structural proteins (S, E, N and M) takes place. These are inserted into endoplasmic reticulum and moves along the ER-Golgi intermediate compartment (ERGIC). The encapsidation of viral genome *via* N-protein also takes place into the membrane of ERGIC. After the assembly, the vesicles containing virions are released by exocytosis [15].

At the molecular level, the viral replication is a complex process that has many stages of viral RNA polymerization, proofreading and capping. The RNA synthesis begins with the formation of replication transcription complex (RTC). The formation of RTC involves the vesicular network of convoluted membranes (CVs) and double membrane vesicles (DMVs) formed from the endoplasmic reticulum [26, 103]. The RTC is associated by the CVs which involve the interaction of nsp3, nsp4 and nsp6. The dsRNA formed after the replication-transcription process is associated with the DMVs. These DMVs protect the dsRNA from its degradation and innate immune response [104]. The polymerization step requires the nsp12 protein that is a polymerase. This large enzyme requires nsp7 and nsp8 as cofactors [81]. The nsp12 has NiRAN and a polymerase domain [88]. The NiRAN (Nidovirus RdRp-associate--Nucleotidyltransferase) is located at the N-terminus and is conserved in all Nidoviruses. It has been shown that this domain is associated with the virus proliferation in SARS-CoV [96]. The C-terminus of nsp12 has RNA polymerase domain [88].

The RNA proofreading and capping is controlled by a bifunctional protein known as nsp14 [26]. The exoribonuclease activity is shown by the N-terminus (ExoN) domain. This domain has three conserved motifs, motif I (DE), motif II (E), motif III (D) and belongs to the superfamily of DEED exonucleases [92]. The ExoN domain has incredibly significant role in nucleic acid repair and prevents the mutations [105]. The viral cap synthesis is performed by the N7-guanin--methyltransferase activity of the C-terminus domain of the nsp14 [86]. The step of capping is important as this provides the stability to viral mRNA and protects it from the viral immune response [106]. The nsp13, nsp14 and nsp16 forms the capping machinery that requires nsp10 as a cofactor [26]. The process of capping starts with the hydrolysis of the 5′γ-phosphate of the RNA, which is initiated by the nsp13 helicases (RNA 5′triphosphatase) [95]. The formation of GpppN-RNA takes place by the transfer of GMP molecule through GTase transferase. The formation of cap-0 (m7GpppN-RNA) takes place by the methylation at the N7 position of the guanosine by the C-terminal N7-MTase domain of Nsp14 using SAM (S-adenosyl methionine) as the methyl donor. In the next step the formation of cap-1 (m7GpppNm-RNA) takes place by the addition of methyl group on the ribose 2-O position at the first transcribed nucleotide by the (SAM)-dependent 2′-O-methyltransferase activity of Nsp16. In all these steps the cofactor nsp10 acts as the allosteric activator [84, 85]. Both the host and viral factors are thus important to initiate, progress and spread of the infection. Therefore, Coronavirus replication is extraordinarily complex and regulated at the molecular levels.

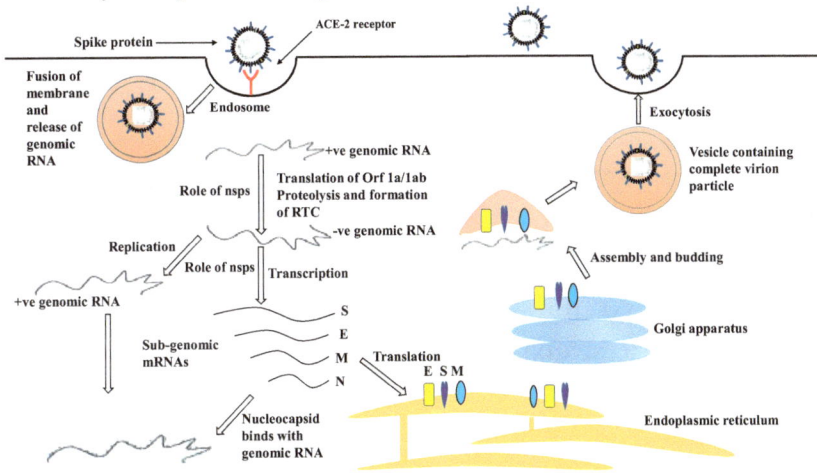

Fig. (4). Replication of the SARS-CoV-2. The virus binds with the host cell membrane *via* its spike protein. This is followed by clathrin mediated endocytosis leading to the viral entry into the host cell. The cleavage of S1 and S2 domain of the spike protein and fusion of membrane are done within the endolytic vesicle. The replication and transcription of viral genomic RNA takes place inside the cytoplasm of the host cell. The genomic RNA forms the structural proteins. The non-structural proteins take part in the viral replication. The assembly and budding of virus particles take place through ERGIC pathway.

CONCLUDING REMARKS

Emergence of coronavirus has created an alarming situation in the last two decades *via* SARS (2002-3), MERS (2013-14) and SARS-CoV-2 (2019-20). The high recombination frequency, elevated mutation rate and wide range of infecting hosts are a major concern for Coronaviruses. The ongoing pandemic of COVID-19 has affected each part of the globe leading to large number of symptomatic and asymptomatic infections. In this report we have depicted the details about the morphology, genomic organization and role of different proteins in viral replication machinery that takes place in the host. An interdisciplinary research involving molecular biologists, virologists, immunologists, biochemists, structural biologists and clinicians is needed to delineate a complete pathway of pathogenesis and viral replication of SARS-CoV-2 in cell lines, animal and human hosts. Description of structure and role of different proteins in viral proliferation will provide insight into formulation of their inhibitors that might act as possible therapeutic agents. In addition, this data will also assist in designing of future vaccines against this viral pathogen.

CONSENT FOR PUBLICATION

Not Applicable.

CONFLICT OF INTEREST

The author declares no conflict of interest, financial or otherwise.

ACKNOWLEDGEMENTS

Arshi Islam and Abu Humza are supported by Research Fellowship by the Indian Council of Medical Research (ICMR), Government of India. Zoya Shafat is supported by Research Fellowship by University Grants Commission (UGC), Government of India. The research in our laboratory is funded by the Council of Scientific and Industrial Research (CSIR), India (37(1697)17/EMR-II) and Central Council for Research in Unani Medicine (CCRUM), Ministry of Ayurveda, Yoga and Naturopathy, Unani, Siddha and Homeopathy (AYUSH) (F.No.3-63/2019-CCRUM/Tech). The authors also extend their appreciation to the Centre of Excellence in Biotechnology Research, Deanship of Scientific Research, King Saud University, Riyadh, Saudi Arabia for support.

REFERENCES

[1]   Shanmugaraj B, Siriwattananon K, Wangkanont K, Phoolcharoen W. Perspectives on monoclonal antibody therapy as potential therapeutic intervention for Coronavirus disease-19 (COVID-19). Asian Pac J Allergy Immunol 2020; 38(1): 10-8.
[PMID: 32134278]

[2]   Banerjee A, Kulcsar K, Misra V, Frieman M, Mossman K. Bats and coronaviruses. Viruses 2019; 11(1): 41.
[http://dx.doi.org/10.3390/v11010041] [PMID: 30634396]

[3]   Masters PS. The molecular biology of coronaviruses. Adv Virus Res 2006; 66: 193-292.
[http://dx.doi.org/10.1016/S0065-3527(06)66005-3] [PMID: 16877062]

[4]   Kruse RL. Therapeutic strategies in an outbreak scenario to treat the novel coronavirus originating in Wuhan, China. F1000 Res 2020; 9: 72.
[http://dx.doi.org/10.12688/f1000research.22211.2] [PMID: 32117569]

[5]   Bai Y, Yao L, Wei T, *et al.* Presumed asymptomatic carrier transmission of COVID-19. JAMA 2020; 323(14): 1406-7.
[http://dx.doi.org/10.1001/jama.2020.2565] [PMID: 32083643]

[6]   Wang D, Hu B, Hu C, *et al.* Clinical characteristics of 138 hospitalized patients with 2019 novel coronavirus–infected pneumonia in Wuhan, China. JAMA 2020; 323(11): 1061-9.
[http://dx.doi.org/10.1001/jama.2020.1585] [PMID: 32031570]

[7]   Lai CC, Shih TP, Ko WC, Tang HJ, Hsueh PR. Severe acute respiratory syndrome coronavirus 2 (SARS-CoV-2) and coronavirus disease-2019 (COVID-19): The epidemic and the challenges. Int J Antimicrob Agents 2020; 55(3): 105924.
[http://dx.doi.org/10.1016/j.ijantimicag.2020.105924] [PMID: 32081636]

[8]   Gralinski LE, Menachery VD. Return of the Coronavirus: 2019-nCoV. Viruses 2020; 12(2): 135.
[http://dx.doi.org/10.3390/v12020135] [PMID: 31991541]

[9]   https://www.worldometers.info/coronavirus/

[10]   Kumar S, Maurya VK, Prasad AK, Bhatt MLB, Saxena SK. Structural, glycosylation and antigenic variation between 2019 novel coronavirus (2019-nCoV) and SARS coronavirus (SARS-CoV). Virusdisease 2020; 31(1): 13-21.
[http://dx.doi.org/10.1007/s13337-020-00571-5] [PMID: 32206694]

[11]   Park WB, Kwon NJ, Choi SJ, *et al.* Virus isolation from the first patient with SARS-CoV-2 in Korea. J Korean Med Sci 2020; 35(7): e84.
[http://dx.doi.org/10.3346/jkms.2020.35.e84] [PMID: 32080990]

[12]   Ashour HM, Elkhatib WF, Rahman MM, Elshabrawy HA. Insights into the recent 2019 novel coronavirus (SARS-CoV-2) in light of past human coronavirus outbreaks. Pathogens 2020; 9(3): 186.
[http://dx.doi.org/10.3390/pathogens9030186] [PMID: 32143502]

[13]   Delmas B, Laude H. Assembly of coronavirus spike protein into trimers and its role in epitope expression. J Virol 1990; 64(11): 5367-75.
[http://dx.doi.org/10.1128/JVI.64.11.5367-5375.1990] [PMID: 2170676]

[14]   Finlay BB, See RH, Brunham RC. Rapid response research to emerging infectious diseases: lessons from SARS. Nat Rev Microbiol 2004; 2(7): 602-7.
[http://dx.doi.org/10.1038/nrmicro930] [PMID: 15197395]

[15]   Fehr AR, Perlman S. Coronaviruses: an overview of their replication and pathogenesis InCoronaviruses. New York, NY: Humana Press 2015; pp. 1-23.
[http://dx.doi.org/10.1007/978-1-4939-2438-7_1] [PMID: 25720466]

[16]   Chang CK, Hou MH, Chang CF, Hsiao CD, Huang TH. The SARS coronavirus nucleocapsid protein--forms and functions. Antiviral Res 2014; 103: 39-50.
[http://dx.doi.org/10.1016/j.antiviral.2013.12.009] [PMID: 24418573]

[17]   Chan JF, To KK, Tse H, Jin DY, Yuen KY. Interspecies transmission and emergence of novel viruses: lessons from bats and birds. Trends Microbiol 2013; 21(10): 544-55.
[http://dx.doi.org/10.1016/j.tim.2013.05.005] [PMID: 23770275]

[18]   Lu R, Zhao X, Li J, *et al.* Genomic characterisation and epidemiology of 2019 novel coronavirus: implications for virus origins and receptor binding. Lancet 2020; 395(10224): 565-74.
[http://dx.doi.org/10.1016/S0140-6736(20)30251-8] [PMID: 32007145]

[19]   Chen Y, Liu Q, Guo D. Emerging coronaviruses: Genome structure, replication, and pathogenesis. J Med Virol 2020; 92(4): 418-23.
[http://dx.doi.org/10.1002/jmv.25681] [PMID: 31967327]

[20]   Luan J, Lu Y, Jin X, Zhang L. Spike protein recognition of mammalian ACE2 predicts the host range and an optimized ACE2 for SARS-CoV-2 infection. Biochem Biophys Res Commun 2020; 526(1): 165-9.

[http://dx.doi.org/10.1016/j.bbrc.2020.03.047] [PMID: 32201080]

[21]   Chan JF, Kok KH, Zhu Z, *et al.* Genomic characterization of the 2019 novel human-pathogenic coronavirus isolated from a patient with atypical pneumonia after visiting Wuhan. Emerg Microbes Infect 2020; 9(1): 221-36.
       [http://dx.doi.org/10.1080/22221751.2020.1719902] [PMID: 31987001]

[22]   Snijder EJ, van der Meer Y, Zevenhoven-Dobbe J, *et al.* Ultrastructure and origin of membrane vesicles associated with the severe acute respiratory syndrome coronavirus replication complex. J Virol 2006; 80(12): 5927-40.
       [http://dx.doi.org/10.1128/JVI.02501-05] [PMID: 16731931]

[23]   Hussain S, Pan J, Chen Y, *et al.* Identification of novel subgenomic RNAs and noncanonical transcription initiation signals of severe acute respiratory syndrome coronavirus. J Virol 2005; 79(9): 5288-95.
       [http://dx.doi.org/10.1128/JVI.79.9.5288-5295.2005] [PMID: 15827143]

[24]   Perlman S, Netland J. Coronaviruses post-SARS: update on replication and pathogenesis. Nat Rev Microbiol 2009; 7(6): 439-50.
       [http://dx.doi.org/10.1038/nrmicro2147] [PMID: 19430490]

[25]   Ziebuhr J, Snijder EJ, Gorbalenya AE. Virus-encoded proteinases and proteolytic processing in the Nidovirales. J Gen Virol 2000; 81(Pt 4): 853-79.
       [http://dx.doi.org/10.1099/0022-1317-81-4-853] [PMID: 10725411]

[26]   Romano M, Ruggiero A, Squeglia F, Maga G, Berisio R. A Structural View of SARS-CoV-2 RNA Replication Machinery: RNA Synthesis, Proofreading and Final Capping. Cells 2020; 9(5): 1267.
       [http://dx.doi.org/10.3390/cells9051267] [PMID: 32443810]

[27]   Dong S, Sun J, Mao Z, Wang L, Lu YL, Li J. A guideline for homology modeling of the proteins from newly discovered betacoronavirus, 2019 novel coronavirus (2019-nCoV). J Med Virol 2020; 92(9): 1542-8.
       [http://dx.doi.org/10.1002/jmv.25768] [PMID: 32181901]

[28]   Ceccarelli M, Berretta M, Venanzi Rullo E, Nunnari G, Cacopardo B. Differences and similarities between Severe Acute Respiratory Syndrome (SARS)-CoronaVirus (CoV) and SARS-CoV-2. Would a rose by another name smell as sweet? Eur Rev Med Pharmacol Sci 2020; 24(5): 2781-3.
       [http://dx.doi.org/10.26355/eurrev_202003_20551] [PMID: 32196628]

[29]   Jeffers SA, Tusell SM, Gillim-Ross L, *et al.* CD209L (L-SIGN) is a receptor for severe acute respiratory syndrome coronavirus. Proc Natl Acad Sci USA 2004; 101(44): 15748-53.
       [http://dx.doi.org/10.1073/pnas.0403812101] [PMID: 15496474]

[30]   Kubo H, Yamada YK, Taguchi F. Localization of neutralizing epitopes and the receptor-binding site within the amino-terminal 330 amino acids of the murine coronavirus spike protein. J Virol 1994; 68(9): 5403-10.
       [http://dx.doi.org/10.1128/JVI.68.9.5403-5410.1994] [PMID: 7520090]

[31]   Hoffmann M, Kleine-Weber H, Schroeder S, *et al.* SARS-CoV-2 cell entry depends on ACE2 and TMPRSS2 and is blocked by a clinically proven protease inhibitor. Cell 2020; 181(2): 271-80.
       [http://dx.doi.org/10.1016/j.cell.2020.02.052] [PMID: 32142651]

[32]   Pillay TS. Gene of the month: the 2019-nCoV/SARS-CoV-2 novel coronavirus spike protein. J Clin Pathol 2020; 73(7): 366-9.
       [http://dx.doi.org/10.1136/jclinpath-2020-206658] [PMID: 32376714]

[33]   He Y, Zhou Y, Liu S, *et al.* Receptor-binding domain of SARS-CoV spike protein induces highly potent neutralizing antibodies: implication for developing subunit vaccine. Biochem Biophys Res Commun 2004; 324(2): 773-81.
       [http://dx.doi.org/10.1016/j.bbrc.2004.09.106] [PMID: 15474494]

[34]   Wrapp D, Wang N, Corbett KS, *et al.* Cryo-EM structure of the 2019-nCoV spike in the prefusion

conformation. Science 2020; 367(6483): 1260-3.
[http://dx.doi.org/10.1126/science.abb2507] [PMID: 32075877]

[35] Qian Z, Dominguez SR, Holmes KV. Role of the spike glycoprotein of human Middle East respiratory syndrome coronavirus (MERS-CoV) in virus entry and syncytia formation. PLoS One 2013; 8(10): e76469.
[http://dx.doi.org/10.1371/journal.pone.0076469] [PMID: 24098509]

[36] Li F. Structure, function, and evolution of coronavirus spike proteins. Annu Rev Virol 2016; 3(1): 237-61.
[http://dx.doi.org/10.1146/annurev-virology-110615-042301] [PMID: 27578435]

[37] Song Z, Xu Y, Bao L, *et al.* From SARS to MERS, thrusting coronaviruses into the spotlight. Viruses 2019; 11(1): 59.
[http://dx.doi.org/10.3390/v11010059] [PMID: 30646565]

[38] Belouzard S, Chu VC, Whittaker GR. Activation of the SARS coronavirus spike protein *via* sequential proteolytic cleavage at two distinct sites. Proc Natl Acad Sci USA 2009; 106(14): 5871-6.
[http://dx.doi.org/10.1073/pnas.0809524106] [PMID: 19321428]

[39] Millet JK, Whittaker GR. Host cell entry of Middle East respiratory syndrome coronavirus after two-step, furin-mediated activation of the spike protein. Proc Natl Acad Sci USA 2014; 111(42): 15214-9.
[http://dx.doi.org/10.1073/pnas.1407087111] [PMID: 25288733]

[40] Millet JK, Whittaker GR. Host cell proteases: Critical determinants of coronavirus tropism and pathogenesis. Virus Res 2015; 202: 120-34.
[http://dx.doi.org/10.1016/j.virusres.2014.11.021] [PMID: 25445340]

[41] Izaguirre G. The proteolytic regulation of virus cell entry by furin and other proprotein convertases. Viruses 2019; 11(9): 837.
[http://dx.doi.org/10.3390/v11090837] [PMID: 31505793]

[42] Coutard B, Valle C, de Lamballerie X, Canard B, Seidah NG, Decroly E. The spike glycoprotein of the new coronavirus 2019-nCoV contains a furin-like cleavage site absent in CoV of the same clade. Antiviral Res 2020; 176: 104742.
[http://dx.doi.org/10.1016/j.antiviral.2020.104742] [PMID: 32057769]

[43] Kuo L, Hurst KR, Masters PS. Exceptional flexibility in the sequence requirements for coronavirus small envelope protein function. J Virol 2007; 81(5): 2249-62.
[http://dx.doi.org/10.1128/JVI.01577-06] [PMID: 17182690]

[44] Arbely E, Khattari Z, Brotons G, Akkawi M, Salditt T, Arkin IT. A highly unusual palindromic transmembrane helical hairpin formed by SARS coronavirus E protein. J Mol Biol 2004; 341(3): 769-79.
[http://dx.doi.org/10.1016/j.jmb.2004.06.044] [PMID: 15288785]

[45] Giri R, Bhardwaj T, Shegane M, *et al.* Understanding COVID-19 *via* comparative analysis of dark proteomes of SARS-CoV-2, human SARS and bat SARS-like coronaviruses. Cell Mol Life Sci 2020; Jul 25: 1-34.
[http://dx.doi.org/10.1007/s00018-020-03603-x] [PMID: 32712910]

[46] Schoeman D, Fielding BC. Coronavirus envelope protein: current knowledge. Virol J 2019; 16(1): 69.
[http://dx.doi.org/10.1186/s12985-019-1182-0] [PMID: 31133031]

[47] Siu YL, Teoh KT, Lo J, *et al.* The M, E, and N structural proteins of the severe acute respiratory syndrome coronavirus are required for efficient assembly, trafficking, and release of virus-like particles. J Virol 2008; 82(22): 11318-30.
[http://dx.doi.org/10.1128/JVI.01052-08] [PMID: 18753196]

[48] DeDiego ML, Álvarez E, Almazán F, *et al.* A severe acute respiratory syndrome coronavirus that lacks the E gene is attenuated *in vitro* and *in vivo*. J Virol 2007; 81(4): 1701-13.
[http://dx.doi.org/10.1128/JVI.01467-06] [PMID: 17108030]

[49] Nieto-Torres JL, DeDiego ML, Verdiá-Báguena C, *et al.* Severe acute respiratory syndrome coronavirus envelope protein ion channel activity promotes virus fitness and pathogenesis. PLoS Pathog 2014; 10(5): e1004077.
[http://dx.doi.org/10.1371/journal.ppat.1004077] [PMID: 24788150]

[50] Hogue BG, Machamer CE. Spike protein recognition of mammalian ACE2 predicts the host range and an optimized ACE2 for SARS-CoV-2 infection. Biochemical and biophysical research communications. 2020 Mar 19.

[51] Venkatagopalan P, Daskalova SM, Lopez LA, Dolezal KA, Hogue BG. Coronavirus envelope (E) protein remains at the site of assembly. Virology 2015; 478: 75-85.
[http://dx.doi.org/10.1016/j.virol.2015.02.005] [PMID: 25726972]

[52] Neuman BW, Kiss G, Kunding AH, *et al.* A structural analysis of M protein in coronavirus assembly and morphology. J Struct Biol 2011; 174(1): 11-22.
[http://dx.doi.org/10.1016/j.jsb.2010.11.021] [PMID: 21130884]

[53] Nal B, Chan C, Kien F, *et al.* Differential maturation and subcellular localization of severe acute respiratory syndrome coronavirus surface proteins S, M and E. J Gen Virol 2005; 86(Pt 5): 1423-34.
[http://dx.doi.org/10.1099/vir.0.80671-0] [PMID: 15831954]

[54] Bos EC, Luytjes W, van der Meulen HV, Koerten HK, Spaan WJ. The production of recombinant infectious DI-particles of a murine coronavirus in the absence of helper virus. Virology 1996; 218(1): 52-60.
[http://dx.doi.org/10.1006/viro.1996.0165] [PMID: 8615041]

[55] Hurst KR, Kuo L, Koetzner CA, Ye R, Hsue B, Masters PS. A major determinant for membrane protein interaction localizes to the carboxy-terminal domain of the mouse coronavirus nucleocapsid protein. J Virol 2005; 79(21): 13285-97.
[http://dx.doi.org/10.1128/JVI.79.21.13285-13297.2005] [PMID: 16227251]

[56] de Haan CA, de Wit M, Kuo L, *et al.* The glycosylation status of the murine hepatitis coronavirus M protein affects the interferogenic capacity of the virus *in vitro* and its ability to replicate in the liver but not the brain. Virology 2003; 312(2): 395-406.
[http://dx.doi.org/10.1016/S0042-6822(03)00235-6] [PMID: 12919744]

[57] Weiss SR, Navas-Martin S. Coronavirus pathogenesis and the emerging pathogen severe acute respiratory syndrome coronavirus. Microbiol Mol Biol Rev 2005; 69(4): 635-64.
[http://dx.doi.org/10.1128/MMBR.69.4.635-664.2005] [PMID: 16339739]

[58] Mortola E, Roy P. Efficient assembly and release of SARS coronavirus-like particles by a heterologous expression system. FEBS Lett 2004; 576(1-2): 174-8.
[http://dx.doi.org/10.1016/j.febslet.2004.09.009] [PMID: 15474033]

[59] Opstelten DJ, Raamsman MJ, Wolfs K, Horzinek MC, Rottier PJ. Envelope glycoprotein interactions in coronavirus assembly. J Cell Biol 1995; 131(2): 339-49.
[http://dx.doi.org/10.1083/jcb.131.2.339] [PMID: 7593163]

[60] Menachery VD, Graham RL, Baric RS. Jumping species-a mechanism for coronavirus persistence and survival. Curr Opin Virol 2017; 23: 1-7.
[http://dx.doi.org/10.1016/j.coviro.2017.01.002] [PMID: 28214731]

[61] Stohlman SA, Lai MM. Phosphoproteins of murine hepatitis viruses. J Virol 1979; 32(2): 672-5.
[http://dx.doi.org/10.1128/JVI.32.2.672-675.1979] [PMID: 228084]

[62] McBride R, van Zyl M, Fielding BC. The coronavirus nucleocapsid is a multifunctional protein. Viruses 2014; 6(8): 2991-3018.
[http://dx.doi.org/10.3390/v6082991] [PMID: 25105276]

[63] Chen CY, Chang CK, Chang YW, *et al.* Structure of the SARS coronavirus nucleocapsid protein RNA-binding dimerization domain suggests a mechanism for helical packaging of viral RNA. J Mol Biol 2007; 368(4): 1075-86.

[http://dx.doi.org/10.1016/j.jmb.2007.02.069] [PMID: 17379242]

[64]   Chang CK, Sue SC, Yu TH, *et al.* Modular organization of SARS coronavirus nucleocapsid protein. J Biomed Sci 2006; 13(1): 59-72.
[http://dx.doi.org/10.1007/s11373-005-9035-9] [PMID: 16228284]

[65]   Hurst KR, Koetzner CA, Masters PS. Identification of *in vivo*-interacting domains of the murine coronavirus nucleocapsid protein. J Virol 2009; 83(14): 7221-34.
[http://dx.doi.org/10.1128/JVI.00440-09] [PMID: 19420077]

[66]   Kuo L, Masters PS. Functional analysis of the murine coronavirus genomic RNA packaging signal. J Virol 2013; 87(9): 5182-92.
[http://dx.doi.org/10.1128/JVI.00100-13] [PMID: 23449786]

[67]   Hurst KR, Koetzner CA, Masters PS. Characterization of a critical interaction between the coronavirus nucleocapsid protein and nonstructural protein 3 of the viral replicase-transcriptase complex. J Virol 2013; 87(16): 9159-72.
[http://dx.doi.org/10.1128/JVI.01275-13] [PMID: 23760243]

[68]   Lei J, Kusov Y, Hilgenfeld R. Nsp3 of coronaviruses: Structures and functions of a large multi-domain protein. Antiviral Res 2018; 149: 58-74.
[http://dx.doi.org/10.1016/j.antiviral.2017.11.001] [PMID: 29128390]

[69]   Stobart CC, Sexton NR, Munjal H, *et al.* Chimeric exchange of coronavirus nsp5 proteases (3CLpro) identifies common and divergent regulatory determinants of protease activity. J Virol 2013; 87(23): 12611-8.
[http://dx.doi.org/10.1128/JVI.02050-13] [PMID: 24027335]

[70]   Lokugamage KG, Narayanan K, Huang C, Makino S. Severe acute respiratory syndrome coronavirus protein nsp1 is a novel eukaryotic translation inhibitor that represses multiple steps of translation initiation. J Virol 2012; 86(24): 13598-608.
[http://dx.doi.org/10.1128/JVI.01958-12] [PMID: 23035226]

[71]   Huang C, Lokugamage KG, Rozovics JM, Narayanan K, Semler BL, Makino S. SARS coronavirus nsp1 protein induces template-dependent endonucleolytic cleavage of mRNAs: viral mRNAs are resistant to nsp1-induced RNA cleavage. PLoS Pathog 2011; 7(12): e1002433.
[http://dx.doi.org/10.1371/journal.ppat.1002433] [PMID: 22174690]

[72]   Tanaka T, Kamitani W, DeDiego ML, Enjuanes L, Matsuura Y. Severe acute respiratory syndrome coronavirus nsp1 facilitates efficient propagation in cells through a specific translational shutoff of host mRNA. J Virol 2012; 86(20): 11128-37.
[http://dx.doi.org/10.1128/JVI.01700-12] [PMID: 22855488]

[73]   Cornillez-Ty CT, Liao L, Yates JR III, Kuhn P, Buchmeier MJ. Severe acute respiratory syndrome coronavirus nonstructural protein 2 interacts with a host protein complex involved in mitochondrial biogenesis and intracellular signaling. J Virol 2009; 83(19): 10314-8.
[http://dx.doi.org/10.1128/JVI.00842-09] [PMID: 19640993]

[74]   Serrano P, Johnson MA, Chatterjee A, *et al.* Nuclear magnetic resonance structure of the nucleic acid-binding domain of severe acute respiratory syndrome coronavirus nonstructural protein 3. J Virol 2009; 83(24): 12998-3008.
[http://dx.doi.org/10.1128/JVI.01253-09] [PMID: 19828617]

[75]   Frieman M, Ratia K, Johnston RE, Mesecar AD, Baric RS. Severe acute respiratory syndrome coronavirus papain-like protease ubiquitin-like domain and catalytic domain regulate antagonism of IRF3 and NF-kappaB signaling. J Virol 2009; 83(13): 6689-705.
[http://dx.doi.org/10.1128/JVI.02220-08] [PMID: 19369340]

[76]   Beachboard DC, Anderson-Daniels JM, Denison MR. Mutations across murine hepatitis virus nsp4 alter virus fitness and membrane modifications. J Virol 2015; 89(4): 2080-9.
[http://dx.doi.org/10.1128/JVI.02776-14] [PMID: 25473044]

[77]   Zhu X, Fang L, Wang D, *et al.* Porcine deltacoronavirus nsp5 inhibits interferon-β production through the cleavage of NEMO. Virology 2017; 502: 33-8.
[http://dx.doi.org/10.1016/j.virol.2016.12.005] [PMID: 27984784]

[78]   Li H, Zhou Y, Zhang M, Wang H, Zhao Q, Liu J. Updated approaches against SARS-CoV-2. Antimicrob Agents Chemother 2020; 64(6): e00483-20.
[http://dx.doi.org/10.1128/AAC.00483-20] [PMID: 32205349]

[79]   Angelini MM, Akhlaghpour M, Neuman BW, Buchmeier MJ. Severe acute respiratory syndrome coronavirus nonstructural proteins 3, 4, and 6 induce double-membrane vesicles. MBio 2013; 4(4): e00524-13.
[http://dx.doi.org/10.1128/mBio.00524-13] [PMID: 23943763]

[80]   Cottam EM, Whelband MC, Wileman T. Coronavirus NSP6 restricts autophagosome expansion. Autophagy 2014; 10(8): 1426-41.
[http://dx.doi.org/10.4161/auto.29309] [PMID: 24991833]

[81]   Kirchdoerfer RN, Ward AB. Structure of the SARS-CoV nsp12 polymerase bound to nsp7 and nsp8 co-factors. Nat Commun 2019; 10(1): 2342.
[http://dx.doi.org/10.1038/s41467-019-10280-3] [PMID: 31138817]

[82]   te Velthuis AJ, van den Worm SH, Snijder EJ. The SARS-coronavirus nsp7+nsp8 complex is a unique multimeric RNA polymerase capable of both de novo initiation and primer extension. Nucleic Acids Res 2012; 40(4): 1737-47.
[http://dx.doi.org/10.1093/nar/gkr893] [PMID: 22039154]

[83]   Egloff MP, Ferron F, Campanacci V, *et al.* The severe acute respiratory syndrome-coronavirus replicative protein nsp9 is a single-stranded RNA-binding subunit unique in the RNA virus world. Proc Natl Acad Sci USA 2004; 101(11): 3792-6.
[http://dx.doi.org/10.1073/pnas.0307877101] [PMID: 15007178]

[84]   Decroly E, Debarnot C, Ferron F, *et al.* Crystal structure and functional analysis of the SARS-coronavirus RNA cap 2'-O-methyltransferase nsp10/nsp16 complex. PLoS Pathog 2011; 7(5): e1002059.
[http://dx.doi.org/10.1371/journal.ppat.1002059] [PMID: 21637813]

[85]   Chen Y, Su C, Ke M, *et al.* Biochemical and structural insights into the mechanisms of SARS coronavirus RNA ribose 2'-O-methylation by nsp16/nsp10 protein complex. PLoS Pathog 2011; 7(10): e1002294.
[http://dx.doi.org/10.1371/journal.ppat.1002294] [PMID: 22022266]

[86]   Ma Y, Wu L, Shaw N, *et al.* Structural basis and functional analysis of the SARS coronavirus nsp14-nsp10 complex. Proc Natl Acad Sci USA 2015; 112(30): 9436-41.
[http://dx.doi.org/10.1073/pnas.1508686112] [PMID: 26159422]

[87]   Bouvet M, Debarnot C, Imbert I, *et al. In vitro* reconstitution of SARS-coronavirus mRNA cap methylation. PLoS Pathog 2010; 6(4): e1000863.
[http://dx.doi.org/10.1371/journal.ppat.1000863] [PMID: 20421945]

[88]   Gao Y, Yan L, Huang Y, *et al.* Structure of the RNA-dependent RNA polymerase from COVID-19 virus. Science 2020; 368(6492): 779-82.
[http://dx.doi.org/10.1126/science.abb7498] [PMID: 32277040]

[89]   Ahn DG, Choi JK, Taylor DR, Oh JW. Biochemical characterization of a recombinant SARS coronavirus nsp12 RNA-dependent RNA polymerase capable of copying viral RNA templates. Arch Virol 2012; 157(11): 2095-104.
[http://dx.doi.org/10.1007/s00705-012-1404-x] [PMID: 22791111]

[90]   Gordon CJ, Tchesnokov EP, Feng JY, Porter DP, Götte M. The antiviral compound remdesivir potently inhibits RNA-dependent RNA polymerase from Middle East respiratory syndrome coronavirus. J Biol Chem 2020; 295(15): 4773-9.

[http://dx.doi.org/10.1074/jbc.AC120.013056] [PMID: 32094225]

[91]   Adedeji AO, Lazarus H. Biochemical characterization of Middle East respiratory syndrome coronavirus helicase. MSphere 2016; 1(5): e00235-16.
[http://dx.doi.org/10.1128/mSphere.00235-16] [PMID: 27631026]

[92]   Ogando NS, Ferron F, Decroly E, Canard B, Posthuma CC, Snijder EJ. The curious case of the nidovirus exoribonuclease: its role in RNA synthesis and replication fidelity. Front Microbiol 2019; 10: 1813.
[http://dx.doi.org/10.3389/fmicb.2019.01813] [PMID: 31440227]

[93]   Zhang L, Li L, Yan L, *et al.* Structural and biochemical characterization of endoribonuclease Nsp15 encoded by Middle East respiratory syndrome coronavirus. J Virol 2018; 92(22): e00893-18.
[http://dx.doi.org/10.1128/JVI.00893-18] [PMID: 30135128]

[94]   Ivanov KA, Hertzig T, Rozanov M, *et al.* Major genetic marker of nidoviruses encodes a replicative endoribonuclease. Proc Natl Acad Sci USA 2004; 101(34): 12694-9.
[http://dx.doi.org/10.1073/pnas.0403127101] [PMID: 15304651]

[95]   Ivanov KA, Thiel V, Dobbe JC, van der Meer Y, Snijder EJ, Ziebuhr J. Multiple enzymatic activities associated with severe acute respiratory syndrome coronavirus helicase. J Virol 2004; 78(11): 5619-32.
[http://dx.doi.org/10.1128/JVI.78.11.5619-5632.2004] [PMID: 15140959]

[96]   Lehmann KC, Gulyaeva A, Zevenhoven-Dobbe JC, *et al.* Discovery of an essential nucleotidylating activity associated with a newly delineated conserved domain in the RNA polymerase-containing protein of all nidoviruses. Nucleic Acids Res 2015; 43(17): 8416-34.
[http://dx.doi.org/10.1093/nar/gkv838] [PMID: 26304538]

[97]   Chen L, Liu W, Zhang Q, *et al.* RNA based mNGS approach identifies a novel human coronavirus from two individual pneumonia cases in 2019 Wuhan outbreak. Emerg Microbes Infect 2020; 9(1): 313-9.
[http://dx.doi.org/10.1080/22221751.2020.1725399] [PMID: 32020836]

[98]   Wang K, Chen W, Zhou YS, *et al.* SARS-CoV-2 invades host cells *via* a novel route: CD147-spike protein. bioRxiv 2020.

[99]   Neveu G, Ziv-Av A, Barouch-Bentov R, Berkerman E, Mulholland J, Einav S. AP-2-associated protein kinase 1 and cyclin G-associated kinase regulate hepatitis C virus entry and are potential drug targets. J Virol 2015; 89(8): 4387-404.
[http://dx.doi.org/10.1128/JVI.02705-14] [PMID: 25653444]

[100]   Baranov PV, Henderson CM, Anderson CB, Gesteland RF, Atkins JF, Howard MT. Programmed ribosomal frameshifting in decoding the SARS-CoV genome. Virology 2005; 332(2): 498-510.
[http://dx.doi.org/10.1016/j.virol.2004.11.038] [PMID: 15680415]

[101]   Brierley I, Digard P, Inglis SC. Characterization of an efficient coronavirus ribosomal frameshifting signal: requirement for an RNA pseudoknot. Cell 1989; 57(4): 537-47.
[http://dx.doi.org/10.1016/0092-8674(89)90124-4] [PMID: 2720781]

[102]   Sethna PB, Hofmann MA, Brian DA. Minus-strand copies of replicating coronavirus mRNAs contain antileaders. J Virol 1991; 65(1): 320-5.
[http://dx.doi.org/10.1128/JVI.65.1.320-325.1991] [PMID: 1985203]

[103]   Sola I, Almazán F, Zúñiga S, Enjuanes L. Continuous and discontinuous RNA synthesis in coronaviruses. Annu Rev Virol 2015; 2(1): 265-88.
[http://dx.doi.org/10.1146/annurev-virology-100114-055218] [PMID: 26958916]

[104]   Knoops K, Kikkert M, Worm SH, *et al.* SARS-coronavirus replication is supported by a reticulovesicular network of modified endoplasmic reticulum. PLoS Biol 2008; 6(9): e226.
[http://dx.doi.org/10.1371/journal.pbio.0060226] [PMID: 18798692]

[105]   Becares M, Pascual-Iglesias A, Nogales A, Sola I, Enjuanes L, Zuñiga S. Mutagenesis of coronavirus

nsp14 reveals its potential role in modulation of the innate immune response. J Virol 2016; 90(11): 5399-414.
[http://dx.doi.org/10.1128/JVI.03259-15] [PMID: 27009949]

[106] Decroly E, Ferron F, Lescar J, Canard B. Conventional and unconventional mechanisms for capping viral mRNA. Nat Rev Microbiol 2011; 10(1): 51-65.
[http://dx.doi.org/10.1038/nrmicro2675] [PMID: 22138959]

CHAPTER 3

Structural Protein Genes of SARS-CoV-2: Comprehensive Molecular Characterization

Zoya Shafat[1], Syed Abuzar Raza Rizvi[2], Mohammad Misbah Urrehmaan[1,2], Ayesha Tazeen[1], Priyanka Sinha[1], Anwar Ahmed[3,4] and Shama Parveen[1,*]

[1] *Centre for Interdisciplinary Research in Basic Sciences, Jamia Millia Islamia, New Delhi, India*

[2] *Department of Biotechnology, School of Chemical & Life Sciences, Jamia Hamdard, New Delhi, India*

[3] *Center of Excellence in Biotechnology Research, College of Science, King Saud University, Riyadh, Saudi Arabia*

[4] *Protein Research Chair, Department of Biochemistry, College of Science, King Saud University, Riyadh, Saudi Arabia*

Abstract: Severe acute respiratory syndrome coronavirus 2 (SARS-CoV-2) is the causative agent of the global pandemic of Coronavirus disease 2019 (COVID-19). Limited information is available on evolutionary aspects of the structural proteins: spike (S), envelope (E), membrane (M) and nucleocapsid (N) of the virus. Therefore, we attempted detailed molecular and genetic characterization of SARS-CoV-2 structural protein genes using nucleotide composition, codon usage patterns, phylogenetic, entropy and selection pressure analyses. The RSCU patterns suggested codon biasness due to preference of U/A-ended over C/G-ended codons. Mutational pressure and natural selection influence the synonymous codon usage of structural protein genes in SARS-CoV-2. Phylogenetic analyses of different coronaviruses for all the four structural genes showed that all 2019-nCoV study sequences were clustered under the SARS-CoV-2 clade which was closest to bat coronaviruses. Additional phylogenetic analyses of SARS-CoV-2 structural protein genes showed discordance in the topology, suggesting different patterns of evolutionary relationships among these genes. Few non-synonymous amino acid mutations, low value of entropy and purifying selection suggested limited variations in the studied genes. However, these variations in the SARS-CoV-2 genome are likely to increase in near future since the virus will try to evade the host immune response to enhance its survival in humans. Thus, we evaluated the genetic diversity of the structural protein genes along with the genomic composition and codon usage patterns of SARS-CoV-2. Thus, present data on molecular characterization of structural protein genes is likely to augment the information about the evolution, biology and adaptation of SARS-CoV-2 in the human host.

---

* **Corresponding author Shama Parveen:** Centre for Interdisciplinary Research in Basic Sciences, Jamia Millia Islamia, New Delhi, India; E-mails: sparveen2@jmi.ac.in and shamp25@yahoo.com

Keywords: Entropy, Gene ontology, Molecular characterization, Mutational pressure, Natural selection, Nucleotide composition, Phylogenetic analysis, SARS-CoV-2, Structural proteins, Synonymous codon usage.

INTRODUCTION

The newest virus that has captured the world's attention is known as "SARS-CoV-2" that causes Coronavirus disease 2019 (COVID-19). It was first recognized to cause human infection at the end of 2019. The initial cases of the infection were linked to seafood and live-animal market in Wuhan, China [1, 2]. These initial cases led to a local epidemic in this region. The viral infection later spread to other geographical regions by travellers and significant human to human transmission. COVID-19 was declared as the pandemic by the WHO on 12th March 2020 [3]. SARS-CoV-2 belongs to the coronavirus family that has other human pathogens, including severe acute respiratory syndrome (SARS) and Middle East Respiratory Syndrome (MERS). The SARS epidemic of 2002-03 and the MERS outbreak 2012-13 have caused significant disease burden in China and Saudi Arabia, respectively [4] [5].

The SARS-CoV-2 are enveloped, positive single-stranded RNA viruses with a genome of approximately 30 Kb in length [6]. The first open reading frame (ORF-1a/b) encompasses two-third of the viral RNA, encodes 16 non-structural proteins (NSPs). The remaining genome encodes for four essential structure proteins: spike (S), small envelope (E), membrane (M), and nucleocapsid (N) and several accessory proteins. Structural proteins have a crucial role in the pathogenicity of the virus as it facilitates assembly and release of the virion [7]. The S glycoprotein of SARS-CoV-2 comprises two subunits; S1, which determines the virus host range and cellular tropism and S2 is involved in the virus-cell membrane fusion activity by HR1 [8, 9] and HR2 [10]. The S2 unit is highly conserved and thus, forms a target for antiviral compounds [10]. The M protein is responsible for the budding process. The proteins E and N interfere with the host immune response [7].

Previous studies have reported the genotype diversity of gene/genomic characterisation and the epidemiology of SARS-CoV-2 proteins [11]. But the comprehensive genetic information on structural proteins of the virus is limited. It may be noted that the phenomenon of codon usage bias pertains to organisms, where one synonymous codon is preferred over others [12, 13]. The codon usage patterns have been reported in a few viruses [14 - 16] and have been extensively studied. However, in SARS-CoV-2, the RSCU patterns have not been implicated for the structural protein genes. Therefore, we performed the composition and codon usage pattern, phylogenetic, entropy and selection pressure analyses of the structural protein genes of this novel coronavirus to gain insight into its basis of molecular evolution.

MATERIALS AND METHODS

Sequences

Nucleotide sequences of SARS-CoV-2 were retrieved from the National Center for Biotechnology Information (NCBI). The retrieval of selected sequences was based on the following inclusion criteria: (a) The strain (GenBank Accession number: NC_001434.1) was used as the new coronavirus (SARS-CoV-2) reference strain; (b) Sequences from the same or different countries at varying time intervals were assembled in order to avoid repetition; (c) Sampling dates were clearly mentioned. Accumulated sequences were edited using the Bioedit v.7.2 sequence analysis software (http://bioedit.software.informer.com/7.2/) to obtain structural gene products spike (S), envelope (E), membrane (M), nucleocapsid (N) proteins. Multiple alignments for SARS-CoV-2 sequences were carried out using the Clustal X2 Algorithm (http://www.clustal.org/clustal2/) [17].

Compositional Properties

Nucleotide composition analysis of the four structural protein genes S, E, M and N of SARS-CoV-2 sequences was calculated using CodonW v.1.4.2 software. The overall nucleotides occurrence frequency (A%, C%, T/U%, and G%) and overall occurrence of nucleotide frequency at the third position of codon (A3%, C3% U3% and G3%) were analysed. The overall GC content at different codon positions was also determined. The termination codons do not encode any amino acid, and Met and Trp are only encoded by AUG and UGG codons, respectively, hence these codons do not exhibit usage bias. Therefore, these five codons (UAG, UGA, UAA, AUG and UGG) were not considered for the analysis.

Relative Synonymous Codon Usage (RSCU)

The ratio between the observed and expected usage frequency of a codon is described as the RSCU value if all synonymous codons are used equally for any specific amino acid [18]. The RSCU index was determined as follows:

$$RSCU = \frac{G_{ij}}{\sum_j^{n_i} G_{ij}} n_i$$

where *RSCU* is the relative synonymous codon usage value, G_{ij} is the observed number of the ith codon for the jth amino acid that has an *"ni"* type of synonymous codon. The RSCU values of the structural coding genes were calculated using

CodonW v.1.4.2 to determine the codon usage characteristics without the effect of amino acid composition and coding sequence length. Codons with RSCU values (> 1.6) and (< 0.6) were considered as "over-represented" and "under-represented" codons, respectively, whereas codons having the RSCU values (1) were regarded as not biased (average level codon).

Physiochemical Characterization

The various physical and chemical parameters for structural proteins of the SARS-CoV-2 prototype strain were also computed using the ProtParam tool on the ExPASY server (https://web.expasy.org/protscale/) [19].

Phylogenetic Analyses

The study sequences of different coronaviruses were retrieved, and three different data sets built were used for comparative phylogenetic analyses. The alignment for all the datasets was achieved using Clustal X2 in BioEdit v.7.2 [20]. The phylogenetic tree was generated in MEGA v.6.06 software [21], using the best-fitting nucleotide substitution model, with the General time reversible model (GTR) and gamma distribution. To evaluate the reliability of a tree, bootstrap analysis was used by setting a value up to 1000 replicates.

Dataset I

The first data set contained 33 full-length sequences of different coronaviruses, (SARS-CoV-2, SARS-1, MERS and bat coronaviruses). A Maximum Likelihood phylogenetic tree was generated in MEGA software using the same algorithm.

Dataset II

The second dataset contained 30 different coronavirus sequences each for S, E, M and N gene proteins, respectively. The Neighbor-Joining phylogenetic trees were constructed and comparative analyses among the four structural protein genes were analysed.

Dataset III

The third dataset contained only SARS-CoV-2 study sequences each for S, E, M and N genes, respectively. Maximum-Likelihood phylogenetic trees based on these gene encoding protein sequences were constructed using the same algorithms implemented in MEGA software and comparative analyses were performed.

Gene Ontology (GO)

CELLO2GO [22], a web-based public system, was used to infer biological function for four structural proteins of SARS-CoV-2 prototype strain with their localization prediction.

Mutational Analysis

PROVEAN (Protein Variation Effect Analyzer) version 1.1 software (http://provean.jcvi.org) [23] was used to predict the effect of the amino acid mutation on the biological function of SARS-CoV-2 study sequences.

Selection Pressure Analysis

The analysis of selective pressure on S, E, M and N gene sequences was carried out to identify codon sites under positive selection. The ratio (ω) of the nonsynonymous (dN) to the silent substitution (dS) rates on a protein-coding gene determines the selection pressure strength. Different methods, including internal fixed effects likelihood (IFEL), single-likelihood ancestor counting (SLAC) and random effects likelihood (REL), were used in this study to measure this ratio under the F81, HKY85 and REV models of nucleotide substitution. These approaches are implemented in the HYPHY package available at datamonkeys.org.

Analysis of Entropy of Amino Acid Sequences

The Shannon entropy analysis of S, E, M and N proteins was carried out for the identification of possible variability/mutability. The entropy of aligned amino acid sequences was calculated at a particular codon position using BioEdit software to comprehend the variation within these proteins.

RESULTS

Nucleotide Composition Analysis

The values for nucleotide composition of all the individual sequences for S, E, M and N were calculated to analyse the impact of nucleotide constraints on codon usage (Table **1**).

Table 1. Nucleotide composition of the structural protein genes of SARS-CoV-2.

Nucleotide	S Gene	E Gene	M Gene	N Gene
A	29.43	21.5	25.56	31.74
C	18.91	19.72	21.82	24.98

(Table 1) cont.....

Nucleotide	S Gene	E Gene	M Gene	N Gene
T(U)	33.25	40.35	31.83	21.04
G	18.39	18.42	20.77	22.22
A1	30.45	23.68	30.04	31.42
U1	16.39	19.71	21.97	24.04
T1	24.25	28.97	21.97	15.00
G1	28.89	27.63	26.00	29.52
A2	30.84	19.76	22.42	33.33
C2	24.40	21.05	20.62	28.31
U2	29.20	47.34	36.77	16.44
G2	15.54	11.84	20.17	21.90
A3	27.00	21.05	24.21	30.48
C3	15.93	18.42	22.88	22.59
U3	46.31	44.73	36.75	31.69
G3	10.75	15.78	16.14	15.23
GC	37.30	38.14	42.59	47.20
GC1	45.28	47.34	47.97	53.56
GC2	39.94	32.89	40.79	50.21
GC3	26.68	34.2	39.02	37.82

[a]The values are represented as percentage.

S Gene

The nucleotides U and A were most abundant in the S coding sequences, with an average of 33.25% and 29.43%, respectively, compared with C (18.91%) and G (18.39%) (Table 1). The most frequent nucleotide at the third position was U3S (46.31), followed by A3S (27.00%), C3S (15.93%) and G3S (10.72%). Thus, synonymous codons at the third position followed the same trend (U3S> A3S> C3S> G3S). The overall GC content and GC% at different positions GC1, GC2 and GC3 were with an average of 37.30%, 45.28%, 39.94% and 26.68%, respectively.

E Gene

The nucleotides U and A were most abundant in the E coding sequences, with an average of 40.35% and 21.50%, respectively, compared with C (19.72%) and G (18.42%) (Table 1). The most frequent nucleotide at the third position was U3S (44.73%), followed by A3S (21.05%), C3S (18.42%) and G3S (15.78%). Thus, synonymous codons at the third position followed the same trend (U3S> A3S>

C3S> G3S). The overall GC content and GC% at different positions GC1, GC2 and GC3 were with an average of 38.14%, 47.34%, 32.89% and 34.2%, respectively.

M Gene

The nucleotides U and A were most abundant in the M coding sequences, with an average of 31.83% and 25.56% (Table 1), respectively, compared with C (21.82%) and G (20.77%). The most frequent nucleotide at the third position was U3S (36.75%), followed by A3S (24.21%), C3S (22.88%) and G3S (16.14%). Thus, synonymous codons at the third position followed the same trend (U3S> A3S> C3S> G3S). The overall GC content and GC% at different positions GC1, GC2 and GC3 were with an average of 42.59%, 47.97%, 40.79% and 39.02%, respectively.

N Gene

The nucleotides A and C were most abundant in the N coding sequences, with an average of 31.74% and 24.98% (Table 1), respectively, compared with G (22.22%) and U (21.04%). The most frequent nucleotide at the third position was U3S (31.69%), followed by A3S (30.48%), C3S (22.59%) and G3S (15.23%). Thus, synonymous codons at the third position were significantly different (U3S> A3S> C3S> G3S). The overall GC content and GC% at different positions GC1, GC2 and GC3 were with an average 47.20%, 53.56%, 50.21% and 37.82%, respectively.

The nucleotide composition results revealed that nucleotides A and U were over-represented; whereas C and G were under-represented in S, E and M genes. However, the nucleotide A was over-represented for the N gene. In all of the genes, %G3 was the lowest.

U- and A-ending Codons are Preferred in Coding Sequences

RSCU analysis was performed to assess the codon usage patterns in the SARS-CoV-2 structural protein genes (Table 2).

Table 2. The relative synonymous codon usage (RSCU) values of structural protein genes of SARS-CoV-2.

Amino Acid	Codon	S Gene	E Gene	M Gene	N Gene
Phe (F)	UUU	1.53	0.8	0.91	0.47
	UUC	0.47	1.20	1.09	1.53
Leu (L)	UUA	1.56	0.44	0.69	0.46

(Table 2) cont.....

Amino Acid	Codon	S Gene	E Gene	M Gene	N Gene
	UUG	1.11	**0.86**	**0.69**	**1.99**
	CUU	**2**	**3**	**2.06**	**1.77**
	CUC	0.67	0	**1.03**	0.44
	CUA	0.5	**0.85**	**0.86**	0.66
	CUG	0.17	**0.86**	**0.69**	0.66
Ile (I)	AUU	**1.74**	1	**1.65**	**1.93**
	AUC	0.55	1	**0.9**	0.86
	AUA	0.71	1	0.45	0.21
Met (M)	AUG	1	1	**1**	**1**
Val (V)	GUU	**1.98**	**2.15**	1	1
	GUC	**0.87**	0.31	0	1.5
	GUA	0.62	**0.92**	**2**	0.5
	GUG	0.54	**0.62**	1	1
Ser (S)	UCU	**2.24**	**3**	0.8	**1.3**
	UCC	0.73	0	1.2	0.49
	UCA	**1.58**	0.75	1.2	**1.45**
	UCG	0.12	0.75	0.4	0.33
	AGU	1.03	0.75	**1.6**	**1.46**
	AGC	0.3	0.75	0.8	0.98
Pro (P)	CCU	**2**	**4**	0.8	1.14
	CCC	0.28	0	0	**1**
	CCA	**1.72**	0	2.4	**1.57**
	CCG	0	0	0.8	0.29
Thr (T)	ACU	**1.81**	1	**1.54**	**2**
	ACC	0.41	0	0.92	0.75
	ACA	**1.65**	**2**	0.92	**1**
	ACG	0.12	1	0.62	0.25
Ala (A)	GCU	**2.13**	1	**2.52**	**2.05**
	GCC	0.41	1	0.43	**0.76**
	GCA	**1.37**	0	**0.84**	**0.86**
	GCG	0.1	**2**	0.21	0.32
Tyr (Y)	UAU	**1.48**	0	**0.89**	0.36
	UAC	0.52	**2**	**1.11**	**1.64**
His (H)	CAU	1.53	0	**1.6**	1.5

(Table 2) cont.....

Amino Acid	Codon	S Gene	E Gene	M Gene	N Gene
	CAC	0.47	0	0.4	0.5
Gln (Q)	CAA	**1.49**	0	1	**1.54**
	CAG	0.51	0	1	**0.46**
Arn (N)	AAU	**1.23**	1.6	0.73	1.45
	AAC	**0.77**	0.4	1.27	0.55
Lys (K)	AAA	**1.25**	2	1.14	1.35
	AAG	**0.75**	0	0.86	0.65
Asp (D)	GAU	1.39	2	0.33	1.17
	GAC	0.61	0	1.67	0.83
Glu (E)	GAA	1.42	1	1.71	1.33
	GAG	0.58	1	0.29	0.67
Cys (C)	UGU	**1.4**	0.67	**2**	0
	UGC	0.6	**1.33**	0	0
	UGG	1	0	**1**	1
Arg (R)	CGU	1.28	2	**2.14**	1.24
	CGC	0.14	0	0.86	1.03
	CGA	0	2	0.43	1.03
	CGG	0.28	0	0	0.41
	AGA	2.86	2	1.29	**2.07**
	AGG	1.43	0	1.29	0.21
Gly (G)	GGU	**2.29**	4	**1.43**	**0.93**
	GGC	0.73	0	0.86	**1.49**
	GGA	0.83	0	**1.71**	**1.21**
	GGG	0.15	0	0	0.37
Average codons		1274	76	223	420

[a]The most frequently used codons are indicated in bold.

S Gene

Out of 24 preferred codons, 21 were U/A-ending (U-ending: 13; A-ending:8) and 3 were C/G-ending (C-ending: 2; G-ending: 1) (Table **2**). Among these preferred ones, 10 had an RSCU value >1.6, while the remaining fourteen preferred codons had RSCU values >0.6 and <1.6.

E Gene

Out of 17 preferred codons, 10 were U/A-ending (U-ending: 6; A-ending:4) and 7 were G/C-ending (G-ending: 4; C-ending: 3) (Table **2**). Among these preferred ones, 8 had RSCU value >1.6, while the remaining 9 had RSCU values >0.6 and <1.6.

M Gene

Out of 30 preferred codons, 19 were U/A-ending (U-ending: 12; A-ending:7) and 11 were C/G -ending (C-ending: 6; G-ending: 5) (Table **2**). Among these preferred ones, 9 had RSCU value >1.6, while the remaining 21 had RSCU values >0.6 and <1.6.

N Gene

Out of 28 preferred codons, 18 codons were U/A-ending and exhibited an equal distribution of U and A (U-ending: 9; A-ending:9) and 10 were C/G -ending (C-ending: 6; G-ending: 4) (Table **2**). Among these, 7 had RSCU value >1.6, while the remaining 20 had RSCU values >0.6 and <1.6.

We found the presence of one underrepresented (RSCU < 0.6) optional synonymous codon for the N gene and absent in the other genes. In line with compositional analysis, the RSCU analysis confirmed the comparatively higher codon usage bias towards U/A ended codons in all the four genes when SARS-CoV-2 coding sequences were not genotypically differentiated among groups.

Analysis of Protein Sequences

Spike Protein

The physiochemical analysis showed that S polypeptide is of 1273 amino acids (141.17 kDa), with an isoelectric point (pI) of 6.24. The instability index was 33.01, which classifies the protein as stable (>40 value implies unstable protein). Further, the Grand Average of Hydropathy (GRAVY) value of -0.079 indicated the hydrophilic nature (positive score indicated hydrophobicity) of the protein.

Envelope Protein

The physiochemical analysis showed that E polypeptide is of 75 amino acids (8.365 kDa), with pI of 8.57. The instability index was 38.68 (stable) and the GRAVY value of 1.128 suggested hydrophobic nature of the protein.

Membrane Protein

The physiochemical analysis showed that M polypeptide is of 222 amino acids (25.146 kDa), with pI 9.51. The instability index was 39.14 (stable) and the GRAVY value of 0.446 suggested hydrophobic nature of the protein.

Nucleocapsid Protein

The physiochemical analysis showed that N polypeptide is of 419 amino acids (45.625 kDa), with pI 10.07. The instability index was 55.09 (unstable) and the GRAVY value (-0.971) indicated the hydrophilic nature of the protein.

Phylogenetic Analysis

Full Genome of Coronaviruses

The phylogenetic analysis of full-length sequences of 33 different coronaviruses sequences suggested that all 2019-nCoV and bat-SL-CoV (MG772934) formed one cluster, as reported in recent publications (data not shown).

Structural Protein Genes of Coronaviruses

In addition, we performed the comparative phylogenetic analyses of the structural gene encoding regions, which included the 30 different coronaviruses sequences. A unique pattern was observed in the phylogenetic tree of the E gene as we witnessed strains of different coronaviruses were clustered under the SARS-CoV-2 clade (Fig. **1**).

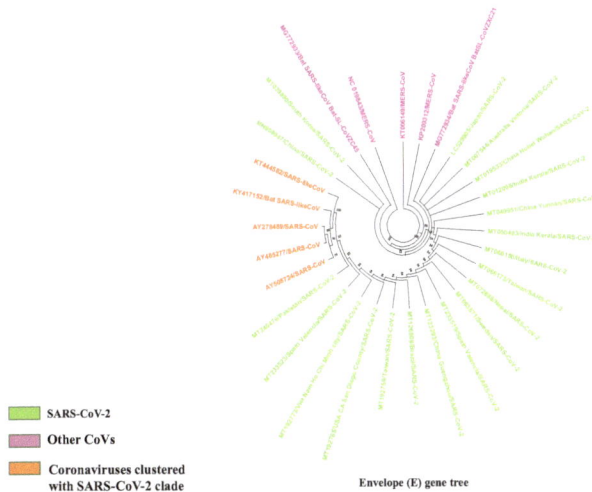

Fig. (1). Neighbor Joining consensus tree of coronaviruses E gene. Bootstrap values are represented by the numbers on nodes generated by 1000 replications.

However, it was evident from the comparative analyses that 2019-nCoV study sequences were clustered in SARS-CoV-2 clade in the other gene trees, *i.e.,* S, M and N (Fig. **2**). The SARS-CoV-2 clades were closest to bat-SL-CoVs (MG772933 & MG772934).

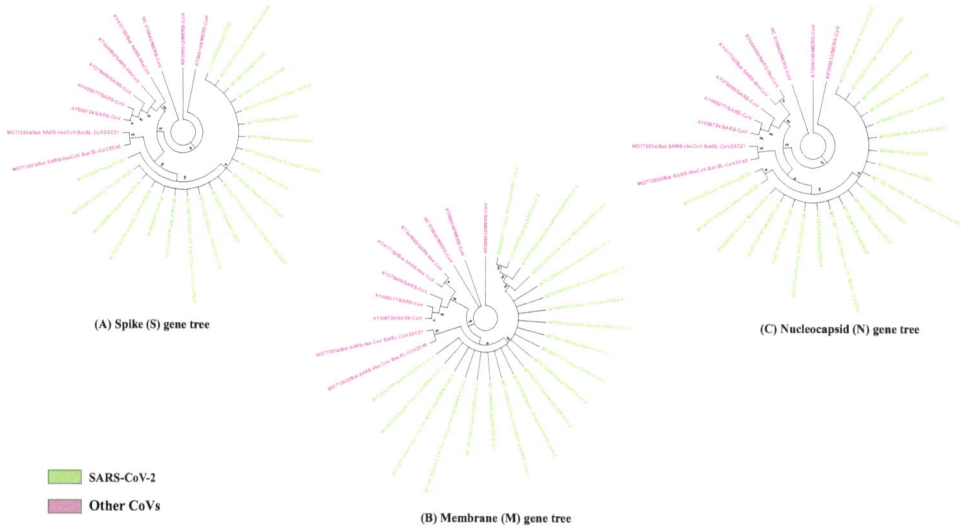

Fig. (2). Neighbor Joining consensus trees of coronaviruses structural protein genes. Panel **(a)** S gene, Panel **(b)** M gene and Panel **(c)** N gene. Bootstrap values are represented by the numbers on nodes generated by 1000 replications.

Structural Protein Genes of Novel Coronaviruses (SARS-CoV-2)

The exploratory phylogenetic analysis of structural protein genes of SARS-CoV-2, from various geographical regions, revealed that both topology and clustering were dissimilar for all four genes S, E, M and N, which suggested that genes followed different patterns of evolutionary relationships (Fig. **3**).

Computer Predicted Features

Subcellular Localization Prediction with Functional Annotation

The S, E and M proteins were predicted to be potential plasma membrane localization while the N protein was predicted to be a potential nuclear localization. Previous reports have suggested the SARS-CoV-2 spike (S) protein involvement in the viral pathogenicity, viral assembly and release, as well as in the fusion with host cell membrane, but extensive data on other protein functions are still limited. Thus, we calculated the detailed GO molecular functions, biological process and cellular components for SARS-CoV-2 (prototype strain) structural protein sequences (Figs. **4 - 7**).

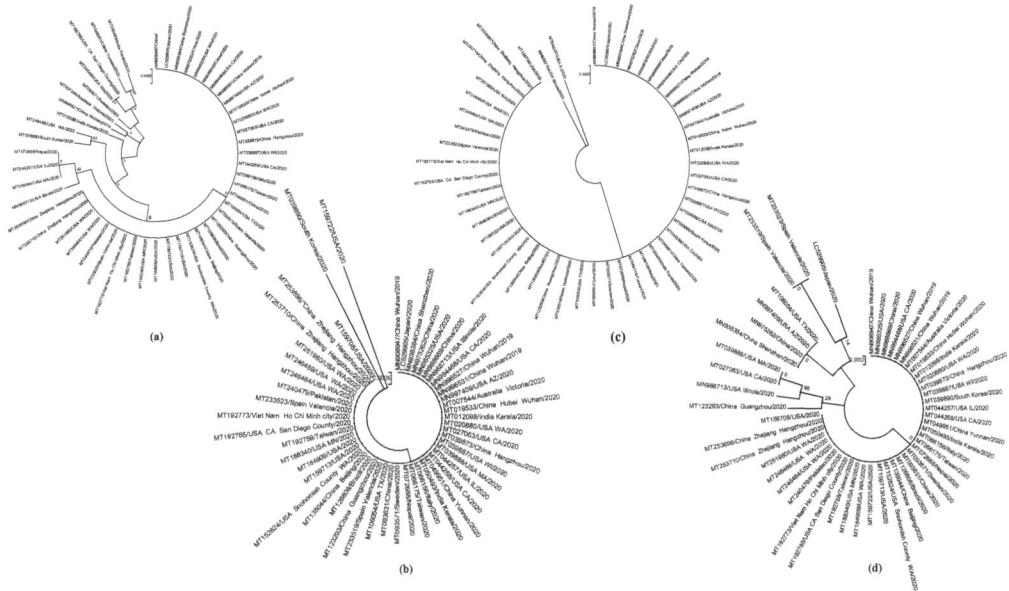

Fig. (3). Maximum Likelihood consensus tree of structural protein genes of SARS-CoV-2. Panel **(a)** S gene, Panel **(b)** E gene, Panel **(c)** M gene and Panel **(d)** N gene .

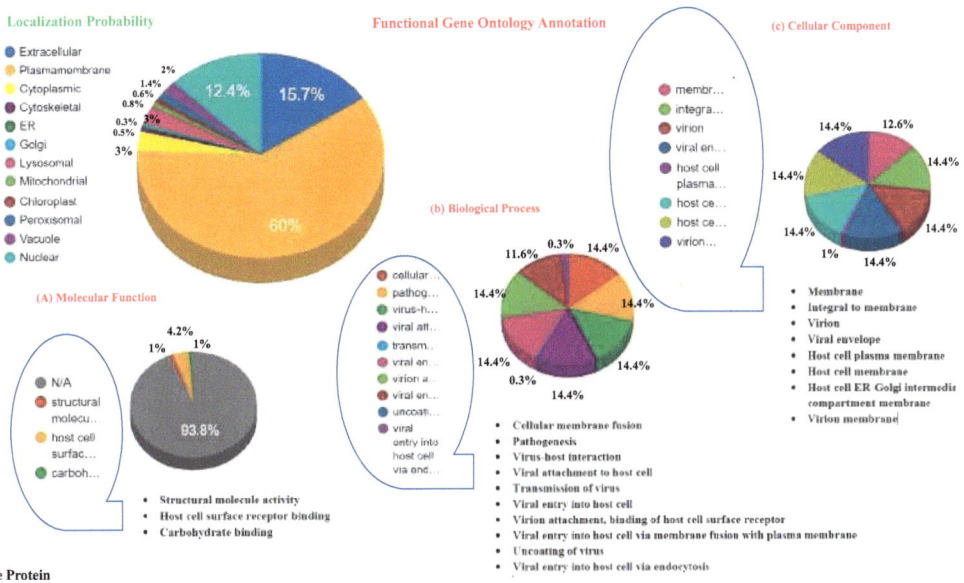

Fig. (4). Functional annotation for the S protein of SARS-CoV-2. The upper left panel shows the subcellular localization. The other pie-charts represents the associated GO annotations in the order **(a)** Molecular function **(b)** Biological process and **(c)** Cellular compartment of the targeted protein.

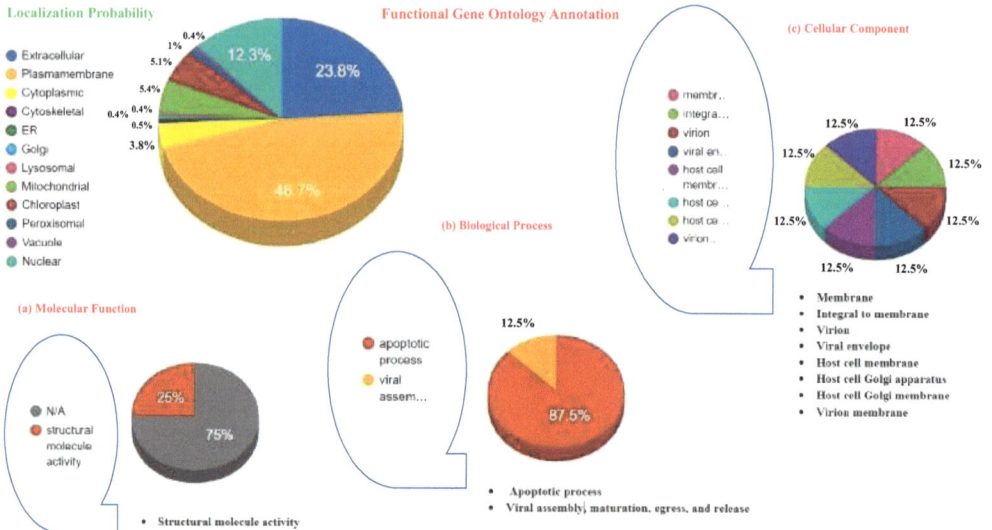

Fig. (5). Functional annotation for the E protein of SARS-CoV-2. The upper left panel shows the subcellular localization. The other pie-charts represents the associated GO annotations in the order **(a)** Molecular function **(b)** Biological process and **(c)** Cellular compartment of the targeted protein.

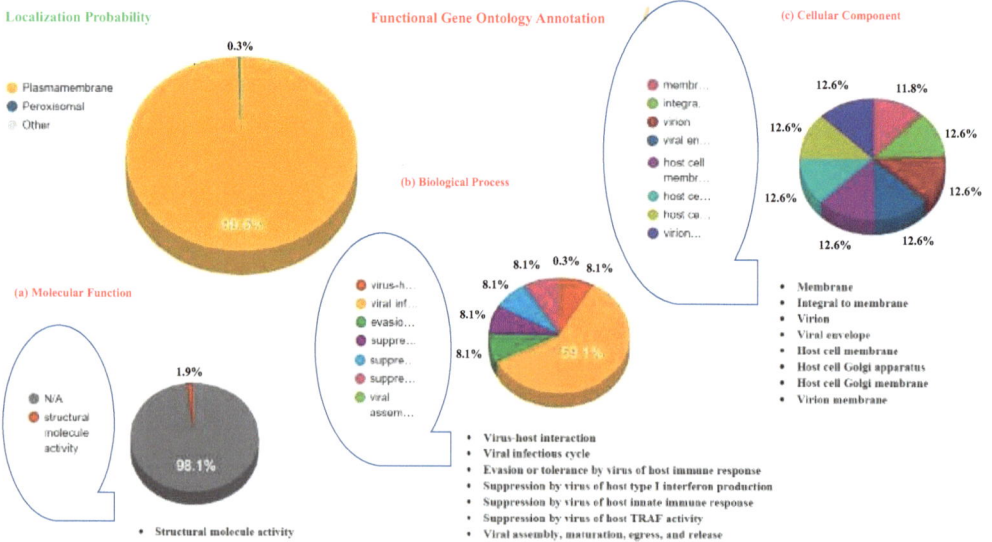

Fig. (6). Functional annotation for the M protein of SARS-CoV-2. The upper left panel shows the subcellular localization. The other pie-charts represents the associated GO annotations in the order **(a)** Molecular function **(b)** Biological process and **(c)** Cellular compartment of the targeted protein.

Fig. (7). Functional annotation for the N protein of SARS-CoV-2. The upper left panel shows the subcellular localization. The other pie-charts represents the associated GO annotations in the order (a) Molecular function (b) Biological process and (c) Cellular compartment of the targeted protein.

Prediction of Effect of Mutations on Protein Function

PROVEAN predicted the effect of mutations on protein function in SARS-CoV-2 study sequences as compared to the prototype strain. The amino acid substitutions with effect on protein functions are summarized in the table (Table **3**).

Table 3. Amino acid mutations with predicted effects on SARS-CoV-2 structural proteins.

Protein	Strain	Variant	PROVEAN Score	Prediction (Cut off = - 2.5)
S	MT049951/ China:Yunnan	Y28N	-0.580	Neutral
S	MT039890/South Korea/2020	S221W	-0.919	Neutral
S	MT007544/Australia: Victoria/2020	S247R	-0.765	Neutral
S	MT012098/India: Kerala/2020	V407I	-0.145	Neutral
S	MT246480/USA: WA/2020	D614G	0.598	Neutral
S	MT192765/USA: CA/2020	D614G	0.598	Neutral
S	MT093571/Sweden/2020	F797C	-2.668	Deleterious
S	MT050493/India: Kerala/2020	A930V	-3.727	Deleterious
E	MT039890/South Korea/2020	L37H	-5.611	Deleterious
N	MT027063/USA: CA/2020	S194L	-4.272	Deleterious
N	MT039888/USA: MA/2020	S194L	-4.272	Deleterious

(Table 3) cont.....

Protein	Strain	Variant	PROVEAN Score	Prediction (Cut off = -2.5)
N	MT233519/Spain: Valencia/2020	S197L	-2.221	Neutral
N	MT233523/Spain: Valencia/2020	S197L	-2.221	Neutral
N	LC529905/Japan/2020	P344S	-4.031	Deleterious

[a]Default threshold is -2.5, that is:
-Variants with a score equal to or below -2.5 are considered "deleterious"
-Variants with a score above -2.5 are considered "neutral"

A total of 9, 1, 1 and 6 amino acid mutations were observed in S, E, M and N gene study sequences. In addition, a total of 26 mutations at the nucleotide level were observed at different sites in the SARS-CoV-2 study sequences. Unknown amino acids were also observed in some of the variants: S (N824X) M (A69X) and N (S194X) (Fig. **9**).

Helical Wheel Plot Analysis

A Helical Wheel is a visual *representation* used to illustrate the arrangement of amino acids in proteins. It plots a peptide sequence in a helical wheel pattern to help in recognizing amphiphilic regions. The helical wheel of the nucleocapsid gene study sequences was drawn since most of the non-synonymous mutations are present in this particular stretch of the protein. It is evident from the wheel plot that in most of the N gene study sequences, serine (hydrophilic) is being replaced by leucine (hydrophobic). This decreases the protein's hydrophilicity character that might affect its structure-function relationship, thus perturbing the environment. A Helical Wheel plot for nucleocapsid protein is depicted in the figure (Fig. **8**).

The non-synonymous mutations present in the S protein gene study sequences are summarized in the figure (Fig. **9**).

Analysis of Positive Selection

S Dataset

IFEL suggested one evidence of negative selection at 921 codon (p-value ≤ 0.25) under the F81 method. Three codon sites (474, 824, 921) were under negative selection by the REL approach using the F81 method. SLAC **found no evidence** of pervasive positive/diversifying selection at all p-values and negative/purifying selection at 1 site at p-value ≤ 0.2 and 2 sites at p-value ≤ 0.25.

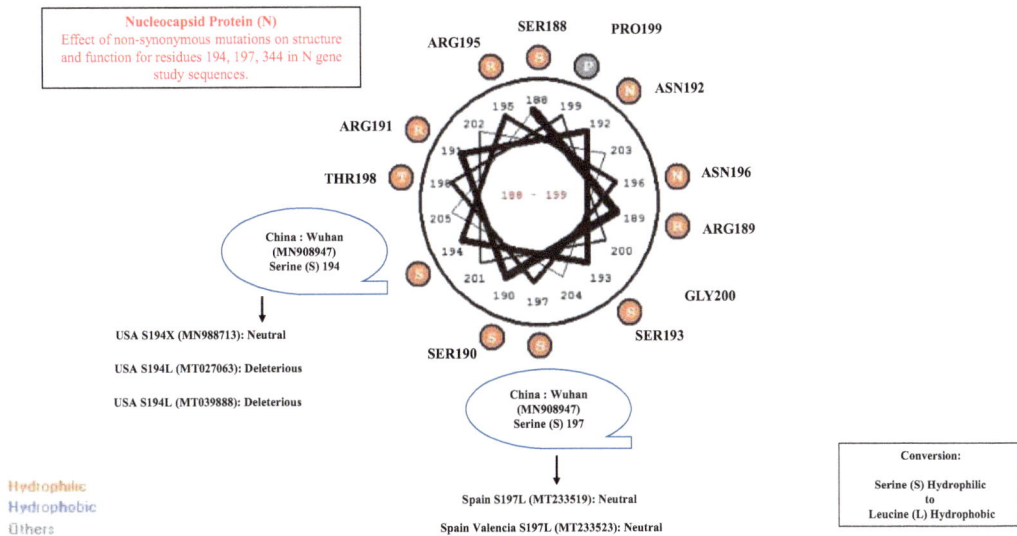

Fig. (8). Helical wheel plot showing the arrangement of amino acid in Nucleocapsid protein. This is shown closest to the circle with respect to the prototype strain (NC_001434) to show the effect of non-synonymous amino acid mutations.

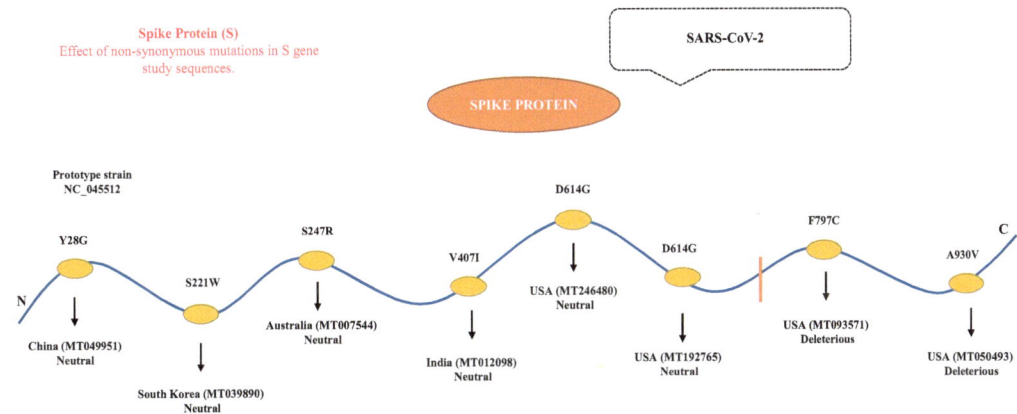

Fig. (9). Diagrammatic representation showing the effect of non-synonymous mutations in S protein. The analysis was done on study sequences with respect to the prototype strain (NC_001434).

E Dataset

IFEL suggested neither positively selected nor negatively selected sites. REL inferred no rates with dN > dS for datasets, suggesting that all sites were under purifying selection. SLAC found no **evidence** of pervasive positive/diversifying selection or negative/purifying selection.

M Dataset

IFEL suggested neither positively selected nor negatively selected sites. REL suggested that all sites were under purifying selection. SLAC found no **evidence** of pervasive positive/diversifying selection or negative/purifying selection.

N Dataset

IFEL found **one evidence** of positive selection at 194 codon under F81 and HKY86 models at all p-values (except p-value ≤ 0.05) and under the REV model (p-value ≤ 0.25). One negatively selected site was observed at 274 codon under the F81 model (p-value 0.25). REL found three codon sites (474, 824, 921) under negative selection using the F81 model. SLAC found **no evidence** of positive/diversifying selection or negative/purifying selection.

No positively selected sites were determined for S, E and M datasets using IFEL, SLAC and REL approaches under all nucleotide substitution models at all p-values, while one positive selection existed in the N dataset.

Analysis of Entropy of Amino Acid Sequences

The entropy score of all the structural protein genes was low since we have compared only the SARS-CoV-2 strains. There is limited variation among different structural proteins of these strains since it is a new virus. A total of 29, 1, 1, 6 sites were identified in S, E, M and N genes, respectively. Out of these, one codon at amino acid at position 614 in the S gene was found to have a slightly higher entropy value 0.17. The entropy percentages for gene sequences were; S: 2.27% (29/1274), E: 1.31 (1/76), M: 0.44% (1/223) and N: 1.42% (6/420) respectively. Therefore, the amino acid sequences of the S gene observed the largest variation and the M gene had the least variation.

DISCUSSION

SARS-CoV-2 has led to a significant disease burden across the globe during the ongoing pandemic. It is imperative to explore the evolutionary dynamics and biology of this emerging viral pathogen to formulate control strategies. Further, inadequate information about the structural proteins of SARS-CoV-2 in literature prompted us to investigate the genetic characteristics of their corresponding genes. The present report describes comparative nucleotide composition, relative codon usage pattern, phylogeny, selection pressure and entropy of structural S, E, M and N genes of circulating coronaviruses with a special focus on SARS-CoV-2.

The amino acids are encoded by more than one synonymous codon. These codons have a specific preference among genomes that is known as codon usage bias

[19]. Mutational bias and natural selection are the two major paradigms that determine the overall codon usage variation. In human RNA viruses, the primary determinant of codon bias is mutational pressure and not translational selection [24]. Investigation of the codon usage patterns is essential for the evolution and efficient expression of viral proteins so that they generate an efficient immune response. Such strategies of codon optimization for preferred codon usage are very useful in vaccine development. Jenkins and Holmes (2003) reported that the codon usage bias can be influenced by overall nucleotide composition or RSCU pattern [24].

The SARS-CoV-2 genomes revealed an overrepresentation of U, with an overall U/A codon bias pattern in the nucleotide composition in the present study. This is an indication of codon bias existence, as revealed in a recent study [25]. It can be correlated with the fact that most of the RNA viruses, either positive or negative stranded, are biased towards a high prevalence of A rather than C. Such A/C biasness in the genomes is also reported for HIV, hepatitis C, rubella viruses [26]. Thus, the overall A/U rich pattern of SARS-CoV-2 structural protein genes is in agreement that nucleotide composition in viruses is correlated with the RSCU patterns. This trend supports the influence of mutational pressure [24]. A recent study has similarly shown that the coronaviruses genomes showed U/A codon bias pattern in the nucleotide composition [27]. This is coherent with earlier investigations, which revealed that the overall AU content was higher than GC content in SARS-CoV-2 [28, 29]. In addition, it is postulated that cytosine deamination and utilization of CpG-suppressed clones are the main features that determine the codon bias in coronavirus genomes [30]. However, we observed that the GC content was least suppressed in the nucleocapsid gene, which is consistent with the previous finding [31]. It has been suggested that the frequencies of nucleotides A and U /T should be equal to that of C and G at the third position of the codon if mutational pressure affects the synonymous codon usage bias [32]. However, huge variations were noted in the nucleotide base composition in the case of all the four structural protein genes, signifying that synonymous codon usage bias could majorly be influenced by natural selection.

Our phylogenetic analysis of full-length genomes of different coronaviruses suggested that ten 2019-nCoV and one bat-SL-CoV (MG772934) formed a cluster, which is consistent with the previous reports, but it was distantly related to SARS as reported earlier [11]. This is in agreement with recent reports that have suggested that bats sold in the seafood market in Wuhan, China, might be the original host of this virus [33]. Thus, the bat is considered as a potential reservoir of many emerging viruses, including coronaviruses. The large availability of gene sequences for different coronaviruses facilitated the comparative phylogenetic studies, by utilising varying portions of the genome (S,

E, M and N genes). The additional phylogenetic analyses revealed that all SARS-CoV-2 sequences were clustered together in the SARS-CoV-2 clade and trees generated from different genes showed different topology due to change in clustering of the sequences.

Natural selection facilitates advantageous mutations while causes a reduction in the deleterious ones. Genes undergoing positive selection phenomena usually has major functions and are promoted by natural selection [34]. Therefore, we inspected the nucleotide and amino acid variations in the structural protein genes. The present study mostly shows changes in structural protein genes which correspond to synonymous mutations, although non-synonymous changes were found to be predominant at few codons. We found such non-synonymous mutations in certain amino acids S (F797C and A930V), E (L37H) and N (S194L and P344S) proteins. The PROVEAN tool considered these mutations as deleterious that might influence the antigenicity, host specificity and cellular tropism of the virus. In line with this, Zhang et al. [35] concluded that SARS-CoV-2 genotypes have been mutated when analysed in different patients in China. However, further detailed experimental investigations, including full genome sequencing of the patient samples and site directed mutagenesis studies are required to ascertain relationships between the mutations and their corresponding functional changes. Furthermore, the gene ontology analysis suggested about the involvement of S protein in the viral fusion, pathogenesis, interaction as well as other functions, which is in accordance with the published reports [7]. Reports have suggested the involvement of other proteins in host immune response as well as in the immunopathology of the virus [10]. Also, the production of type 1 interferon (IFNα/β) in response to the virus-host interaction has been previously reported [36], which is clearly shown by our results. Thus, we concluded that our gene ontology results showed consistency with the previous studies. This can be used as an initial platform for further research in order to determine the structural characteristics of different proteins of SARS-CoV-2 and their interaction during viral pathogenesis.

Selection pressure analysis of the structural protein genes revealed purifying or negative selection. One positively selected site was observed in the N gene. The entropy is one useful method of quantification of diversity in amino acid sequences [37]. Structurally or functionally important amino acid variations are correlated with high scoring entropy values [38]. These amino acid variations play an important role in the evolution of viruses. Few mutations, purifying selection and low entropy value suggest limited variation in this pathogen. However, these mutations, especially in the S protein, are likely to increase in the near future since the virus will try to evade the host immune response to enhance its survival in the new host. Therefore, it can be interpreted that in the present scenario, the microevolution of SARS-CoV-2 is mainly driven by the negative selection, which is also in agreement with the nucleotide base composition of structural protein genes. These results probably suggest that these genomic regions are essential for the viability of the virus particles. In addition, gene ontology findings also indicated that the structural protein genes play fundamental roles in the pathogenesis of SARS-CoV-2.

CONCLUDING REMARKS

The present report describes the detailed molecular characterization of the structural protein genes (S, E, M and N) of SARS-CoV-2. The present study is thus envisaged to infer the evolution, adaptation and biology of SARS-CoV-2 via specific codon preferences driven by genetic diversity and negative selection. Further investigations are needed on codon optimization of individual genes and full genomes of human coronaviruses (SARS, SARS-CoV-2 and MERS) for high protein expression. This data might be utilized for designing broad-spectrum vaccines against these emerging viral pathogens.

CONSENT FOR PUBLICATION

Not Applicable.

CONFLICT OF INTEREST

The author declares no conflict of interest, financial or otherwise.

ACKNOWLEDGEMENTS

Zoya Shafat and Ayesha Tazeen are supported by Research Fellowship by the University Grant Commission (UGC), Government of India. Priyanka Sinha is supported by Fellowship from Indian Council of Medical research (ICMR), Government of India. The research in our laboratory is funded by the Council of Scientific and Industrial Research (CSIR), India (37(1697)17/EMR-II) and Central Council for Research in Unani Medicine (CCRUM), Ministry of Ayurveda, Yoga and Naturopathy, Unani, Siddha and Homeopathy (AYUSH), India (F.No.3-63/2019-CCRUM/Tech). The authors also extend their appreciation to the Centre of Excellence in Biotechnology Research, Deanship of Scientific Research, King Saud University, Riyadh, Saudi Arabia, for support.

REFERENCES

[1]   Tan W, Zhao X, Ma X, *et al.* A novel coronavirus genome identified in a cluster of pneumonia cases—Wuhan, China 2019. CCDC Weekly 2020; 2(4): 61-2.
         [http://dx.doi.org/10.46234/ccdcw2020.017]

[2]   Zhu N, Zhang D, Wang W, *et al.* A novel coronavirus from patients with pneumonia in China, 2019. N

Engl J Med 2020; 382(8): 727-33.
[http://dx.doi.org/10.1056/NEJMoa2001017] [PMID: 31978945]

[3] World Health Organization. WHO Virtual press conference on COVID-19

[4] Chan-Yeung M, Xu RH. SARS: epidemiology. Respirology 2003; 8 (Suppl.): S9-S14.
[http://dx.doi.org/10.1046/j.1440-1843.2003.00518.x] [PMID: 15018127]

[5] Zaki AM, van Boheemen S, Bestebroer TM, Osterhaus AD, Fouchier RA. Isolation of a novel coronavirus from a man with pneumonia in Saudi Arabia. N Engl J Med 2012; 367(19): 1814-20.
[http://dx.doi.org/10.1056/NEJMoa1211721] [PMID: 23075143]

[6] Fehr AR, Perlman S. Coronaviruses: an overview of their replication and pathogenesis. In Coronaviruses Humana Press 2015.

[7] Guo YR, Cao QD, Hong ZS, *et al.* The origin, transmission and clinical therapies on coronavirus disease 2019 (COVID-19) outbreak–an update on the status. Mil Med Res 2020; 7(1): 1-0.
[http://dx.doi.org/10.1186/s40779-020-00240-0] [PMID: 31928528]

[8] Xia S, Zhu Y, Liu M, *et al.* Fusion mechanism of 2019-nCoV and fusion inhibitors targeting HR1 domain in spike protein. Cell Mol Immunol 2020; 17(7): 765-7.
[http://dx.doi.org/10.1038/s41423-020-0374-2] [PMID: 32047258]

[9] Yu F, Du L, Ojcius DM, Pan C, Jiang S. Measures for diagnosing and treating infections by a novel coronavirus responsible for a pneumonia outbreak originating in Wuhan. China: Microb Infect 2020; 22(2): 74-9.
[http://dx.doi.org/10.1016/j.micinf.2020.01.003]

[10] Cascella M, Rajnik M, Cuomo A, Dulebohn SC, Di Napoli R. Features, evaluation and treatment coronavirus (COVID-19) InStatpearls. StatPearls Publishing 2020.

[11] Lu R, Zhao X, Li J, *et al.* Genomic characterisation and epidemiology of 2019 novel coronavirus: implications for virus origins and receptor binding. Lancet 2020; 395(10224): 565-74.
[http://dx.doi.org/10.1016/S0140-6736(20)30251-8] [PMID: 32007145]

[12] Grantham R, Gautier C, Gouy M, Mercier R, Pavé A. Codon catalog usage and the genome hypothesis. Nucleic Acids Res 1980; 8(1): r49-62.
[http://dx.doi.org/10.1093/nar/8.1.197-c] [PMID: 6986610]

[13] Shackelton LA, Parrish CR, Holmes EC. Evolutionary basis of codon usage and nucleotide composition bias in vertebrate DNA viruses. J Mol Evol 2006; 62(5): 551-63.
[http://dx.doi.org/10.1007/s00239-005-0221-1] [PMID: 16557338]

[14] Makhija A, Kumar S. Analysis of synonymous codon usage in spike protein gene of infectious bronchitis virus. Can J Microbiol 2015; 61(12): 983-9.
[http://dx.doi.org/10.1139/cjm-2015-0418] [PMID: 26452019]

[15] Morla S, Makhija A, Kumar S. Synonymous codon usage pattern in glycoprotein gene of rabies virus. Gene 2016; 584(1): 1-6.
[http://dx.doi.org/10.1016/j.gene.2016.02.047] [PMID: 26945626]

[16] Das M, Kumar S. Analysis of codon usage pattern of infectious laryngotracheitis virus immunogenic glycoproteins and its biological implications. Infect Genet Evol 2018; 62: 53-9.
[http://dx.doi.org/10.1016/j.meegid.2018.04.009] [PMID: 29654923]

[17] Thompson JD, Gibson TJ, Higgins DG. Multiple sequence alignment using ClustalW and ClustalX. Curr Protoc Bioinformatics 2003; 1: 2-3.
[http://dx.doi.org/10.1002/0471250953.bi0203s00] [PMID: 18792934]

[18] Sharp PM, Li WH. Codon usage in regulatory genes in Escherichia coli does not reflect selection for 'rare' codons. Nucleic Acids Res 1986; 14(19): 7737-49.
[http://dx.doi.org/10.1093/nar/14.19.7737] [PMID: 3534792]

[19] ExPASY server https://web.expasy.org/protscale/

[20]   Hall TA. BioEdit v 7.2. 3. Biological sequence alignment editor for Win 95/98/NT/2K/XP7.

[21]   Tamura K, Stecher G, Peterson D, Filipski A, Kumar S. MEGA6: molecular evolutionary genetics analysis version 6.0. Mol Biol Evol 2013; 30(12): 2725-9.
       [http://dx.doi.org/10.1093/molbev/mst197] [PMID: 24132122]

[22]   Yu CS, Cheng CW, Su WC, et al. CELLO2GO: a web server for protein subCELlular LOcalization prediction with functional gene ontology annotation. PLoS One 2014; 9(6): e99368.
       [http://dx.doi.org/10.1371/journal.pone.0099368] [PMID: 24911789]

[23]   Choi Y, Chan AP. PROVEAN web server: a tool to predict the functional effect of amino acid substitutions and indels. Bioinformatics 2015; 31(16): 2745-7.
       [http://dx.doi.org/10.1093/bioinformatics/btv195] [PMID: 25851949]

[24]   Jenkins GM, Holmes EC. The extent of codon usage bias in human RNA viruses and its evolutionary origin. Virus Res 2003; 92(1): 1-7.
       [http://dx.doi.org/10.1016/S0168-1702(02)00309-X] [PMID: 12606071]

[25]   Dilucca M, Forcelloni S, Georgakilas AG, Giansanti A, Pavlopoulou A. Codon Usage and Phenotypic Divergences of SARS-CoV-2 Genes. Viruses 2020; 12(5): 498.
       [http://dx.doi.org/10.3390/v12050498] [PMID: 32366025]

[26]   Auewarakul P. Composition bias and genome polarity of RNA viruses. Virus Res 2005; 109(1): 33-7.
       [http://dx.doi.org/10.1016/j.virusres.2004.10.004] [PMID: 15826910]

[27]   Tort FL, Castells M, Cristina J. A comprehensive analysis of genome composition and codon usage patterns of emerging coronaviruses. Virus Res 2020; 283: 197976.
       [http://dx.doi.org/10.1016/j.virusres.2020.197976] [PMID: 32294518]

[28]   Gu W, Zhou T, Ma J, Sun X, Lu Z. Analysis of synonymous codon usage in SARS Coronavirus and other viruses in the Nidovirales. Virus Res 2004; 101(2): 155-61.
       [http://dx.doi.org/10.1016/j.virusres.2004.01.006] [PMID: 15041183]

[29]   Zhou T, Gu W, Ma J, Sun X, Lu Z. Analysis of synonymous codon usage in H5N1 virus and other influenza A viruses. Biosystems 2005; 81(1): 77-86.
       [http://dx.doi.org/10.1016/j.biosystems.2005.03.002] [PMID: 15917130]

[30]   Woo PC, Wong BH, Huang Y, Lau SK, Yuen KY. Cytosine deamination and selection of CpG suppressed clones are the two major independent biological forces that shape codon usage bias in coronaviruses. Virology 2007; 369(2): 431-42.
       [http://dx.doi.org/10.1016/j.virol.2007.08.010] [PMID: 17881030]

[31]   Gu H, Chu DK, Peiris M, Poon LL. Multivariate analyses of codon usage of SARS-CoV-2 and other betacoronaviruses. Virus Evol. 2020;6(1): veaa032.
       [http://dx.doi.org/10.1093/ve/veaa032] [PMID: 32431949]

[32]   Zhang Z, Dai W, Wang Y, Lu C, Fan H. Analysis of synonymous codon usage patterns in torque teno sus virus 1 (TTSuV1). Arch Virol 2013; 158(1): 145-54.
       [http://dx.doi.org/10.1007/s00705-012-1480-y] [PMID: 23011310]

[33]   Chan JF, Kok KH, Zhu Z, et al. Genomic characterization of the 2019 novel human-pathogenic coronavirus isolated from a patient with atypical pneumonia after visiting Wuhan. Emerg Microbes Infect 2020; 9(1): 221-36.
       [http://dx.doi.org/10.1080/22221751.2020.1719902] [PMID: 31987001]

[34]   Tang X, Li G, Vasilakis N, et al. Differential stepwise evolution of SARS coronavirus functional proteins in different host species. BMC Evol Biol 2009; 9(1): 52.
       [http://dx.doi.org/10.1186/1471-2148-9-52] [PMID: 19261195]

[35]   Zhang L, Shen FM, Chen F, Lin Z. Origin and evolution of the 2019 novel coronavirus. Clin Infect Dis 2020; 71(15): 882-3.
       [http://dx.doi.org/10.1093/cid/ciaa112] [PMID: 32011673]

[36]   Kawai T, Akira S. The role of pattern-recognition receptors in innate immunity: update on Toll-like receptors. Nat Immunol 2010; 11(5): 373-84.
[http://dx.doi.org/10.1038/ni.1863] [PMID: 20404851]

[37]   Pan K, Deem MW. Quantifying selection and diversity in viruses by entropy methods, with application to the haemagglutinin of H3N2 influenza. J R Soc Interface 2011; 8(64): 1644-53.
[http://dx.doi.org/10.1098/rsif.2011.0105] [PMID: 21543352]

[38]   Wang K, Samudrala R. Incorporating background frequency improves entropy-based residue conservation measures. BMC Bioinformatics 2006; 7(1): 385.
[http://dx.doi.org/10.1186/1471-2105-7-385] [PMID: 16916457]

CHAPTER 4

Codon Based Characterization of S2 Subunit of Severe Acute Respiratory Syndrome-Related Coronaviruses

Arshi Islam[1], Nazish Parveen[1], Md. Shakir Hussain Haider[1], Ravins Dohare[1], Anwar Ahmed[2,3], Sher Ali[1,4] and Shama Parveen[1,*]

[1] *Centre for Interdisciplinary Research in Basic Sciences, Jamia Millia Islamia, New Delhi, India*

[2] *Centre of Excellence in Biotechnology Research, College of Science, King Saud University, Riyadh, Saudi Arabia*

[3] *Protein Research Chair, Department of Biochemistry, College of Science, King Saud University, Riyadh, Saudi Arabia*

[4] *School of Basic Sciences and Research, Department of Life Sciences, Sharda University, Greater Noida, India*

Abstract: The emergence of a global pandemic, COVID-19 is caused by the newly identified SARS-CoV-2. The current situation warrants us to understand the molecular basis of the evolution of this emerging pathogen. In this context, we conducted a comparative codon-based characterization of the viruses within the species *Severe acute respiratory syndrome-related coronavirus* (SARSr-CoV). We attempted phylogenetic analysis, and codon-based characterization by employing selection pressure and Shannon entropy analyses in the S2 subunit gene sequences of SARS-CoV, Bat-SL-CoV and SARS-CoV-2. Further, the pattern of N-linked/O-linked glycosylation was analyzed within the SARS-CoV species. The phylogenetic analysis and pairwise distance calculations showed high similarities in the S2 subunit of SARS-CoV-2 with Bat-SL-CoVs. Our findings uncovered the low mean value of dN/dS, suggesting purifying selection, but certain codon positions were found to be under positive selection. The entropy analyses showed 71 codon positions having its high score. Three codon positions (160, 244 and 562) were identified to be positively selected with high entropy value suggesting that they are more prone to mutations. Further, the analysis revealed a conserved pattern in N-linked glycosylation though the discrepancies were found within the O-linked glycosylation pattern. Our findings may help in predicting the signature sequences based on the codon-based model of molecular evolution. Further, this approach may provide information on the evolutionary dynamics of this pathogen, facilitating much-desired control strategies against COVID-19.

[*] **Corresponding author Shama Parveen:** Centre for Interdisciplinary Research in Basic Sciences, Jamia Millia Islamia, New Delhi, India; E-mails: sparveen2@jmi.ac.in and shamp25@yahoo.com

Keywords: Bat-SL-CoV, Coronavirus, N-linked and O-linked glycosylation, SARS-CoV, SARS-CoV-2, Selection pressure analysis, Shannon entropy analysis.

INTRODUCTION

Coronavirus disease 2019 (COVID-19) has resulted in a major pandemic across the world. The disease, caused by a novel coronavirus, is known to be originated from the Wuhan city of China in late 2019 [1]. On the basis of phylogeny and taxonomy, *Coronaviridae* Study Group (CGS) recognized this novel identified viral strains forming a sister clade to severe acute respiratory syndrome coronaviruses of the humans and bats (SARS-CoVs), which belongs to the species *Severe acute respiratory syndrome-related coronavirus* (SARSr-CoV). The uncharacterized strains were thus named SARS-CoV-2 [2].

The recent classification of coronaviruses (CoVs) includes 39 species, 27 subgenera, 5 genera and 2 subfamilies. The virus belongs to the family *Coronaviridae* and suborder *Cornidovirineae*. The order and realm are *Nidovirales* and *Riboviria*, respectively [2]. On the basis of serology and phylogenetic clustering, *Coronaviridae* are further categorized into four alpha, beta, gamma and delta CoVs groups [3]. Seven human coronaviruses have been discovered, with the last one being SARS-CoV-2 (https://www.cdc.gov/corona virus/types.html). The four human CoVs: HCoV-229E, HCoV-NL63, HCoV-OC43 and HCoV-HKU1 have been found to cause mild infections in humans [4]. SARS-CoVs and MERS-CoVs both were identified as the main cause of severe human respiratory illness in China (2002-03) and Saudi Arabia (2012), respectively [3].

The coronavirus (CoV) consists of 4 structural proteins: spike (S), envelope (E), membrane (M), and nucleocapsid (N). The outermost spike protein is classified into class I viral fusion protein. This protein is initially synthesized as a single chain precursor of approximately 1,300 amino acid residues [5]. The protein trimerizes upon folding [5]. The S protein forms a crown on the surface of CoVs and is the key target of neutralizing antibodies upon infection [5]. The amino acid sequence representing S protein of SARS-CoV-2 showed homologies of 76% and 79-80% with SARS-CoV and Bat-SL-CoVs, respectively [6]. The receptor-binding domain (RBD)of the SARS-CoV-2's S protein supports strong interaction with human ACE2 molecules like that of S-protein of SARS-CoVs, despite sequence variation between the two [7]. Thus, it maybe postulated that SARS-CoV-2 transmission poses a risk to human health *via* the S protein–ACE2 interaction pathway [7].

Further, there are two subunits of S glycoprotein. The S1 subunit of S glycoprotein consists of a signal peptide, the N-terminal domain (NTD) and the receptor-binding domain (RBD). The S2 subunit of the spike protein contains fusion peptide (FP), which is conserved in nature and the heptad repeats: HR 1 and HR2, a transmembrane domain, (TM), and the cytoplasmic domain (CP) [8]. A study has reported 99% similarity of the S2 subunit sequences of SARS-CoV-2 to that of Bat-SL-CoVs [8]. Owing to this conservation in the S2 subunit of the variable S protein gene, the present study was conceptualized to attain an understanding of the codon bias phenomena *via* selection pressure and Shannon entropy analysis and to understand its N-linked and O-linked glycosylation pattern. We also analyzed the similarities at the nucleotides and amino acid levels amongst the sequences of the SARSr-CoVs. The codon-based model of molecular evolution of the SARSr-CoVs may be predicted using this data, which is envisaged to assist in designing antiviral peptides against S2 subunit of SARS-CoV-2. This may prove to be a significant preventive measure towards the treatment of COVID-19.

METHODOLOGY

Data Collection and Sequence Alignment

The whole-genome sequences of the SARS-CoV, Bat-SL-CoV and SARS-CoV-2 of the species *Severe acute respiratory syndrome-related coronavirus* were retrieved from the GenBank. Sequences from different isolates like wtic-MB isolate P3pp23, ExoN1 isolate P3pp37, BJ202, *etc.* and from different hosts encompassing bat, civet and humans were included in the present study. The multiple sequence alignment of the full genome of SARS-and SARS-like CoVs was done using ClustalW in Bioedit (v.7.2) software. The S2 subunit gene sequences were extracted from the full genome sequence and used for analyses.

Phylogenetic Analysis

The phylogenetic tree of the S2 subunit sequences was generated by using MEGA6 (v.6.06) software. The evolutionary history of the tree was deduced using the Maximum Likelihood method. This approach was based on the Tamura-Nei model. The numbers on nodes represent bootstrap values. These values were produced by 1000 replications. Genetic distances were calculated using the nucleotide and amino acid alignment of 5 sequences consisting of two sequences of SARS-CoV-2 (MN938384/HKU-SZ-002a 2020 and MN975262/HKU-S--005b 2020), two Bat-SL-CoVs (MG772934/bat-SL-CoVZXC21 and MG772933/bat-SL-CoVZC45) and one SARS-CoV (NC004718/SARS-CoV).This analysis was conducted using the Poisson correction model in MEGA6 software.

Selection Pressure Analyses

The selection pressure analysis was scrutinized at the individual codon position of the S2 subunit sequences using online web-server Datamonkey (http://www. datamonkey.org). Three different analytical methods involving Internal fixed effects likelihood (IFEL), mixed-effects model of episodic selection (MEME) and Random effects likelihood (REL); each with different nucleotide substitutions model HKY85, F81and REV were explored to determine the ratio of non-synonymous mutations to synonymous ones (dN/dS). The average or mean dN/dS of the aligned sequences of S2 subunit and dN/dS per codon positions were calculated. The genomic region was considered as negatively, neutral or positively selected according to the ratio of mean dN/dS. A ratio <1 indicates purifying or negative selection and if the ratio is equal to (=) 1, the region is recognized to be under the neutral selection. The genomic region was considered as positively selected if the ratio of mean dN/dS was greater than (>) 1. In this study, we have considered those codon positions under positive selection, which possessed dN/dS value greater than 1 by a minimum of two different analytical methods. Two significant values, one is P-value (0.05–0.25) for IFEL and MEME methods and the other one is Bayes factor (25–125) for the REL approach were used to define a codon position under the positive selection.

Analysis of Shannon Entropy

The Shannon entropy analysis was carried out using BioEdit (v.7.2.) software. A high entropy score of a particular site means an increased likelihood of variation at that position in an amino acid or in a protein sequence. Values that were obtained through various calculations in the BioEdit software were transferred into a Microsoft Excel sheet to generate the Shannon entropy graph.

Glycosylation Analysis

N-linked and O-linked glycosylation pattern in the S2 subunit amino acid sequences of spike glycoprotein was envisaged by the online tools. One is NetNGlyc 1.0 (http://www.cbs.dtu.dk/services/NetNGlyc/) server for N-glycosylation and the other is NetOGlyc 4.0 server (http://www.cbs.dtu.dk/ services/NetOGlyc/) for O-linked glycosylation. The possible N-linked and O-linked glycosylation sites in a protein sequence were defined as Asn-Xaa-Ser/Thr (where Xaa is not proline) and serine/threonine, respectively.

RESULTS

Phylogenetic Analysis and Genetic Distance Estimation

The analysis involved 18, 14 and 13 nucleotide sequences (n=45) of SARS-CoV, Bat-SL- CoV and SARS-CoV-2, respectively. The S2 subunit of 1764bp (588 amino acids: 668-1255 of S gene of reference genome: NC004718 SARS-CoV) was used for the construction of the phylogenetic tree. The tree was drawn to scale with branch lengths measured in the number of substitutions per site. The phylogenetic analysis revealed a highly conserved nature of S2 subunit gene sequences of spike glycoprotein of SARS-CoV-2 with Bat-SL-CoVZXC21 and Bat-SL-CoVZC45 than its sister sequences of SARS-CoVs (Fig. **1**).

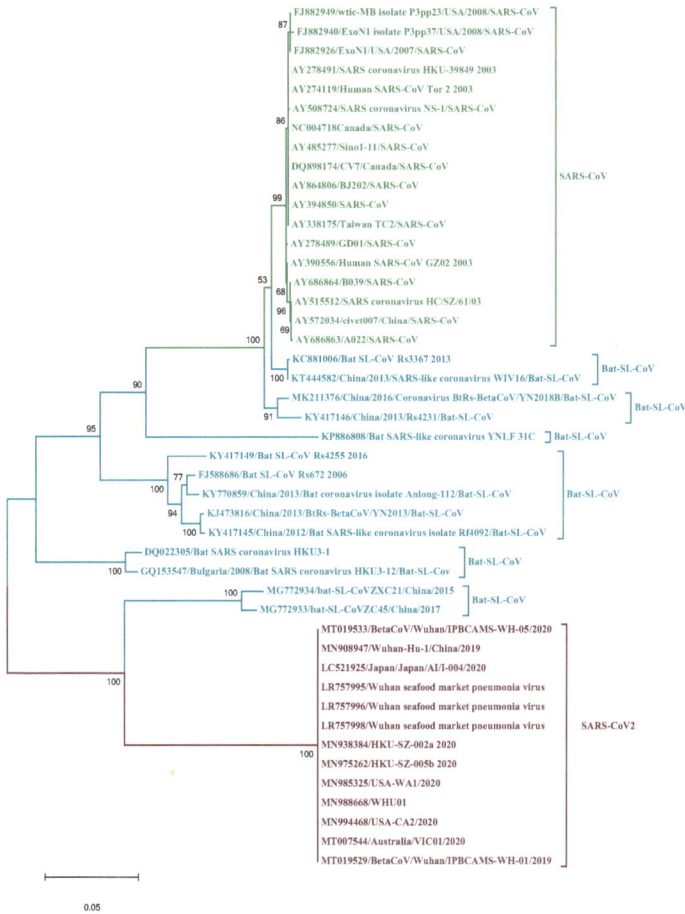

Fig. (1). Phylogenetic tree of S2 subunit gene sequences of *Severe acute respiratory syndrome-related coronaviruses*. The taxon name is described with the accession number and the strain names. There were a total of 1764 positions in the final dataset.

Genetic distance was calculated using nucleotides and amino acid alignment of the five sequences. The amino acid alignment used for the calculation of pairwise distances is represented in Fig. (**2**).

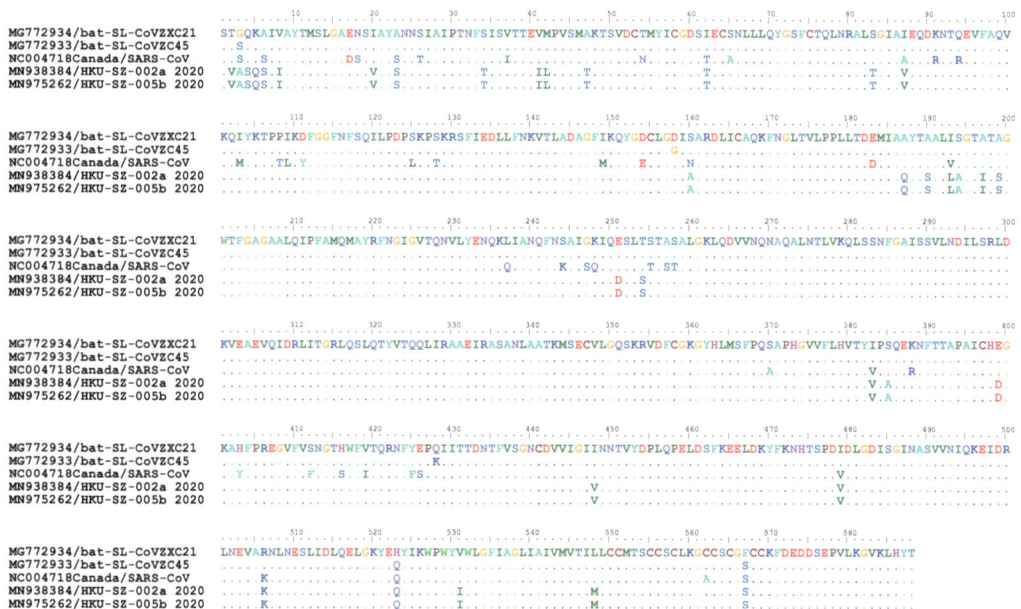

```
                    10        20        30        40        50        60        70        80        90       100
                ....|....|....|....|....|....|....|....|....|....|....|....|....|....|....|....|....|....|....|....|
MG772934/bat-SL-CoVZXC21  STGQKAIVAYTMSLGAENSIAYANNSIAIPTNFSISVTTEVMPVSMAKTSVDCTMYICGDSIECSNLLLQYGSFCTQLNRALSGIAIEQDKNTQEVFAQV
MG772933/bat-SL-CoVZC45   ..S.................................................................................................
NC004718Canada/SARS-CoV   ..S..S.........DS...S..T.........I...............N.......T..A...............A...R..R......
MN938384/HKU-SZ-002a 2020 .VASQS.I...........V..S.........T.....IL....T.........T.............T...V..........
MN975262/HKU-SZ-005b 2020 .VASQS.I...........V..S.........T.....IL....T.........T.............T...V..........

                    110       120       130       140       150       160       170       180       190       200
                ....|....|....|....|....|....|....|....|....|....|....|....|....|....|....|....|....|....|....|....|
MG772934/bat-SL-CoVZXC21  KQIYKTPPIKDFGGFNFSQILPDPSKPSKRSFIEDLLFNKVTLADAGFIKQYGDCLGDISARDLICAQKFNGLTVLPPLLTDEMIAAYTAALISGTATAG
MG772933/bat-SL-CoVZC45   ...............................................................G...................................
NC004718Canada/SARS-CoV   .M...TL.Y..........L..T.............M...E....N......................D.......V...
MN938384/HKU-SZ-002a 2020 ..........................................A.....................Q..S..LA..I.S.
MN975262/HKU-SZ-005b 2020 ..........................................A.....................Q..S..LA..I.S.

                    210       220       230       240       250       260       270       280       290       300
                ....|....|....|....|....|....|....|....|....|....|....|....|....|....|....|....|....|....|....|....|
MG772934/bat-SL-CoVZXC21  WTFGAGAALQIPFAMQMAYRFNGIGVTQNVLYENQKLIANQFNSAIGKIQESLTSTASALGKLQDVVNQNAQALNTLVKQLSSNFGAISSVLNDILSRLD
MG772933/bat-SL-CoVZC45   ..................................................................................................
NC004718Canada/SARS-CoV   ..............................Q.....K..SQ.....T.ST....................................
MN938384/HKU-SZ-002a 2020 ...............................................D..S................................
MN975262/HKU-SZ-005b 2020 ...............................................D..S................................

                    310       320       330       340       350       360       370       380       390       400
                ....|....|....|....|....|....|....|....|....|....|....|....|....|....|....|....|....|....|....|....|
MG772934/bat-SL-CoVZXC21  KVEAEVQIDRLITGRLQSLQTYVTQQLIRAAEIRASANLAATKMSECVLGQSKRVDFCGKGYHLMSFPQSAPHGVVFLHVTYIPSQEKNFTTAPAICHEG
MG772933/bat-SL-CoVZC45   ..................................................................................................
NC004718Canada/SARS-CoV   .......................................................A......V..R...........
MN938384/HKU-SZ-002a 2020 .......................................................V.A................D.
MN975262/HKU-SZ-005b 2020 .......................................................V.A................D.

                    410       420       430       440       450       460       470       480       490       500
                ....|....|....|....|....|....|....|....|....|....|....|....|....|....|....|....|....|....|....|....|
MG772934/bat-SL-CoVZXC21  KAHFPREGVFVSNGTHWFVTQRNFYEPQIITTDNTFVSGNCDVVIGIINNTVYDPLQPELDSFKEELDKYFKNHTSPDIDLGDISGINASVVNIQKEIDR
MG772933/bat-SL-CoVZC45   ..........................K.......................................................
NC004718Canada/SARS-CoV   .Y......F..S..I....FS..............................V...........
MN938384/HKU-SZ-002a 2020 .................................V.................V...........
MN975262/HKU-SZ-005b 2020 .................................V.................V...........

                    510       520       530       540       550       560       570       580
                ....|....|....|....|....|....|....|....|....|....|....|....|....|....|....|....|
MG772934/bat-SL-CoVZXC21  LNEVARNLNESLIDLQELGKYEHYIKWPWYVWLGFIAGLIAIVMVTILLCCMTSCCSCLKGCCSCGFCCKFDEDDSEPVLKGVKLHYT
MG772933/bat-SL-CoVZC45   ......................Q.......................................S...........
NC004718Canada/SARS-CoV   ....K.................Q........................A...S...........
MN938384/HKU-SZ-002a 2020 ....K.................Q.......I...........M.......S...........
MN975262/HKU-SZ-005b 2020 ....K.................Q.......I...........M.......S...........
```

Fig. (2). Comparison of amino acid sequences of S2 subunit of *Severe acute respiratory syndrome-related coronaviruses*. The analysis includes a total of 5 sequences: 1 sequence of SARS-CoV (NC004718 Canada/SARS-CoV), 2 sequences of Bat-SL-CoV (MG772934/bat-SL-CoVZXC21 and MG772933/bat-S--CoVZC45) and 2 sequences of SARS-CoV-2 (MN938384/HKU-SZ-002a 2020 and MN975262/HKU-S--005b 2020). The substitutions are shown by amino acid symbols at the respective positions and similarities are represented by the dots.

The results of the sequence identities estimated *via* pairwise distance calculation are summarized in Table **1**.

Table1. Sequence identities amongst S2 subunit of *Severe acute respiratory syndrome-related coronaviruses*.

Sequence Name	Nucleotide Identity (%)	Amino Acid Identity (%)	Nucleotide Identity (%)	Amino Acid Identity (%)
SARS-CoV-2	HKU-SZ-002a 2020	HKU-SZ-002a 2020	HKU-SZ-005b 2020	HKU-SZ-005b 2020
Bat-SL-CoVZXC21	83.3	94	83.3	94
Bat-SL-CoVZC45	83.6	94	83.6	94
NC004718 SARS-CoV	77.5	89.4	77.5	89.4

Selection Pressure Analysis

The analysis was carried out for sequence alignment (n=45) consisting of S2 subunit gene sequences of SARS-CoV-2 (n=13), SARS-CoV (n=18) and Bat-SL-CoVs (n=14). The identified codon positions under positive selection are summarized in Table **2**. The results were interpreted for codon positions under positive selection by the use of different parameters such as the ratio of dN/dS and significant values (p-values and Bayes factor) by employing different nucleotide substitution methods and bias models. No site was identified under positive selection using SLAC hence it is not shown in the given table. The mean dN/dS was calculated as 0.0526 suggesting that codons in the S2 subunit are under purifying or negative selection. However, individual codon positions 160, 244 and 562 were found to be under positive selection (dN/dS>1) employing more than one nucleotide substitution method.

Table 2. Selection pressure analysis of S2 subunit of *Severe acute respiratory syndrome-related coronaviruses*.

Nucleotide Substitution Method	IFEL						MEME			REL					
Nucleotide Substitution Bias Model	F81		HKY85		REV		F81	HKY85	REV	F81		HKY85		REV	
Positively Selected Codon	P value	dN/dS	P Value	dN/dS	P Value	dN/dS	P Value	P Value	P Value	B-Factor	dN/dS	B-Factor	dN/dS	B-Factor	dN/dS
1	-	-	-	-	-	-	0.0595	0.0595	0.595	-	-	-	-	-	-
2	-	-	-	-	-	-	-	-	-	248.05	0.6582	39.64	0.4041	35.48	0.6455
23	-	-	-	-	0.2493	0.6952	0.2482	0.2482	0.2482	-	-	-	-	-	-
47	-	-	-	-	-	-	-	-	-	55.83	0.4262	30.96	0.3394	41.19	0.5215
76	-	-	-	-	-	-	0.0587	0.0587	0.0587	-	-	-	-	-	-
87	-	-	-	-	-	-	-	-	-	34.76	0.3682	-	-	-	-
91	-	-	-	-	-	-	0.1593	-	-	-	-	-	-	-	-
95	-	-	-	-	-	-	0.2107	0.2107	0.2107	-	-	-	-	-	-
98	-	-	-	-	-	-	0.0825	0.0825	0.0825	-	-	-	-	-	-
108	-	-	-	-	-	-	-	-	-	34.32	0.2835	-	-	-	-
111	-	-	-	-	-	-	-	0.0363	0.0363	-	-	-	-	-	-
127	-	-	-	-	-	-	0.0337	0.0337	0.0337	-	-	-	-	-	-
154	-	-	-	-	-	-	-	-	-	88.80	0.4581	105.25	0.6545	108.62	0.8076
159	-	-	-	-	-	-	0.1897	0.1897	0.1897	-	-	-	-	-	-
160	-	-	-	-	0.1885	4.0983	-	-	-	205.57	0.6196	133.75	0.7611	169.02	0.9635
244	-	-	0.2023	1.1928	0.1750	1.6842	0.0247	0.0247	0.0247	-	-	-	-	-	-
253	-	-	-	-	-	-	0.1855	0.1855	0.1855	-	-	-	-	-	-
334	-	-	-	-	-	-	0.0243	0.0243	0.0243	-	-	-	-	-	-
349	-	-	-	-	-	-	0.1454	0.1454	0.1454	-	-	-	-	-	-

(Table 2) cont.....

Nucleotide Substitution Method	IFEL						MEME			REL					
Nucleotide Substitution Bias Model	F81		HKY85		REV		F81	HKY85	REV	F81		HKY85		REV	
Positively Selected Codon	P value	dN/dS	P Value	dN/dS	P Value	dN/dS	P Value	P Value	P Value	B-Factor	dN/dS	B-Factor	dN/dS	B-Factor	dN/dS
413	-	-	-	-	-	-	0.0181	0.0181	0.0181	-	-	-	-	-	-
428	-	-	-	-	-	-	0.1640	0.1640	0.1640	-	-	-	-	-	-
461	-	-	-	-	-	-	0.0650	0.0650	0.0650	-	-	-	-	-	-
496	-	-	-	-	-	-	0.0715	0.0715	0.0715	-	-	-	-	-	-
499	-	-	-	-	-	-	0.0140	0.0140	0.0140	-	-	-	-	-	-
559	-	-	-	-	-	-	0.2015	0.2015	0.2015	-	-	-	-	-	-
562	-	-	-	-	-	-	0.0558	0.0558	0.0558	154	0.5587	47.59	0.5431	55.11	0.6612

dN/dS — ratio of non-synonymous to synonymous mutation.
B-Factor — Bayes factor
Positively selected sites: Codon position 160, 244 and 562 (bold in the table)

Shannon Entropy Analysis

The Shannon entropy analysis (n=45) was carried out to identify the variable sites among the S2 subunit amino acid sequences of the SARS-CoV (n=18), Bat-S--CoVs (n=14) and SARS-CoV-2 (n=13). Various codon positions and their respective entropy score are represented in Shannon entropy (Hx) plot (Fig. **3**).

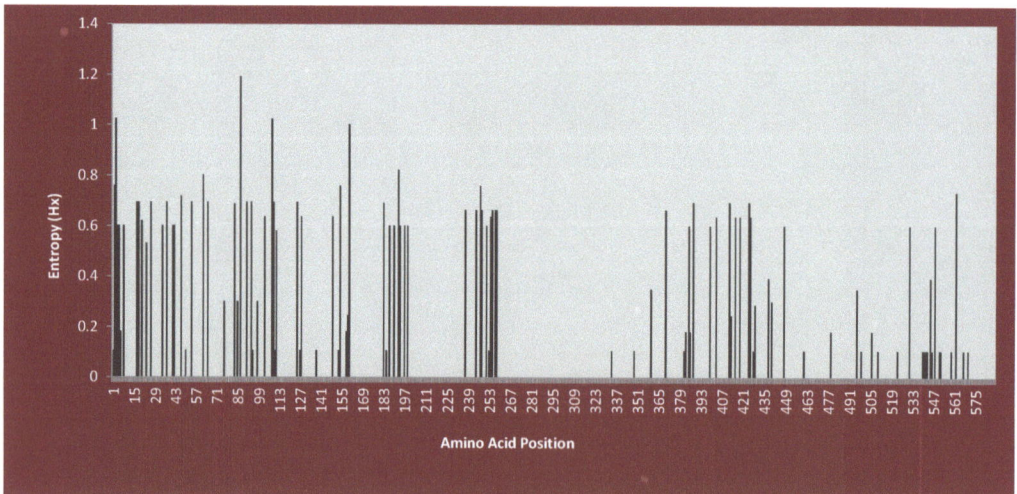

Fig. (3). Shannon entropy plot of S2 subunit of *Severe acute respiratory syndrome-related coronaviruses*. The plot is derived from a total of 45 amino acid sequences. An entropy score greater than the threshold (0.2) signifies increased likelihood of variation at that position in the amino acid sequence of the S2 subunit.

The threshold value of 0.2 entropy score was used for the selection of codon positions that are prone to mutations. A total of 71 variable sites (entropy score >0.2) were identified. The three codon positions that were positively selected by more than one nucleotide substitution method (160, 244 and 562) have also shown entropy score more than 0.5 (1.0, 0.66 and 0.73 respectively) indicating high probability of mutation at these sites. Other, set of four codon positions (3, 87, 108 and 160) was found where each of them showed very high entropy score (greater than or equal to 1), indicating that these sites were prone to mutation. The codon positions with substitutions are shown in Fig. (**2**). The sites with entropy score of more than 0.2 are given in Table **3**.

Table 3. **Codon positions with high entropy score along with the substitutions in the S2 subunit of S protein of** *Severe acute respiratory syndrome-related coronaviruses.*

S.No.	Codon Positions	Entropy Score	Substitutions Between SARS-CoV and SARS-CoV-2	Substitutions Between Bat-SL-CoVs and SARS-CoV-2
1	2	0.75	T2V	T2V
2	3	1.02	S3A	G3A (ZXC21), S3A (ZC45)
3	4	0.60	Q4S	Q4S
4	5	0.60	K5Q	K5Q
5	8	0.60	V8I	V8I
6	17	0.69	D17E	-
7	18	0.69	S18N	-
8	20	0.61	I20V	I20V
9	23	0.52	-	A23S
10	26	0.69	T26S	-
11	34	0.60	S34T	S34T
12	37	0.69	I37V	-
13	41	0.60	V41I	V41I
14	42	0.60	M42L	M42L
15	47	0.71	A47T	A47T
16	54	0.69	N54T	-
17	62	0.80	-	I62T
18	65	0.69	A65S	-
19	83	0.68	S83T	S83T
20	85	0.29	-	-
21	87	1.19	A87V	I87V

(Table 3) cont.....

S.No.	Codon Positions	Entropy Score	Substitutions Between SARS-CoV and SARS-CoV-2	Substitutions Between Bat-SL-CoVs and SARS-CoV-2
22	91	0.69	R91K	-
23	94	0.69	R94Q	-
24	98	0.29	-	-
25	103	0.63	M103I	-
26	108	1.02	T108P	-
27	109	0.69	L109I	-
28	111	0.57	Y111D	-
29	125	0.69	L125S	-
30	128	0.63	T128S	-
31	149	0.63	M149I	-
32	154	0.75	E154D	-
33	159	0.24	-	-
34	160	1.00	N160A	S160A
35	183	0.69	D183E	-
36	187	0.60	A187Q	A187Q
37	190	0.60	A190S	A190S
38	193	0.82	V193L	I193L
39	194	0.60	S194A	S194A
40	199	0.60	A199S	A199S
41	237	0.66	Q237L	-
42	244	0.66	K244S	-
43	247	0.75	S247G	-
44	248	0.66	Q248K	-
45	251	0.60	E251D	E251D
46	254	0.63	T254S	T254S
47	255	0.66	T255S	-
48	257	0.66	S257A	-
49	258	0.66	T258S	-
50	360	0.34	-	-
51	370	0.66	A370S	-
52	385	0.60	S385A	S385A
53	388	0.69	R388K	-
54	399	0.60	E399D	E399D

(Table 3) cont.....

S.No.	Codon Positions	Entropy Score	Substitutions Between SARS-CoV and SARS-CoV-2	Substitutions Between Bat-SL-CoVs and SARS-CoV-2
55	400	0.63	-	-
56	403	0.63	Y403H	-
57	412	0.69	F412S	-
58	413	0.24	-	-
59	416	0.63	S416H	-
60	419	0.63	I419V	-
61	425	0.69	F425Y	-
62	426	0.63	S426E	-
63	429	0.28	-	-
64	438	0.39	-	-
65	440	0.29	-	-
66	448	0.34	I448V	I448V
67	496	0.34	-	-
68	531	0.60	V531I	V531I
69	545	0.39	-	-
70	548	0.60	L548M	L548M
71	562	0.73	A562C	-

N-linked and O-linked Glycosylation

The N- and O-linked glycosylation pattern was analyzed for the S2 subunit sequences of spike glycoprotein of the species *Severe acute respiratory syndrome-related coronavirus* which includes SARS-CoV-2, SARS-CoV and Bat-SL-CoV. N-glycosylation is known to take place on Asn residues in Asn-Xaa-Ser/Thr stretch (where Xaa represents any amino acid but not Proline). The sequences had three N glycosylation sites at positions 32, 116 and 509. All the identified positions have glycosylation potential more than the threshold value of 0.5. The sites at these codon positions (32, 116 and 509) were conserved among all the strains included for the present study (n=45). Similarly, the analysis of O-glycosylation revealed two Ser sites at codon positions 125 and 257. The glycosylation potential at Ser 257 was identified only in SARS-CoV whereas some of the Bat-SL-CoVs have shown glycosylation potential at position 125 as well. The Bat-SL-CoVs MG772934/bat-SL-CoVZXC21 and MG772933/bat-S--CoVZC45 like the sequences of SARS-CoV-2 have not shown any probability for O-linked glycosylation. Moreover, the analysis revealed that Ser at position 125 and 257 is not conserved in the species of *Severe acute respiratory syndrome-related coronavirus.* The results of N-linked and O-linked are glycosylation are shown in Fig. (**4**).

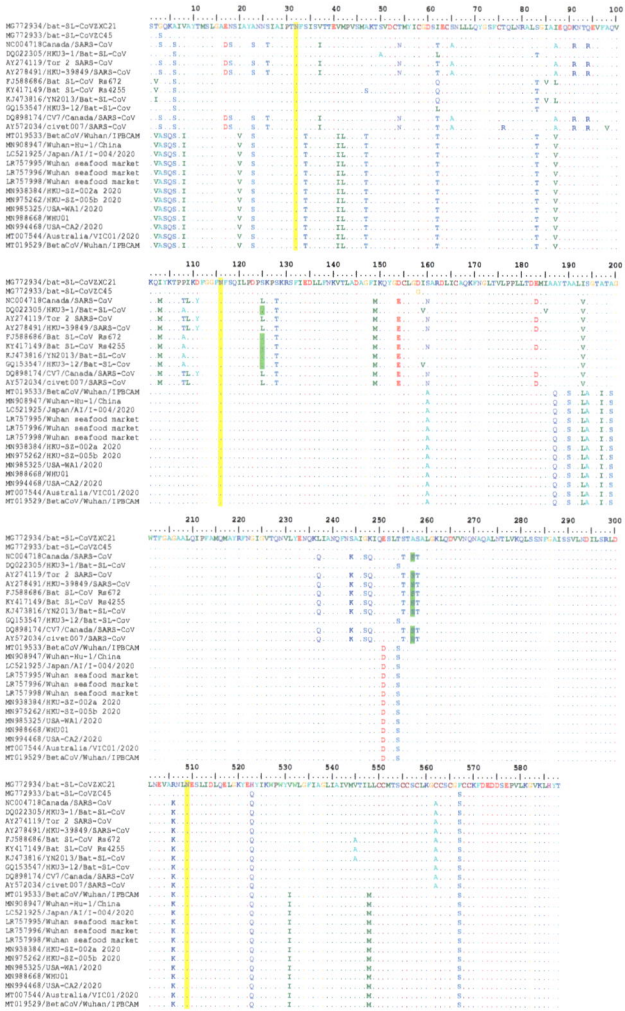

Fig. (4). N-linked and O-linked glycosylation pattern in S2 subunit of *Severe acute respiratory syndrome-related coronaviruses.* The N-linked and O-linked glycosylation sites are highlighted in yellow and green respectively.

*Note: The glycosylation analysis was done using all the 45 sequences. However, the alignment in Fig. (**4**) is depicting only some of the selected sequences of SARS-CoV, Bat-SL-CoVand SARS-CoV-2 to avoid repetition of the similar identifications.

DISCUSSION

The availability of the full-length genome sequence of SARS-CoV-2 within a small duration of time has equipped the scientific community to undertake its molecular characterization. This will assist towards the development of diagnostic tests against COVID-19. The spike surface glycoprotein (S protein) binds with the receptor present on the host cell [9]. The most conserved region in highly variable S protein gene is its S2 subunit [8]. It was demonstrated in a study that SARS-CoV S murine polyclonal antibodies inhibit SARS-CoV-2 S mediated entry into cells. This suggests that cross-neutralizing antibodies targeting the S epitopes can be elicited upon vaccination [10].Therefore, the S2 subunit can be the best candidate for targeting antiviral peptides against SARS-CoV-2. To gain an insight into the molecular characteristics of this potential region, we conducted comparative codon based analyses of the S2 subunit of S glycoprotein of *Severe acute respiratory syndrome-related coronaviruses* encompassing SARS-CoV, Bat-SL-CoV and SARS-CoV-2.

The phylogenetic analyses revealed that S2-subunit of SARS-CoV-2 is more similar to Bat-SL-CoV than its counterpart SARS-CoV. The estimation of evolutionary divergence between S2 subunit of SARS-CoV-2 and Bat-SL-CoVs showed about 94% amino acid sequence similarity and 83% nucleotides sequence similarity. Similarly, 89% and 78% sequence similarity were found between SARS-CoV-2 and SARS-CoV at the amino acid and nucleotide level, respectively.

As phylogeny suggested the origin of a newly identified strain, the natural selection played an important role in shaping its genetic composition. To delineate the biological taxa, the study on the molecular adaptations becomes crucial [11]. The identification of non-synonymous mutations in a protein coding sequence helps greatly in understanding the evolutionary biology of taxa as it may affect the fitness and thus in turn survival of an organism in a population. If these non-synonymous mutations at particular codon positions in a protein sequence has an insignificant or no effect on expression that would not affect the fitness of the organism. In such a scenario, the rates of non-synonymous substitutions (dN) can be compared to the rates of synonymous ones (dS), since this site tend to evolve neutrally [11]. In the present study, a value of mean dN/dS less than 1 indicates purifying selection in the S2 subunit of the *Severe acute respiratory syndrome-related coronavirus*es. However, the individual codon positions 160, 244 and 562 were found under positive selection by more than one nucleotide substitution methods. These sites were further verified by the Shannon entropy analysis. This way, seventy-one sites were identified having entropy score greater than the threshold value (0.2). The Shannon entropy analysis were carried out at amino acid level and thus can identify the positions even with low value of dN/dS to be under selection because this approach does not consider substitutions at the nucleotide level [12].

It has been known that glycoproteins undergo post-translational modifications which include the addition of oligosaccharides in two ways the N-linked and O-linked glycosylation [13, 14]. In our study, three N-linked glycosylation sites (32, 116 and 509) were identified in all the sequences of SARS-CoV, Bat-SL-CoV and SARS-CoV-2 . This suggests the conservative nature of N-linked glycosylation pattern within the S2 subunit of the S glycoprotein. However, variations were found in O-linked glycosylation. In the sequences of SARS-CoV, the Ser residue at the position 257 showed the O-linked glycosylation capability. The same position was identified in some of the sequences of Bat-SL-CoV. The Ser at 125 was found in the sequences of Bat-SL-CoV but not in all the sequences that were included for the analysis. Some sequences of Bat-SL-CoVs were identified at both the sites 125 and 257, that are capable of O-linked glycosylation. The two Bat-SL-CoVs: Bat-SL-CoVZXC21 and Bat-SL-CoVZC45 did not show any sites for O-linked glycosylation in the S2 subunit. Similarly, no O-linked glycosylation sites were identified in any of the sequences of SARS-CoV-2. This pattern of O-linked glycosylation of the two sequences of Bat-SL-CoV and that of SARS-CoV-2 showed the high level of genomic similarities. Nonetheless, role of these glycosylation sequences needs to be investigated in the antigenicity and resultant pathogenicity studies.

A virus possesses unique genomic features that requires investigations to ascertain the roles of its structural and non-structural proteins and nail down the cause of its devastating virulence property. Our approach is based on estimating the relative rates of non-synonymous (dN) and synonymous (dS) substitutions of the homologous sequence alignment. We envisage that, this study on codon-based models of molecular evolution will help to uncover the signatures of selection sequences. Further, the entropy analyses with less computational time can effectively select regions of the genome that may prove to be good markers to establish phylogenetic relationships, thus, making the large phylogenies more accessible. Further, delineation of unique signature sequences based on codon based approach on the full genomes of the SARS and SARS-like viruses is envisaged to provide the information on evolutionary trajectory and virulency of this emerging SARS-CoV-2 pathogen. Such data is likely to bring us closer to a broad spectrum anti-viral therapeutic agent against the S2 subunit of *Severe acute respiratory syndrome-related coronaviruses*. Moreover, the bioinformatics or computational analyses suggest, a multi-epitope vaccine structurally stable as it can induce specific immune responses against SARS-CoV-2 [15].

CONCLUDING REMARKS

Some of the individual codon positions of the S2 subunit were found to be under positive selection suggesting that such substitutional replacement would increase the fitness of SARS-CoV-2 in the host population. Since the pandemic is still ongoing, the mutation rates may modulate with significant substitution in the future viral strains of SARS-CoV-2. The pattern of N-linked glycosylation is conserved in S2 subunit of spike glycoprotein. However, discrepancies were found within the O-linked glycosylation pattern. The information obtained from these analyses may be helpful in understanding the evolutionary dynamics of *Severe acute respiratory syndrome-related coronaviruses* that may assist in designing the antiviral therapeutic remedies.

CONSENT FOR PUBLICATION

Not Applicable.

CONFLICT OF INTEREST

The authors declare no conflict of interest, financial or otherwise.

ACKNOWLEDGEMENTS

Arshi Islam is supported by Senior Research Fellowship of Indian Council of Medical Research (ICMR), Government of India. The research in our laboratory is funded by Central Council for Research in Unani Medicine (CCRUM), Ministry of Ayurveda, Yoga and Naturopathy, Unani, Siddha and Homeopathy (AYUSH) (F.No.3-63/2019-CCRUM/Tech). Professor Sher Ali is grateful for financial support from DBT (BT/PR12828/AAQ/1/622/2015), New Delhi and JC Bose award (SR/S2/JCB-49/2011) from SERB-DST, New Delhi. The authors also extend their appreciation to the Centre of Excellence in Biotechnology Research, King Saud University, Riyadh, Saudi Arabia for support.

REFERENCES

[1]   Islam A, Ahmed A, Naqvi IH, Parveen S. Emergence of deadly severe acute respiratory syndrome coronavirus-2 during 2019–2020. VirusDis 2020; Apr 8;31(2):1-9.
[http://dx.doi.org/10.1007/s13337-020-00575-1] [PMID: 32292802]

[2]   Gorbalenya AE, Baker SC, Baric RS, *et al.* The species *Severe acute respiratory syndrome-related coronavirus*: classifying 2019-nCoV and naming it SARS-CoV-2. Nat Microbiol 2020; 5(4): 536-44.
[http://dx.doi.org/10.1038/s41564-020-0695-z] [PMID: 32123347]

[3]   Fehr AR, Perlman S. Coronaviruses: an overview of their replication and pathogenesis. Methods Mol Biol 2015; 1282: 1-23.
[http://dx.doi.org/10.1007/978-1-4939-2438-7_1] [PMID: 25720466]

[4]   Cui J, Li F, Shi ZL. Origin and evolution of pathogenic coronaviruses. Nat Rev Microbiol 2019; 17(3): 181-92.
[http://dx.doi.org/10.1038/s41579-018-0118-9] [PMID: 30531947]

[5]   Walls AC, Tortorici MA, Snijder J, *et al.* Tectonic conformational changes of a coronavirus spike glycoprotein promote membrane fusion. Proc Natl Acad Sci USA 2017; 114(42): 11157-62.
[http://dx.doi.org/10.1073/pnas.1708727114] [PMID: 29073020]

[6]   Lu R, Zhao X, Li J, *et al.* Genomic characterisation and epidemiology of 2019 novel coronavirus: implications for virus origins and receptor binding. Lancet 2020; 395(10224): 565-74.
[http://dx.doi.org/10.1016/S0140-6736(20)30251-8] [PMID: 32007145]

[7]   Xu X, Chen P, Wang J, *et al.* Evolution of the novel coronavirus from the ongoing Wuhan outbreak and modeling of its spike protein for risk of human transmission. Sci China Life Sci 2020; 63(3): 457-60.
[http://dx.doi.org/10.1007/s11427-020-1637-5] [PMID: 32009228]

[8]   Chan JF, Kok KH, Zhu Z, *et al.* Genomic characterization of the 2019 novel human-pathogenic coronavirus isolated from a patient with atypical pneumonia after visiting Wuhan. Emerg Microbes Infect 2020; 9(1): 221-36.
[http://dx.doi.org/10.1080/22221751.2020.1719902] [PMID: 31987001]

[9]   Li F. Structure, function, and evolution of coronavirus spike proteins. Annu Rev Virol 2016; 3(1): 237-61.
[http://dx.doi.org/10.1146/annurev-virology-110615-042301] [PMID: 27578435]

[10]   Walls AC, Park YJ, Tortorici MA, Wall A, McGuire AT, Veesler D. Structure, function, and antigenicity of the SARS-CoV-2 spike glycoprotein. Cell 2020; 181(2): 281-292.e6.
[http://dx.doi.org/10.1016/j.cell.2020.02.058] [PMID: 32155444]

[11]   Poon AF, Frost SD, Pond SL. Detecting signatures of selection from DNA sequences using Datamonkey. Methods Mol Biol 2009; 537: 163-83.
[http://dx.doi.org/10.1007/978-1-59745-251-9_8] [PMID: 19378144]

[12]   Pan K, Deem MW. Quantifying selection and diversity in viruses by entropy methods, with application to the haemagglutinin of H3N2 influenza. J R Soc Interface 2011; 8(64): 1644-53.
[http://dx.doi.org/10.1098/rsif.2011.0105] [PMID: 21543352]

[13]   Kornfeld R, Kornfeld S. Assembly of asparagine-linked oligosaccharides. Annu Rev Biochem 1985; 54(1): 631-64.
[http://dx.doi.org/10.1146/annurev.bi.54.070185.003215] [PMID: 3896128]

[14]   Bagdonaite I, Nordén R, Joshi HJ, *et al.* A strategy for O-glycoproteomics of enveloped viruses--the O-glycoproteome of herpes simplex virus type 1. PLoS Pathog 2015; 11(4): e1004784.
[http://dx.doi.org/10.1371/journal.ppat.1004784] [PMID: 25830354]

[15]   Ka T, Narsaria U, Basak S, *et al.* A Candidate multi-epitope vaccine against SARS-CoV-2. Sci Rep. 2020 Jul 2;10(1): 10895.
[http://dx.doi.org/10.1038/s41598-020-67749-1] [PMID: 32616763]

CHAPTER 5

Global Epidemiology and Transmission of COVID-19

Md. Wasim Khan[1,#], Sajda Ara[1,#], Farah Deeba[1], Ayesha Tazeen[1], Nasir Salam[2], Irshad H. Naqvi[3] and Shama Parveen[1,*]

[1] *Centre for Interdisciplinary Research in Basic Sciences, Jamia Millia Islamia, New Delhi, India*

[2] *Department of Microbiology, Central University of Punjab, Bathinda, Panjab, India*

[3] *Dr. M. A. Ansari Health Centre, Jamia Millia Islamia, New Delhi, India*

Abstract: Coronavirus Disease 2019 (COVID-19) is a viral infection caused by severe acute respiratory syndrome coronavirus 2 (SARS-CoV-2). It started as an outbreak in Wuhan, China, at the end of 2019. But within a few months, it took the form of a deadly pandemic affecting millions of people in more than 216 countries. Transmission *via* a large number of asymptomatic cases and international travel played a pivotal role in the spread of infection to different geographical regions. In the present chapter, we have given the chronological details about the spread of the infection across the globe. The countries with the greatest international connectivity showed a large number of cases. Further, the countries that suspended international travelling and sealed their borders are the ones that have managed the spread impressively. Subsequently, we have summarized the emergence of human Coronaviruses (SARS, SARS-CoV-2 and MERS) in humans. We have also described the different modes of human to human transmission of SARS-CoV-2. However, the infectivity is undercounted as many patients with mild or no symptoms are not getting tested. The present chapter summarizes the origin, global epidemiology and modes of transmission of the infection. Comprehensive hospital and community-based surveillance and detailed interpretation of full genomes of SARS-CoV-2 need to be carried out across different geographical regions. This data will assist in the demarcation of mutation rates and resultant evolutionary trajectory of this emerging viral pathogen. Preventive measures like social distancing, wearing masks and good hygiene should be followed religiously to prevent the spread of the contagion.

Keywords: COVID-19, Epidemiology, Origin, Pandemic, SARS-CoV-2, Transmission.

---

* **Corresponding author Shama Parveen:** Centre for Interdisciplinary Research in Basic Sciences, Jamia Millia Islamia, New Delhi, India; E-mails: sparveen2@jmi.ac.in and shamp25@yahoo.com
# Both authors contributed equally.

INTRODUCTION

The world entered the year 2020, witnessing the second pandemic of this century in the form of infectious Coronavirus Disease 2019 (COVID-19). This is a novel infection of the respiratory tract, which may develop into fulminant pneumonia-like disease that is similar to severe acute respiratory syndrome (SARS). This pathogen was named severe acute respiratory syndrome coronavirus 2 (SARS-CoV-2) by World Health Organization (WHO) since its genome is similar to SARS. It has affected millions of people across the world in the last one year, and the cases are still increasing exponentially. On January 9, 2020, the WHO issued a statement that the Chinese CDC (Centre for Disease Control and Prevention) has reported the causative agent of this viral infection to be Coronavirus and submitted the whole genome sequence in the GenBank [1].

COVID-19 began with the first report from Wuhan, China, on 31st December 2019. The Municipal Health Commission of Wuhan city reported several pneumonia-like cases with unknown etiology and their common link to Wuhan Hanan Seafood wholesale market. Due to several links with a common seafood market, it was originally believed to have originated from the market [2]. However, there were reports of infection with no direct or indirect interaction with the Hanan seafood market. The virus was probably transferred to humans from a spillover event in a bat virus through an unknown mediator [3]. Various studies in late April 2020 strongly suggested this mediator is probably Pangolins since coronavirus genomes in these animals were found to have a close similarity with the SARS-CoV-2 [4]. However, the convincing source of this viral infection among humans is still not understood.

The virus was initially underappreciated with many asymptomatic infections and a long incubation period. Thus, enormous air travel and the rapid rate of transmission led to its spread worldwide. Eventually, in a span of a few months, the virus moved across the entire globe leading to the current pandemic situation. The spread started with parts of the world connected with China through travelers due to business or tourism purposes. SARS-CoV-2 has many modes of transmission, such as respiratory droplets from the mouth and nose of the infected person, the aerosol transmission, including others [5]. Around 80% of the cases do not develop the severe form of the disease and show only mild signs and symptoms of seasonal flu. These patients recover easily without any major treatment. However, the estimated incidence rate is much higher and is in the range of 20–60% compared to the flu with 8% incidence. A preliminary observation concluded that those with severe disease conditions need hospitalization for a period twice as much as that for acute flu [6].

We have analyzed the sequential events that have led to the spread of the infection across the globe (Fig. **1**). This is followed by a discussion of the probable zoonotic origin of the pathogen along with a comparison of epidemiological features among the three human Coronaviruses (SARS, SARS-CoV-2 and MERS). Later in the chapter, we had discussed different modes of transmission of this viral infection.

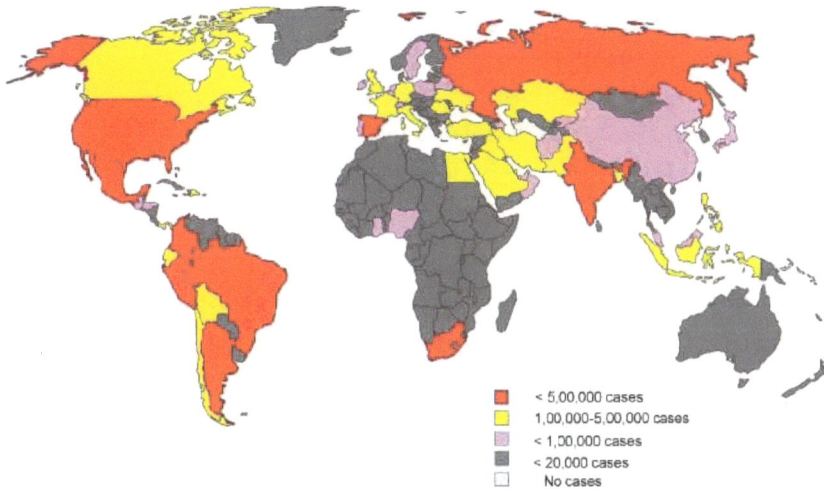

Fig. (1). A map showing distribution of Covid-19 cases in the affected regions of the world till 31st August 2020. The freely editable version of the world map was taken (http://All-free-download.com/ free-vector/simple-world-map-vector.html).

THE SPREAD

- The first few cases of SARS-CoV-2 infection were speculated to have originated at the end of 2019 from Wuhan, Hubei Province, China. Of all suspected cases from China, 80% were from the Wuhan district, and it was the epicenter of the initial outbreak.
- The first death reported was of a 61-year-old male patient admitted to a hospital with respiratory failure and severe pneumonia and other co-morbidities.
- The first case reported outside China was from Thailand, where a 61-year-old Chinese woman had travelled to Wuhan.
- The virus then briefly entered Japan and marked its 3rd country on January 16th, 2020, where a 30-year-old man with a travel history to Wuhan developed pneumonia-like condition. However, Japan is one of the few countries that recorded the lowest death rate per capita and managed the spread very well.
- On January 15th 2020, the first known travel-related confirmed case was reported from Washington, United States.
- By the end of January, it took the shape of a pandemic affecting Russia, North America, South America, Southeast Asia, Pacific and Middle East countries.

- On 29th January, Finland reported an imported case from Wuhan, and on 30th January, India reported its first case from Kerala.
- The initial cases of COVID-19 from different countries suggested that in most of the cases, the patients had a travel history to Wuhan or some direct or familial contact with the traveler.
- On 31st January, WHO Director-General declared the SARS-CoV-2 outbreak a "Public Health Emergency of International Concern" with a total number of 9826 confirmed cases and 213 deaths. Of all the confirmed cases till then, China had accounted for around 99% of the patients [7].
- By February, the number of active cases started rising exponentially.
- The Diamond Princess cruise ship stranded in the Pacific Ocean carrying 3,711 persons, including passengers and cabin crew, departed from Port of Yokohama on 20th January for a round trip of South-East Asia during the Lunar New Year period [8].
- The cruise reported a cluster of 10 individuals infected with the virus on 5th February. The passengers were subsequently quarantined in closed spaces on board. By early March, the number of active cases in the ship reached 696, with 14 deaths.
- By 11th February, in a span of 10 days, the number of confirmed cases and deaths quadrupled and increased around five-folds, respectively.
- By the end of February, Brazil, in South America and Algeria in Africa reported their first confirmed cases.
- Further, in just one day, seven European countries reported their first cases on 27th February.
- On 27th February, 621 confirmed cases and 61 deaths were reported from Europe.
- USA started declaring restricted travel bans with China on 2nd February, Iran on 2nd March, European countries in the Schengen area on 13th March, whereas the United Kingdom and Ireland on 16th March.
- By 16th March, for the first time, the number of active cases and deaths surpassed altogether outside China.
- On March 16th, WHO declared SARS-CoV-2 a pandemic.
- The number of active cases reached 2,00,000 on 19th March. Further, the time taken for doubling the cases to 2 million was sharply reduced to 12 days.
- Apart from common citizens, the British and Russian Prime Ministers were also confirmed for the Coronavirus infection.
- Wuhan, the epicenter of the outbreak, reported no new active case on 19th March, whereas, by March 22nd, the number of global deaths exceeded 30,000.
- On 25th March, the United Nation launched a $2 billion global humanitarian response plan appeal to assist poor and vulnerable countries to fight against the COVID-19 pandemic.

- By 26th March, the global active cases of COVID-19 surpassed 6,00,000.
- Meanwhile, by the end of March, Spain and Italy were the most affected countries with 832 and 889 deaths, respectively.
- Botswana, a country in South Africa, reported its first active case on 30th March.
- Following this, many African countries reported the viral infection, although the number of active cases and mortality rates remained significantly low.
- The month of April started with the number of active cases and deaths drastically increasing even after taking harsh precautionary measures like strict lockdown with all kinds of social gatherings terminated in various countries. These included European Union countries with Spain, France and Italy being the worst affected.
- With the highest number of death tolls from Spain, it reported a total of 11,744 deaths and 1,24,736 active cases and was the worst-hit country by pandemic hitherto.
- On 3rd April, Asian Development Bank estimated a global economic impact of COVID-19 to be around $ 2-4 trillion [9].
- USA joined the fleets too with 8,162 cases and 3,00,915 confirmed cases by 4th April.
- Soon the USA became the most affected country with the highest number of cases in the world that is twice the number of cases in Italy, which was the second most affected country after USA.
- The worldwide death toll from the pandemic was increased to 1,37,500, with more than 20,83,320 declared cases in 193 countries by mid of April.
- However, China lifted the lockdown on Wuhan, the epicenter of the outbreak on 8th April for the first time since the outbreak begun.
- Whereas on 10th April, the global number of deaths reached 1,00,000. Meanwhile, war-torn Yemen reported its first positive confirmed case on the same day [10].
- The number of positive cases in the African subcontinent surpassed 15,000.
- On 12th April, USA recorded the highest death rate for any country during this pandemic in a single day, which accounted for nearly 2,000 people. In the month of April, the number of active cases as well as deaths increased exponentially.
- On 16th April, Saudi Arabia funded $500 million to the global response.
- Additionally, a sharp increase in the number of positive cases due to lack of Personal Protection Equipment in African countries was recorded.
- On 19th April, the death toll in Europe due to COVID-19 crossed 1,00,000, with the death rate reaching nearly 9% [11].
- By 21st April, there were 2.5 million global cases.
- Whereas, by 25th April, the global deaths surpassed 2,00,000, of which the USA accounted for 29% of the total deaths alone.
- WHO launched a COVID-19 tool accelerator. The main motive behind this tool

was to speed up the production of therapeutic vaccines [12].

- On 6th April, Australia launched a Bluetooth based surveillance voluntary tracking application to monitor active cases.
- By 27th April, the number of global cases reached up to 3 million.
- While New Zealand after reporting no active cases in the country decided to ease the lockdown measures and opened most of its business' outlets.
- However, on April 28th, the global number of cases in UK exceeded more than a million (1/3 of total cases). Additionally, on the same day number of deaths exceeded 58,000 in USA alone.
- On May 2nd, India recorded a new spike in the number of positive cases, 2,933 cases in a single day.
- Similarly, Russia recorded the highest one-day spike of 9,623 cases. According to the Moscow mayor, around 2% of the Moscow population was infected by this time.
- On 3rd May, random testing of 500 suspected peoples in Afghanistan revealed that more than 150 people were infected.
- By 9th May, global cases reached 4 million.
- Wuhan reported a fresh new case on 10th May, nearly after a month after lifting the lockdown [13].
- By 14th May, global deaths reached 3,00,000.
- May 20th witnessed 1,06,200 fresh global cases; this accounted for the highest single-day spike recorded till then.
- The COVID-19 hits reached about 5 million global cases by 21st May.
- By 22nd May, Brazil overtook Russia with the highest number of cases following USA. Indigenous people in Brazil were found to be at higher risk of infection and had a high mortality rate.
- By 26th May, the number of confirmed global cases reached 5.5 million.
- In the next five days, COVID-19 cases touched 6 million worldwide, with 1,00,000 deaths in USA alone.
- By 1st June, Brazil reached a new peak in the number of cases and crossed the mark of 5,00,000.
- The worldwide cases increased from 6 to 6.5 million on June 4th and to 7 million by June 8th within a span of 2 days. The number of global death crosses 4,00,000.
- By 10th June, the African continent marked 2,00,000 infected cases.
- It took 98 days to reach 1,00,000 cases in Africa, while only 18 additional days to stretch up to 2,00,000 cases.
- Till 20th June 2020, COVID-19 had spread across 188 countries, with the total number of active cases jumped above 8 million (8,666,697), with global deaths reaching half a million (4,60,066).
- By June 21st, infected cases in Brazil increased beyond 1 million, with the death

toll reaching 50,000.

- Number of active COVID-19 cases crossed 9 million soon. On June 24th, the situation in USA was still critical as it reported the highest daily new cases.
- India also recorded its highest single-day peak of nearly about 16,000 cases.
- By the end of June, USA, Brazil and Russia documented to be first, second and third highly affected countries, respectively.
- On the other hand, India observed a continuous exponential rise of daily cases, making it the fourth-worst affected country by this time.
- By June 24th, the number of globally active cases stands at 9,295,365 and the total deaths worldwide reported hitherto was 4,78,285 [14].
- By June 28th, around 6 months after the first reported case of COVID-19, the total number of confirmed global cases crossed 10 million, and death toll reached 5,00,000.
- New Zealand on 30th June confirmed no new cases of COVID-19 after two travelers returned from UK were tested positive until a few weeks ago.
- By 2nd July, the number of active cases in India surpassed 6,00,000, with 15,834 deaths.
- Columbia, too joined the fleet of countries with 1,00,000 active cases.
- US recorded a sharpest one-day spike in the number of confirmed cases with 50,000 cases since the outbreak of pandemic.
- By 3rd July, Brazil remained the second-highest affected country with the total number of cases being 1.5 million. India reported another highest single-day spike of 20,903 cases. The number of active cases surpassed 11 million, and it took only five days from the mark of 10 million.
- A study published in Lancet reported that around 5% of Spain's population developed antibodies for SARS-CoV-2 [15].
- By 6th July, India overtook Russia being the third most affected country after a single-day spike in the number of cases with 25,000 cases and 613 deaths in the last 24 hours [16].
- By 7th July, the number of active cases and deaths in UK observed a sharp decline for the first time.
- By 8th July, the number of active global cases surpassed 12 million. The number of confirmed cases in USA reached 3 million, with 1,30,000 deaths [17].
- WHO observed the highest single-day spike of 2,28,102 active cases in 24 hours on 10th July 2020.
- The number of active cases is increasing at an exponential rate (Fig. **2**).
- By 12th July, 23,000 new cases were reported from 10 different countries.
- By 15th July, the number of confirmed cases and deaths reached 13,512,693 and 5,83,359, respectively.
- By 18th July, the number of confirmed global cases surpassed 17 million and confirmed death reached 600,000.

- Pan American Health Organization warned that three out of ten people in America are at increased risk of developing COVID-19 infection [18].
- Number of active COVID-19 cases surpassed 15 million on 22nd July.
- By 26th July, the number of cases surpassed 16 million.
- By 5th August confirmed global death surpassed 700,000 and the number of confirmed cases reached 18 million.
- African subcontinent surpassed 1 million COVID-19 cases on 7th August.
- By 8th August, the number of cases in America reached 5 million.
- Number of confirmed cases surpassed 20 million worldwide on 10th August.
- New Zealand reported new COVID cases in a family with no record of travel overseas. This announcement came soon after the government celebrated 100 days of no community transmission on 12th August [19].
- Hongkong reported its first new reinfection of COVID-19 in a 33-year-old man on 24th August.
- The number of confirmed cases surpassed 24 million globally by August 27.
- On 30th August, India reported its highest single-day spike of any country during the pandemic with 78,761 new cases.
- By 31st August, the number of cases in USA surpassed 6 million [20].
- Total global cases were 24.854,140 million and deaths were 0.8,38,924 by 31st August 2020.
- The timeline of events of the COVID-19 pandemic till 31st August 2020 is shown in (Fig. **3**).

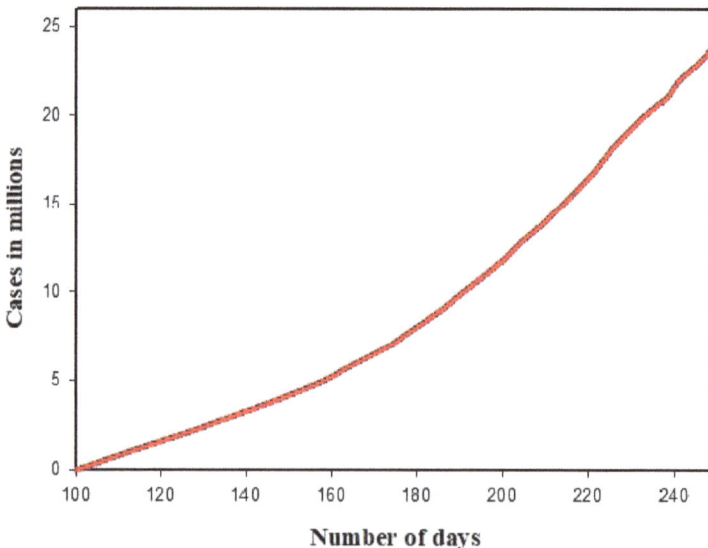

Fig. (2). The graph showing the increase in number of COVID-19 cases with respect to time till 31st August 2020.

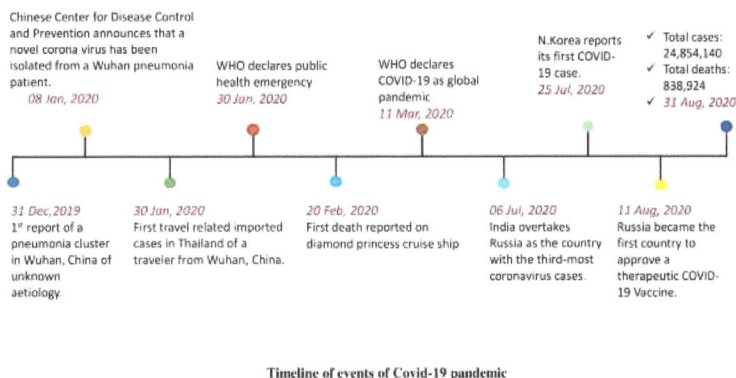

Timeline of events of Covid-19 pandemic

Fig. (3). Timeline of events of the COVID-19 pandemic till 31st August 2020.

INCREASE IN INFECTIVITY OF SARS-COV-2

Coronaviruses are the largest positive-stranded, enveloped RNA viruses belonging to the family *Coronoviridae*. Their genome is approximately 26-32 kb in length. RNA viruses, unlike DNA viruses, have the potential for mutations at a much higher rate since the RNA polymerase does not have proofreading activity to take care of the incorrectly incorporated bases [2]. Higher mutation rates lead to variations and viral evolution, thus enabling pathogens to escape host immunity and develop drug resistance. Ever since the release of the SARS-CoV-2 full genome, scientists all over the world started following it for the meaningful alterations in its genome. A group of researchers showed a sequence similarity of 96% between SARS-CoV-2 and bat coronavirus at the genome level [22]. The study comprised random 95 complete genome sequences from GenBank till 5th April 2020, and concluded that there were a total of 116 mutations or unique variants [22]. Phylogenetic networking of around 1400 SARS-CoV-2 genomes available at NCBI till 7th May 2020 (Fig. **4**) clustered around 1200 sequences mostly from China, USA and initial sequences from India all together showing the high similarity between these strains. However, the continuous presence of the virus in these regions led to the emergence of related strains with different mutations branching out from the main cluster in the network.

The three most common mutations reported are 29095C>T in the N gene, 8782C>T in the ORF1ab gene and 28144T>C in the ORF8 gene [22]. The replicase/transcriptase genes are also called ORF1a and ORF1b. Evidence of modifications in the coding sequence of ORF1ab in the SARS and other Coronaviruses indicates that ORF1ab proteins probably have a significant function in the viral pathogenesis, and it might be directly involved in the replication of the virus [23]. The reverse genetic study showed that ORF1ab proteins might be involved in the modification of cellular gene expression and cellular signaling [23]. In another study, 558 complete genome sequences of infected COVID-19 patients were retrieved from the GISAID database and were analyzed using bioinformatics tools like multiple sequence alignment and SNP genotyping. It was found that these strains showed large mutational diversity. Some high-frequency mutations were seen in the single nucleotide polymorphism (SNP) profiles of many SARS-CoV-2 strains. Thus, these high-frequency mutations possibly contributed to the increased transmissibility of SARS-CoV-2 [24].

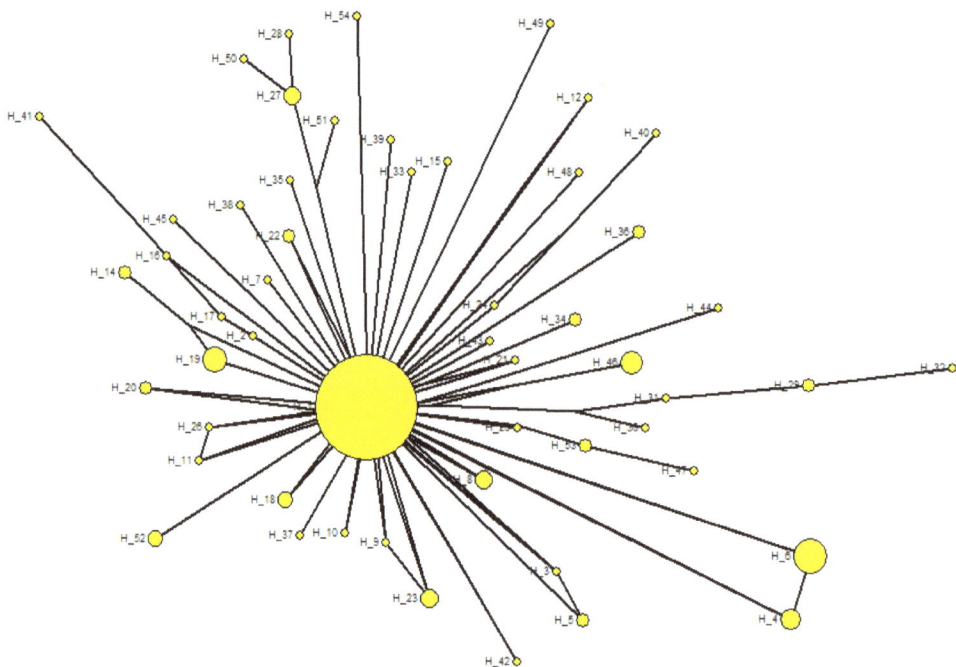

Fig. (4). Phylogenetic network of 1400 full genomes of SARS-CoV-2.

Similarly, in a recent publication, bioinformatics analysis was carried out on 351 full genome sequences from SARS-CoV-2 patients, retrieved from the GISAID database. The results showed many mutations in non-structural (NS) proteins, which play a major role in Coronavirus RNA synthesis and processing. Mutations were seen mainly in two NS proteins, NSP6 and an amino acid region near ORF10. NSP6 is found in both alpha and beta coronaviruses in humans as well as in animals. A literature survey has shown that the presence of several phenylalanine residues in the NSP6 outer membrane region favors the affinity between this region and the endoplasmic membrane. This induces a more stable binding of the protein to the endoplasmic membrane. In addition, this binding might help in infection by reducing the capability of autophagosomes to deliver viral particles in the lysosomes for degradation. Therefore, its role will be hindered only to the autophagosomes growth, and hence it may favor viral replication [25].

In another study, the genome analysis of five different isolates of SARS-CoV-2, among which two samples each from China and from India, US and Italy, were compared with the reference sequence of SARS-CoV-2003. It was found out that the envelope protein has a high amount of valine among SARS-CoV-2 sequences. It was also observed that the gene sequences coding for E protein of SARS-CoV-2 has high GC (40%) content as compared to the SARS-CoV-2003. Further, the in-depth analysis showed that the length of the envelope protein of SARS-CoV-2003 (231bp) is 3bp longer than the SARS-CoV-2 (228bp). Hence, there is a deletion of one amino acid, i.e., valine, in this case. It is now apparent that there are point mutations as well as deletions occurring in a specific region of SARS-CoV-2 [26]. Some important mutations have been documented in spike protein as well. The spike (S) protein protrudes from the surface of the virus and mediates binding and fusion of viral and cellular membranes. There are two domains in S protein- S1 and S2. A mutation at residue number 614 (D to G) was observed in the initial stages of the pandemic, with G almost completely replacing the D with the rapid spread of the virus [27]. It has been speculated that this mutation promotes an open configuration of S protein, which is more susceptible to ACE2 receptor association with higher affinity and hence an increase in infectivity of the virus.

Numerous mutations are reported in SARS-CoV-2 based on the 48,635 full genome sequences submitted in GISAID from different countries in a recent study [28]. The authors estimated a rate of 7.3 mutations/sample with respect to the prototype strain of China. SNPs were observed over short deletion/ insertion across the global sequences. Classification of SARS-CoV-2 mutation was done according to their type:

- C>T transition contributed to around 55.1% of all the global mutations.

- A>G transition is the second most common change that contributed towards 14.8% changes in Europe, America and Africa.

- G>T is the third most frequent transition that resulted in 12% changes.

The strains were classified into 5 clades based on the specific mutations i.e G, GH, GR, S and V. The clade G is based on a mutation in the S protein (S-D614G), the clade V (variant of the ORF3a coding protein NS3-G251), and clade S (variant ORF8-L84S).

Clade G: The most prevalent mutation in the sequenced SARS-CoV-2 genomes worldwide is a transversion affecting the 23,403rd nucleotide, adenosine that is mutated to guanosine (A23403G). This mutation causes a D614G (aspartate to glycine at amino acid position 614 in the S protein that defines the G-clade. It is prevalent in Europe (that has reported the maximum SARS-CoV-2 genomes), Oceania, South America, and Africa.

The second most common amino acid mutation is P314L, which affects the NSP12 that code for the viral RNA-dependent RNA polymerase. The two derivatives of G clade are GR and GH that report other mutations in addition to the D614G change.

Clade GR: This carries the combination of spike D614G and nucleocapsid RG203KR mutations. It is currently the most common representative of the viral population worldwide.

Clade GH: This reports the ORF3a:Q57H mutation in addition to D614G.

Clade S: This clade is named after the mutation in ORF8 L84S, and it is also described by a silent mutation, C8782T.

Clade V: It is defined by the ORF3a:G251V mutation, mostly co-existing with the NSP6:L37F change [28].

THE SPILLOVER ZOONOTIC EVENTS

Before the COVID-19 pandemic, there were two other outbreaks in the last two decades, which led to the crossover of animal beta-corona viruses to humans leading to outbreaks. In 2002-03, a *Betacoronavirus* of bat origin jumped to humans through the intermediary host, civet cats in the Guangdong province, China. This virus was named SARS, which infected 8422 individuals principally in China before being contained [29]. It has caused around 916 deaths, with an 11% mortality rate. Nearly after a decade, in 2012, another Coronavirus originated from the bats *via* dromedary camels as an intermediate host in Saudi Arabia. This coronavirus was named the Middle East respiratory syndrome coronavirus (MERS-CoV), which affected around 2494 individuals with 858 mortalities [30].

The question about the origin of SARS-CoV-2 was answered by many scientists, each suggesting that bat is the probable host [31]. But the question about the intermediate host remains still unanswered, although many researches strongly suggest that pangolins are more likely to be the intermediate host [32]. Apart from having a similar zoonotic origin, these three viruses belong to the same virus family and share almost similar clinical symptoms. In addition, SARS-CoV-2 shares 51% and 79% genomic similarity with the MERS-CoV and SARS-CoV, respectively. Fig. (**5**) depicts the origin of Covid-19 and its emergence into human to human spread. Table **1** shows a comparative detail about emergence, hosts, and key biologic as well as epidemiologic features of these three Coronaviruses.

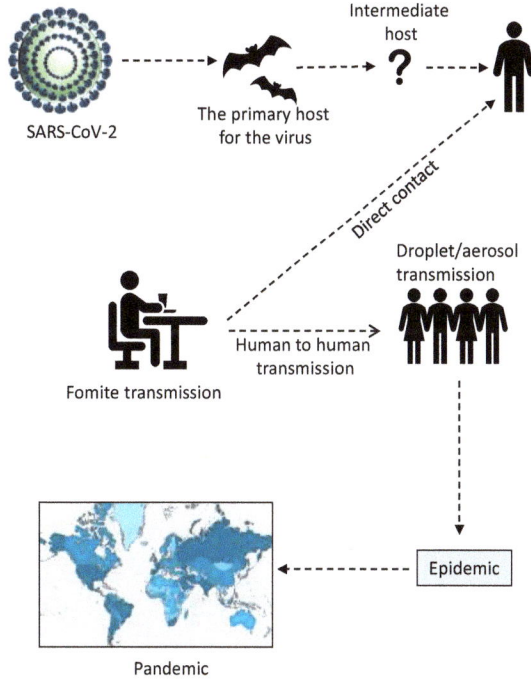

Fig. (5). The origin and transmission of SARS-CoV-2, leading to the COVID-19 pandemic. The world map was taken from the WHO site.

Table 1. Comparison of origin, hosts, epidemiological and biological features of SARS-CoV, MERS-CoV and SARS-CoV-2.

Features	SARS-CoV-2	MERS-CoV	SARS-CoV	Reference
Emergence date	December 2019	April 2012	November 2002	[33, 34]
Area	Wuhan, China	Jeddah, Saudi Arabia	Guangdong, China	[29, 30]
Hosts	Bats, Pangolins	Bats, camel	Bats, palm civets and raccoon dogs	[31, 35, 36]
Type of virus	Positive-sense single-stranded RNA	Positive-sense single-stranded RNA	Positive-sense single-stranded RNA	[32, 33, 35]
Entry receptor in humans	ACE2	DPP4	ACE2	[35, 37]
Clinical manifestation	Fever, dry cough, shortness of breath, tiredness, nausea, vomiting, acute respiratory syndrome	Fever, cough, shortness of breath, nausea diarrhoea	Fever, malaise, myalgia, cough headache, diarrhoea, shivering	[38, 39]

(Table 1) cont.....

Features	SARS-CoV-2	MERS-CoV	SARS-CoV	Reference
Transmission rate	High	Low	Moderate	[33 - 35]
Transmission mode	Aerosol droplets, physical contact, nosocomial transmission	Respiratory and aerosol, limited nosocomial and human-to-human transmission	Aerosol droplets, nosocomial, fecal-oral	[32, 60, 61, 63]
Total cases	24,854,140 cases till 31st August 2020	2494 cases	8906 cases	[38, 40]
Total deaths	838,924 till 31st August 2020	858 cases	744 cases	[38, 40]
Number of countries affected	216 till 31st August 2020	27	26	[38, 40]

TRANSMISSION

Although animals were involved in the initial cases of the viral infection, human to human transmission of SARS-CoV-2 is like that of SARS CoV and MERS CoV. Several human to human modes of transmission of SARS CoV-2 are being updated on a regular basis. There are many expected and observed modes of the human to human transmission of COVID-19, such as contact and droplet transmission [41]. Nonetheless, analysis of all the possible modes of transmission is essential to control the community transmission of the COVID-19. The clinical manifestation of COVID-19 resembles SARS-CoV infection with symptoms such as dry cough, fever, and shortness of breath as the acute respiratory distress syndrome in most of the cases. An infected individual with critical illness shows symptoms of septic shock, respiratory failure, and organs failure, which need medical care [42, 43].

A brief overview of the observed modes of transmission of COVID-19 based on different studies across the world is given below (Table **2**).

Table 2. Possible modes of Transmission of COVID-19.

Mode of transmission	Details	References
Droplet & aerosol mediated transmission	Infected people spread virus when they sneeze/cough/ talk/breathe. Virus encapsulated in saliva/mucous forms larger **droplets** that splash at nearby places, whereas smaller particles evaporate in **aerosols** and are carried to distant places *via* air. SARS-CoV-2 was identified in aerosols for hours. SARS-CoV-2 was detected in stool and probable exposure to aerosols.	[41, 76]

(Table 2) cont.....

Mode of transmission	Details	References
Airborne transmission	Viruses are embedded in aerosols transported to distant places *via* air. SARS-CoV-2 was detected in air samples collected from rooms of COVID-19 treatment areas.	[77]
Faecal-oral transmission	Live SARS-CoV-2 was detected in faeces, suggesting possible faecal oral transmission. Rectal swabs were positive for SARS-CoV-2 by RT-PCR when nasopharyngeal samples were negative. Sewage samples were positive for SARS-CoV-2.	[73, 78]
Air pollution to human transmission	Highly polluted cities in China and Italy had large number of COVID cases.	[76, 79]
Fomite transmission	SARS-CoV-2 was detected on surfaces like personal objects, floor surfaces, waste containers, and toilet. The virus was identified on plastic, copper, stainless steel, ceramics, wood, aluminum, glass, etc. Elevator push buttons and door handles have also contributed significantly to the infections.	[41, 77, 80]
Familial transmission	Familial clusters have been reported frequently.	[72]
Nosocomial transmission	Hospital based infection especially of the health care workers have added to the disease burden.	[73 - 75]

Droplet and Aerosol Mediated Transmission

Infected individuals can spread the virus whenever they sneeze, cough, talk, or even breathe. These viral particles are encapsulated in the water, globs of saliva, and mucus and their fate in the environment depend on their size. The larger ones drop down faster than they evaporate thus, they splash down in droplets form in nearby places [44]. The smaller ones evaporate faster in aerosols form and linger in the air, and further drifts away than the droplets do.

Based on the particle size, specifically aerodynamic diameter, these respiratory particles can be categorized as droplets or aerosols. It can be concluded that aerosols may spread the virus among susceptible hosts who are far away from the point of origin and thus pose a greater risk. However, it is a fact that the viral disease outbreaks by aerosol transmission are comparatively less severe due to dilution and inactivation of viral particles lingered for a longer time period in the air [45]. After several disagreements for the particle size of aerosols and droplets, the WHO and CDC postulated that particles size of less than 5 μm are considered as aerosols or droplet nuclei and more than 5 μm are considered droplets [45, 46]. On the other hand, some other postulations stated that particles with aerodynamic diameter of 10 to 20 μm or lesser must be considered as aerosols on the basis of their ability to hang in the air for a longer time and reachability for the lung alveolar region [47]. Smaller aerosol particles can be inhaled more deeply into the lungs, which may cause alveolar tissue infection in the lower respiratory tract, whereas the larger droplets get trapped in the upper respiratory tract region [48].

In simple terms, aerosol particles are suspensions of liquid or solid present in the air which are created by either anthropogenic or natural phenomena [49]. The transmission of droplets occurs when an infected patient coughs, sneezes, or talks, thus directly spraying the droplets in the mucous membranes or conjunctiva of the susceptible host. On the other hand, contact transmission may also take place when an infected individual physically touches the susceptible host, or there is indirect contact with infected secretions on fomites (contaminated surfaces) [50]. Scientists have postulated that both aerosols and droplets created from violent and non-violent expirations of infected persons can be the cause for airborne transmission of COVID-19. Still, more research must be done to understand the infected droplets and aerosols behavior in different environments, particularly in the enclosed spaces, to fully ascertain the COVID-19 transmission in the environment.

Airborne Transmission

The spread of infection through the dissemination of the infecting agent in the form of aerosols that suspends in the air for a long time and can travel from one place to another with the air is called an airborne infection. The scientific community and WHO, both are regularly observing and evaluating the chances of COVID-19 being an airborne infection [51]. A study by Gou and colleagues concluded that air samples were positive at different locations in wards dedicated to COVID-19 patients in hospitals [52]. These studies include limitations like different stages of the disease at the time of sampling as well as a variety of procedures used. Thus, incomplete information is available on airborne transmission, including viability of the virus in air samples. Another query in this context is that are the viral loads in the air samples high enough to cause infection in the individuals? Still, prior to answering these questions and obtaining evidence for it, it is logical and important to take precautions for possible airborne mediated transmission of disease.

A previous study generated aerosols of infectious samples under controlled laboratory conditions using high-powered jet nebulizers. The RNA of SARS-CoV-2 was detected in air samples within aerosols for up to 3 hours in a study and for 16 hours in another, which also found viable replication-competent virus [53, 54]. These findings were from experimentally induced aerosols that do not reflect normal human cough conditions. Some studies performed in health care centers where symptomatic COVID-19 patients were treated, reported the presence of

RNA of SARS-CoV-2 in air samples [55 - 58]. While some other studies in both health care and non-healthcare centers reported the absence of RNA of SARS-CoV-2 and no study reported the viable virus in air samples [58 - 62].

Faecal Transmission

Many researchers have concluded that faecal samples of the infected patients showed the presence of the virus. Therefore, it can also be considered a probable mode of transmission of COVID-19. The sewage samplings from various areas have also reported positive samples for SARS-CoV-2. In the case of a community, the sewage samplings can play a big role in the transmission of disease. Therefore, even if digested sputum or gastrointestinal involvements are the reason for the presence of virus in stool, it gives a good reason to maintain personal hygiene for protective measures to avoid SARS-CoV-2 infection [40].

Vertical Transmission

The trans-placental or intrauterine transmission from the infected pregnant female to the foetus could be another probable mode of transmission. However, according to various studies on the pregnant female with positive SARS-CoV-2 infection, no indications of intrauterine transmission were found [63]. These studies also highlighted that the COVID-19 course was normal in pregnant females compared to the MERS and SARS [64].

Apart from different modes of transmission of the SARS-CoV-2, various settings in the common lifestyle have also been shown to have a significant role in COVID-19 transmission. These include the following situations:

Fomites Transmission

Contact with fomites followed by touching of nose, mouth, or eyes, although not main yet are important modes of viral transmission [65]. The fomites get contaminated by the deposition of sputum, aerosols, droplets or faeces. It may get contaminated either directly or by touching an object with the skin of an infected person, etc. The transmission risks *via* contact depend on the viral concentration, viability on the selected surfaces over time. The contact transmission depends on the concentration and viability of virus particles on the surface over a period of time [65].

Frequently touched surfaces by several infected people, such as elevator push buttons or door handles, might be more significant transmission *via* fomites as compared to less frequently touched surfaces or objects. Surface transmission can be significant in the case of COVID wards in the hospitals and COVID care centers. Routine cleaning, hand hygiene and surface disinfection reduce the probability of contact transmission. Washing and rinsing hands for a minimum of 20 seconds with soap can help in emulsification of the lipid layer of viral particle making it non-viable. This diffuses the virus particles reducing its spread. Sanitizer is an alternative for washing hands wherever soap is unavailable. Chemical disinfectants such as sodium hypochlorite can be used on the surfaces to inactivate the virus, especially in clinical settings and hospitals. Various guidelines have been formulated for the disinfectants list approved for hard surfaces. In addition, special guidelines have also been formulated for cleaning and disinfecting of public spaces as a precautionary measure to prevent SARS-CoV-2 transmission [65 - 71].

Familial Transmission

There are many reports of the familial clusters getting infected with the COVID-19. The transmission of the infection through an infected family member to other persons of the same family or the closed ones has added to the significant disease burden. In most cases, the familial transmission has occurred through an asymptomatic infected person. It is particularly important to take precautions within the family members if any of the members have a travel history to an infected area or has met a symptomatic person or himself has showed any symptoms [72].

Nosocomial Transmission

The frequency of nosocomial infections is very high in COVID-19 disease. Nurses, doctors, paramedical staff and other health care workers are at higher risk of getting an infection. A study showed that health workers accounted for 3.8% SARS-CoV-2 infections and 5 deaths from a total of 44,672 patients [53]. In addition, both symptomatic and asymptomatic patients must take full protective measures such as wearing masks and shortening the stay in the hospital during their visit. In addition, the common people visiting clinics/hospitals for some other treatment should also take appropriate precautions since they are also at high risk of getting an infection. Efforts to advertise the information about COVID-19 control, prevention, risk of nosocomial infection and early warning signs of the disease are necessary to manage the infection [73, 74].

The chain of transmission could be broken by either avoiding exposure to the virus or developing immunity to the virus. This will require exposure to this virus either naturally or in the form of a vaccine, which seems like a distant possibility right now despite extensive global efforts. This would create a level of herd immunity required to contain the pandemic, which is desirable, especially for the high-risk population [75]. However, acquiring herd immunity by natural exposure to the virus will have devastating consequences for the elderly and people with comorbidities. Vaccination is the only safe way to achieve herd immunity. Until such time when a vaccine is available, exposure to the virus must be avoided.

CONCLUDING REMARKS

The origin of COVID-19 in China and its transformation into a pandemic has led to a significant disease burden across the globe. The researchers are leaving no stone unturned to reveal the mechanism of its global spread. The viral infection has also raised serious concerns about its effective community transmission and a large number of asymptomatic cases. Evolution of the pathogen over time in terms of mutations, especially in the structural proteins, is likely to assist the pathogen towards an increase in its infectivity and to evade the host immune response. Detailed investigation of the epidemiological and transmission dynamics of SARS-CoV-2 is likely to assist in the formulation of measures towards containment of the ongoing pandemic.

CONSENT FOR PUBLICATION

Not Applicable.

CONFLICT OF INTEREST

The author declares no conflict of interest, financial or otherwise.

ACKNOWLEDGEMENT

Sajda Ara acknowledges the Research Fellowship assistance by Council of Scientific and Industrial Research (CSIR), Government of India. Farah Deeba is supported by Research Fellowship by Indian Council of Medical Research (ICMR), Government of India. Ayesha Tazeen is supported by Research Fellowship by University Grants Commission (UGC), Government of India. The research in our laboratory is funded by Council of Scientific and Industrial Research (CSIR), India (37(1697)17/EMR-II) and Central Council for Research in Unani Medicine (CCRUM), Ministry of Ayurveda, Yoga and Naturopathy, Unani, Siddha and Homeopathy (AYUSH), India (F.No.3-63/2019-CCRUM/Tech).

REFRENCES

[1]   WHO Statement regarding cluster of pneumonia cases in Wuhan, China. Available at: https://www.who.int/china/news/detail/09-01-2020-who-statement-regarding-clu-ter-of-pneumonia-cases-in-wuhan-china

[2]   Gill RS, Dogra M. COVID-19: A Geo-Anthropogenic Analysis. J Sci Technol 2020; 9(4): 1555-66. [http://dx.doi.org/10.21275/SR20422233916]

[3]   Li X, Zai J, Zhao Q, *et al.* Evolutionary history, potential intermediate animal host, and cross-species analyses of SARS-CoV-2. J Med Virol 2020; 92(6): 602-11. [http://dx.doi.org/10.1002/jmv.25731] [PMID: 32104911]

[4]   Zhang T, Wu Q, Zhang Z. Probable Pangolin Origin of SARS-CoV-2 Associated with the COVID-19 Outbreak. Curr Biol 2020; 30(7): 1346-1351.e2. [http://dx.doi.org/10.1016/j.cub.2020.03.022] [PMID: 32197085]

[5]   Chan JF, Yuan S, Kok KH, *et al.* A familial cluster of pneumonia associated with the 2019 novel coronavirus indicating person-to-person transmission: a study of a family cluster. Lancet 2020; 395(10223): 514-23. [http://dx.doi.org/10.1016/S0140-6736(20)30154-9] [PMID: 31986261]

[6]   The Lenski Lab Health Plan for the New Coronavirus Outbreak | Telliamed Revisited. (Cited 18 July 2020). Available from: https://telliamedrevisited.wordpress.com/2020/02/29/the-lenski-lab-hea-th-plan-for-the-new-coronavirus-outbreak/

[7]   Organization WH. Coronavirus disease 2019 (COVID-19] Situation Report – 11. WHO Bull. 2020;1–7.

[8]   Mizumoto K, Kagaya K, Zarebski A, Chowell G. Estimating the asymptomatic proportion of coronavirus disease 2019 (COVID-19) cases on board the Diamond Princess cruise ship, Yokohama, Japan, 2020. Euro Surveill 2020; 25(10): 2000180. [http://dx.doi.org/10.2807/1560-7917.ES.2020.25.10.2000180] [PMID: 32183930]

[9]   Developing Asia Growth to Fall in 2020 on COVID-19 Impact | Asian Development Bank. [Cited 26 Jun 2020]. Available from: https://www.adb.org/news/developing-asia-growth-fall-2020-co-id-19-impact

[10]   Yemen: Authorities confirm first COVID-19 case April 10 /update 3. [Cited 2020 Jun 26]. Available from: https://www.garda.com/crisis24/news-alerts/331216/yemen-authorities-confirm-first-co-id-19-case-april-10-update-3

[11]   Worldometer. Coronavirus Cases. Worldometer. 2020 [cited 18 Jul 2020]. p. 1–22. Available from: https://www.worldometers.info/coronavirus/

[12]   Access to COVID-19 Tools [ACT] Accelerator. [Cited 26 Jun 2020]. Available from: https://www.who.int/publications/m/item/access-to-covid-19-tools-[act]-accelerator

[13]   Wuhan Sees First New Coronavirus Cases Since Lockdown Lifted | Time. [cited 26 Jun 2020]. Available from: https://time.com/5835175/wuhan-new-coronavirus-cases/

[14]   COVID-19 Map - Johns Hopkins Coronavirus Resource Center. https://coronavirus.jhu.edu/map.html

[15]   Pollán M, Pérez-Gómez B, Pastor-Barriuso R, *et al.* Prevalence of SARS-CoV-2 in Spain (ENE-COVID): a nationwide, population-based seroepidemiological study. Lancet 2020; 396(10250): 535-44. [http://dx.doi.org/10.1016/S0140-6736(20)31483-5] [PMID: 32645347]

[16]   Coronavirus disease [COVID-19] Situation report-6 July. [Cited 12 Jul 2020]. Available from: https://learn.arcgis.com/en/paths/goarn

[17]   Coronavirus disease [COVID-19] Situation Report-170.

[18]   Pan American Health Organisation (PAHO). https://www.paho.org/en/news/21-7-2020-three-o-

t-10-people-americas-are-increased-risk-severe-covid-19-because-underlying#:-
:text=Next-
,Three%20out%20of%2010%20people%20in%20the%20Americas%20are%20at,underlying%20condi
tions%2C%20PAHO%20Director%20says&text=Diabetes%2C%20kidney%20disease%2C%20hypert
ension%2C,risk%20for%20more%20severe%20disease

[19]   COVID-19. Current cases https://www.health.govt.nz/our-work/diseases-and-conditions/covi-
-19-novel-coronavirus/covid-19-current-situation/covid-19-current-cases

[20]   Coronavirus disease (COVID-19): Weekly Epidemiological Update. Available at:
https://www.who.int/docs/default-source/coronaviruse/situation-reports/202008-
1-weekly-epi-update-3.pdf?sfvrsn=d7032a2a_4

[21]   Zhou P, Yang XL, Wang XG, *et al.* A pneumonia outbreak associated with a new coronavirus of
probable bat origin. Nature 2020; 579(7798): 270-3.
[http://dx.doi.org/10.1038/s41586-020-2012-7] [PMID: 32015507]

[22]   Graham RL, Sparks JS, Eckerle LD, Sims AC, Denison MR. SARS coronavirus replicase proteins in
pathogenesis. Virus Res 2008; 133(1): 88-100.
[http://dx.doi.org/10.1016/j.virusres.2007.02.017] [PMID: 17397959]

[23]   Snijder EJ, Decroly E, Ziebuhr J. The nonstructural proteins directing coronavirus rna synthesis and
processing. Advances in Virus Research. Academic Press Inc. 2016; pp. 59-126.
[http://dx.doi.org/10.1016/bs.aivir.2016.08.008] [PMID: 27712628]

[24]   Yin C. Genotyping coronavirus SARS-CoV-2: methods and implications. Genomics 2020; 112(5):
3588-96.
[http://dx.doi.org/10.1016/j.ygeno.2020.04.016] [PMID: 32353474]

[25]   Benvenuto D, Angeletti S, Giovanetti M, *et al.* Evolutionary analysis of SARS-CoV-2: how mutation
of Non-Structural Protein 6 (NSP6) could affect viral autophagy. J Infect 2020; 81(1): e24-7.
[http://dx.doi.org/10.1016/j.jinf.2020.03.058] [PMID: 32283146]

[26]   Chatterjee S. Understanding the nature of variations in structural sequences coding for coronavirus
spike, envelope, membrane and nucleocapsid proteins of SARS-CoV-2. SSRN Electron J 2020.
[http://dx.doi.org/10.2139/ssrn.3562504]

[27]   Zhang L, Jackson CB, Mou H. The D614G mutation in the SARS-CoV-2 spike protein reduces S1
shedding and increases infectivity. bioRxiv. 2020.
[http://dx.doi.org/10.1101/2020.06.12.148726]

[28]   Mercatelli D, Giorgi FM. Geographic and genomic distribution of SARS-CoV-2 mutations. Front
Microbiol 2020; 11: 1800.
[http://dx.doi.org/10.3389/fmicb.2020.01800] [PMID: 32793182]

[29]   Chan-Yeung M, Xu RH. SARS: epidemiology. Respirology 2003; 8 (Suppl.): S9-S14.
[http://dx.doi.org/10.1046/j.1440-1843.2003.00518.x] [PMID: 15018127]

[30]   Memish ZA, Perlman S, Van Kerkhove MD, Zumla A. Middle East respiratory syndrome. Lancet
2020; 395(10229): 1063-77.
[http://dx.doi.org/10.1016/S0140-6736(19)33221-0] [PMID: 32145185]

[31]   Forster P, Forster L, Renfrew C, Forster M. Phylogenetic network analysis of SARS-CoV-2 genomes.
Proc Natl Acad Sci USA 2020; 117(17): 9241-3.
[http://dx.doi.org/10.1073/pnas.2004999117] [PMID: 32269081]

[32]   Liu P, Jiang JZ, Wan XF, *et al.* Are pangolins the intermediate host of the 2019 novel coronavirus
(SARS-CoV-2)? PLoS Pathog 2020; 16(5): e1008421.
[http://dx.doi.org/10.1371/journal.ppat.1008421] [PMID: 32407364]

[33]   Hui DSI, I Azhar E, Madani TA, *et al.* The continuing 2019-nCoV epidemic threat of novel
coronaviruses to global health - The latest 2019 novel coronavirus outbreak in Wuhan, China. Int J
Infect Dis 2020; 91: 264-6.

[http://dx.doi.org/10.1016/j.ijid.2020.01.009] [PMID: 31953166]

[34]   Huang C, Wang Y, Li X, *et al.* Clinical features of patients infected with 2019 novel coronavirus in Wuhan, China. Lancet 2020; 395(10223): 497-506.
       [http://dx.doi.org/10.1016/S0140-6736(20)30183-5] [PMID: 31986264]

[35]   Lu R, Zhao X, Li J, *et al.* Genomic characterisation and epidemiology of 2019 novel coronavirus: implications for virus origins and receptor binding. Lancet 2020; 395(10224): 565-74.
       [http://dx.doi.org/10.1016/S0140-6736(20)30251-8] [PMID: 32007145]

[36]   Bolles M, Donaldson E, Baric R. SARS-CoV and emergent coronaviruses: viral determinants of interspecies transmission. Curr Opin Virol 2011; 1(6): 624-34.
       [http://dx.doi.org/10.1016/j.coviro.2011.10.012] [PMID: 22180768]

[37]   Chan JF-W, Yuan S, Kok K-H, *et al.* A familial cluster of pneumonia associated with the 2019 novel coronavirus indicating person-to-person transmission: a study of a family cluster. Lancet 2020; 395(10223): 514-23.
       [http://dx.doi.org/10.1016/S0140-6736(20)30154-9] [PMID: 31986261]

[38]   WHO. 2020. www.who.int/emergencies/diseases/novel-coronavirus-2019

[39]   Cui J, Li F, Shi ZL. Origin and evolution of pathogenic coronaviruses. Nat Rev Microbiol 2019; 17(3): 181-92.
       [http://dx.doi.org/10.1038/s41579-018-0118-9] [PMID: 30531947]

[40]   Yeo C, Kaushal S, Yeo D. Enteric involvement of coronaviruses: is faecal-oral transmission of SARS-CoV-2 possible? Lancet Gastroenterol Hepatol 2020; 5(4): 335-7.
       [http://dx.doi.org/10.1016/S2468-1253(20)30048-0] [PMID: 32087098]

[41]   Jayaweera M, Perera H, Gunawardana B, Manatunge J. Transmission of COVID-19 virus by droplets and aerosols: A critical review on the unresolved dichotomy. Environ Res 2020; 188: 109819.
       [http://dx.doi.org/10.1016/j.envres.2020.109819] [PMID: 32569870]

[42]   Chen Y, Liu Q, Guo D. Emerging coronaviruses: Genome structure, replication, and pathogenesis. J Med Virol 2020; 92(4): 418-23.
       [http://dx.doi.org/10.1002/jmv.25681] [PMID: 31967327]

[43]   Chen N, Zhou M, Dong X, *et al.* Epidemiological and clinical characteristics of 99 cases of 2019 novel coronavirus pneumonia in Wuhan, China: a descriptive study. The Lancet. 2020 Feb 15;395(10223): 507-13.
       [http://dx.doi.org/10.1016/S0140-6736(20)30211-7]

[44]   Grayson SA, Griffiths PS, Perez MK, Piedimonte G. Detection of airborne respiratory syncytial virus in a pediatric acute care clinic. Pediatr Pulmonol 2017; 52(5): 684-8.
       [http://dx.doi.org/10.1002/ppul.23630] [PMID: 27740722]

[45]   Shiu EYC, Leung NHL, Cowling BJ. Controversy around airborne versus droplet transmission of respiratory viruses: implication for infection prevention. Curr Opin Infect Dis 2019; 32(4): 372-9.
       [http://dx.doi.org/10.1097/QCO.0000000000000563] [PMID: 31259864]

[46]   World Health Organization (WHO). Infection Prevention and Control of Epidemic and Pandemic Prone Acute Respiratory Infections in Healthcare–WHO Guidelines
       https://www.who.int/csr/bioriskreduction/infection_control/publication/en/

[47]   Gralton J, Tovey E, McLaws ML, Rawlinson WD. The role of particle size in aerosolised pathogen transmission: a review. J Infect 2011; 62(1): 1-13.
       [http://dx.doi.org/10.1016/j.jinf.2010.11.010] [PMID: 21094184]

[48]   Thomas RJ. Particle size and pathogenicity in the respiratory tract. Virulence 2013; 4(8): 847-58.
       [http://dx.doi.org/10.4161/viru.27172] [PMID: 24225380]

[49]   Judson SD, Munster VJ. Nosocomial transmission of emerging viruses *via* aerosol-generating medical procedures. Viruses 2019; 11(10): 940.

[http://dx.doi.org/10.3390/v11100940] [PMID: 31614743]

[50]   Boone SA, Gerba CP. Significance of fomites in the spread of respiratory and enteric viral disease. Appl Environ Microbiol 2007; 73(6): 1687-96.
[http://dx.doi.org/10.1128/AEM.02051-06] [PMID: 17220247]

[51]   Advice on the use of masks in the context of COVID-19. Interim guidance. Geneva: World Health Organization; 2020. Available at: https://www.who.int/publications/i/item/advice-on-the-us--of-masks-in-the-community-during-home-care-and-in-healthcare-settings-in-t-e-context-of-the-novel-coronavirus-(2019-ncov)-outbreak

[52]   Guo ZD, Wang ZY, Zhang SF, *et al.* Aerosol and surface distribution of severe acute respiratory syndrome coronavirus 2 in hospital wards, Wuhan, China, 2020. Emerg Infect Dis 2020; 26(7): 1583-91.
[http://dx.doi.org/10.3201/eid2607.200885] [PMID: 32275497]

[53]   van Doremalen N, Bushmaker T, Morris DH, *et al.* Aerosol and surface stability of SARS-CoV-2 as compared with SARS-CoV-1. N Engl J Med 2020; 382(16): 1564-7.
[http://dx.doi.org/10.1056/NEJMc2004973] [PMID: 32182409]

[54]   Fears AC, Klimstra WB, Duprex P, *et al.* Persistence of Severe Acute Respiratory Syndrome Coronavirus 2 in Aerosol Suspensions. Emerg Infect Dis 2020; 26(9): 2168-71.
[http://dx.doi.org/10.3201/eid2609.201806] [PMID: 32568661]

[55]   Chia PY, Coleman KK, Tan YK. Detection of air and surface contamination by SARS-CoV-2 in hospital rooms of infected patients. Nat Comm 2020; 11(1).
[http://dx.doi.org/10.1038/s41467-020-16670-2]

[56]   Ma J, Qi X, Chen H, Li X, Zhan Z, Wang H, *et al.* Exhaled breath is a significant source of SARS-CoV-2 emission (pre-print). MedRxiv 2020.
[http://dx.doi.org/10.1101/2020.05.31.20115154]

[57]   Liu Y, Ning Z, Chen Y, *et al.* Aerodynamic analysis of SARS-CoV-2 in two Wuhan hospitals. Nature 2020; 582(7813): 557-60.
[http://dx.doi.org/10.1038/s41586-020-2271-3] [PMID: 32340022]

[58]   https://www.who.int/news-room/commentaries/detail/transmission-of-sars-cov-2-implicati-ns-for-infection-prevention-precautions

[59]   Faridi S, Niazi S, Sadeghi K, *et al.* A field indoor air measurement of SARS-CoV-2 in the patient rooms of the largest hospital in Iran. Sci Total Environ 2020; 725: 138401.
[http://dx.doi.org/10.1016/j.scitotenv.2020.138401] [PMID: 32283308]

[60]   Cheng VC-C, Wong S-C, Chan VW-M, *et al.* Air and environmental sampling for SARS-CoV-2 around hospitalized patients with coronavirus disease 2019 (COVID-19). Infect Control Hosp Epidemiol 2020; 41(11): 1258-65.
[http://dx.doi.org/10.1017/ice.2020.282] [PMID: 32507114]

[61]   Ong SWX, Tan YK, Chia PY, *et al.* Air, surface environmental, and personal protective equipment contamination by severe acute respiratory syndrome coronavirus 2 (sars-cov-2) from a symptomatic patient. JAMA 2020; 323(16): 1610-2.
[http://dx.doi.org/10.1001/jama.2020.3227] [PMID: 32129805]

[62]   Wu S, Wang Y, Jin X, Tian J, Liu J, Mao Y. Environmental contamination by SARS-CoV-2 in a designated hospital for coronavirus disease 2019. Am J Infect Control 2020; S0196-6553(20): 30275-3.
[http://dx.doi.org/10.1016/j.ajic.2020.05.003] [PMID: 32407826]

[63]   Schwartz DA. An analysis of 38 pregnant women with COVID-19, their newborn infants, and maternal-fetal transmission of SARS-CoV-2: maternal coronavirus infections and pregnancy outcomes. Arch Pathol Lab Med 2020.
[http://dx.doi.org/10.5858/arpa.2020-0901-SA] [PMID: 32180426]

[64]   Dashraath P, Wong JLJ, Lim MXK, *et al.* Coronavirus disease 2019 (COVID-19) pandemic and pregnancy. Am J Obstet Gynecol 2020; 222(6): 521-31.
[http://dx.doi.org/10.1016/j.ajog.2020.03.021] [PMID: 32217113]

[65]   World Health Organisation. Modes of transmission of virus causing COVID-19: implications for IPC precaution recommendations 2020. https://www.who.int/news-room/commentaries/detail/modes--f-transmission-of-virus-causing-COVID-19-implications-for-ipc-precaution-recommendations

[66]   Boyce JM, Pittet D. Healthcare infection control practices advisory committee; HICPAC/SHEA/APIC/IDSA hand hygiene task force; Society for healthcare epidemiology of america/association for professionals in infection control/infectious diseases society of America. Guideline for hand hygiene in health-care settings. recommendations of the healthcare infection control practices advisory committee and the hicpac/shea/apic/idsa hand hygiene task force. MMWR Recomm Rep 2002; 51(RR-16): 1-45.
[PMID: 12418624]

[67]   US Centers for Disease Control and Prevention. Handwashing: clean hands save lives 2020. https://www.cdc.gov/handwashing/show-me-the-science-handwashing.html

[68]   US Centers for Disease Control and Prevention. When & How to Use Hand Sanitizer in Community Settings 2020. https://www.cdc.gov/handwashing/show-me-the-science-hand-sanitizer.html

[69]   Health Canada. 2020. https://www.canada.ca/en/health-canada/services/drugs-health-products/disinfectants/COVID-19/list.html

[70]   US Environmental Protection Agency. 2020. https://www.epa.gov/pesticide-registration/list-n-disinfectants-use-against-sars-cov-2

[71]   Public Health Agency of Canada. 2020. https://www.canada.ca/en/public-health/services/publications/diseases-conditions/cleaning-disinfecting-public-spaces.html

[72]   Li P, Fu JB, Li KF, *et al.* Transmission of COVID-19 in the terminal stages of the incubation period: A familial cluster. Int J Infect Dis 2020; 96: 452-3.
[http://dx.doi.org/10.1016/j.ijid.2020.03.027] [PMID: 32194239]

[73]   Wang D, Hu B, Hu C, *et al.* Clinical characteristics of 138 hospitalized patients with 2019 novel coronavirus infected pneumonia in Wuhan, China. JAMA 2020; 323: 1061-9.
[http://dx.doi.org/10.1001/jama.2020.1585]

[74]   The novel coronavirus pneumonia emergency response epidemiology team. Vital surveillances: the epidemiological characteristics of an outbreak of 2019 novel coronavirus diseases (COVID-19)—China, 2020. China CDC Weekly 2020; 2: 113-22.
[http://dx.doi.org/10.46234/ccdcw2020.032]

[75]   Randolph HE, Barreiro LB. Herd immunity: understanding COVID-19. Immunity 2020; 52(5): 737-41.
[http://dx.doi.org/10.1016/j.immuni.2020.04.012] [PMID: 32433946]

[76]   Coccia M. Diffusion of covid-19 outbreaks: the interaction between air pollution- to-human and human-to-human transmission dynamics in hinterland regions with cold weather and low average wind speed. Working Paper CocciaLab N. 48/ 2020. CNR - National Research Council of Italy. Available at: https://doi.org/10.2139/ssrn.3567841.

[77]   Santarpia JL, Rivera DN, Herrera V, *et al.* Transmission potential of SARS-CoV-2 in viral shedding observed at the University of Nebraska Medical Center. MedRxIV 2020; 200: 39446.
[http://dx.doi.org/10.1101/ 2020.03.23.20039446]

[78]   Xu Y, Li X, Zhu B, *et al.* Characteristics of pediatric SARS-CoV-2 infection and potential evidence for persistent fecal viral shedding. Nat Med 2020; 26(4): 502-5.
[http://dx.doi.org/10.1038/s41591-020-0817-4] [PMID: 32284613]

[79]   Frontera A, Martin C, Vlachos K, Sgubin G. Regional air pollution persistence links to covid19

infection zoning. J Infect 2020; 81(2): 318-56.
[http://dx.doi.org/10.1016/j.jinf.2020.03.045] [PMID: 32283151]

[80]   Enyoh CE, Verla AW, Qingyue W, Yadav DK, Chowdhury AH, Isiuku BO, *et al.* Indirect exposure to novel coronavirus (SARS-CoV-2): An overview of current knowledge. Preprints 2020; 040460.
[http://dx.doi.org/10.20944/preprints202004.0460.v1]

CHAPTER 6

Risk Factors for Severe Covid-19 Disease

Mohammad Misbah Urrehmaan[1,2], Abu Hamza[2], Zoya Shafat[2], Saba Parveen[2], Saima Wajid[1,*] and Shama Parveen[2,*]

[1] *Department of Biotechnology, School of Chemical & Life Sciences, Jamia Hamdard, New Delhi, India*

[2] *Centre of Interdisciplinary Research in Basic Sciences, Jamia Millia Islamia, New Delhi, India*

Abstract: Coronavirus disease 2019 (COVID-19) has spread to almost every part of the globe. Numerous risk factors have been identified for predisposition to severe infection. Age is reportedly an incredibly significant risk factor due to high fatality in the elderly population. Further, the infection is more predominant in males as compared to females, probably due to the difference in immunity, hormones, and some specific habits (smoking, drinking) that may influence the viral infection. Correlation of blood group with SARS-CoV-2 infection is also reported as individuals with type A blood group are probably more susceptible to the infection since it is native form. Type O blood group is an evolved form, and thus individuals with this group may be less susceptible to the infection. In addition, existing comorbid conditions like hypertension, diabetes, cardiovascular, endocrine, and chronic respiratory diseases are also associated with an increased risk of severe COVID-19. Obesity has also been reported to have a huge impact on the infection rate and post-infection results. There is also an apprehension of vertical transmission from pregnant females to foetus, but this aspect needs to be analysed in detail in future studies. This review summarizes the effects of different risk factors like age, gender, comorbidities, blood group and prenatal transmission on SARS-CoV-2 infection. The correlation of viral infection with genetic predisposition is another factor that can be explored in future studies. Detailed clinical studies involving large patient groups are required across the globe and on different ethnic populations to clearly define the role of risk factors to COVID-19.

Keywords: Age, Blood group, COVID-19, Diabetes and obesity, Gender, Hypertension, Risk factors.

INTRODUCTION

Severe acute respiratory syndrome coronavirus 2 (SARS-CoV-2) has created a ravaging situation of Coronavirus disease 2019 (COVID-19) around the world in

---

* **Corresponding author Saima Wajid and Shama Parveen:** Department of Biotechnology, School of Chemical & Life Sciences, Jamia Hamdard, New Delhi, India and Centre for Interdisciplinary Research in Basic Sciences, Jamia Millia Islamia, New Delhi, India; E-mails: swajid@jamiahamdard.ac.in and sparveen2@jmi.ac.in, shamp25@yahoo.com

a matter of a few months. Transmission of the virus from an infected to a normal person occurs by means of respiratory droplets *via* the respiratory or gastrointestinal tract. Most of the cases initially are mild, but people with pre-existing diseases and the elderly are more susceptible to severe illness. World Health Organization (WHO) had declared the outbreak of the COVID-19 infection as a pandemic on 11th March 2020 since it had spread to a major part of the globe [1]. The outbreak started from Wuhan, China, which went on to spread in more than 200 countries. Until 31st of August 2020, the number of confirmed cases in the world has crossed 25.6 million [2]. By 31st August 2020, the worst affected country in the world was the USA, which reported more than 6.2 million cases and nearly 190,000 deaths. Brazil has second-most deaths with a tally of 3.9 million cases, and more than 121,000 deaths have occurred due to the novel coronavirus [2]. In the past three months, India has seen a logarithmic increase in COVID-19 cases and has reported more than 3.6 million cases, and more than 65000 people have died [2]. Most countries have undergone complete lockdown to contain the viral outbreak and have imposed various security measures such as restricted international travel *etc.* to make sure that the citizens are in the least possible contact with each other. It is to be noted that the pandemic took 3 months to reach 100,000 confirmed cases and just 12 days to reach the next 100,000 [3]. Within the next 26 days, the numbers increased to 1 million and further crossed the 10 million mark on 27th June 2020, just after 86 days of crossing 1 million [2].

The disease originated in China in late 2019. In mid-December 2019, many patients had reported to hospitals with pneumonia in the Wuhan region of China. Many of these patients had visited the seafood market at least once in the past one or two weeks. Etiological investigation was done on the patients showing similar symptoms in this unexplained viral pneumonia. After investigation of the lavage of the patients from the infected place, it was hypothesised that the novel CoV was transmitted from a zoonotic agent and had further spread to people due to human-to-human interaction [4]. On February 11th, 2020, the novel CoV was named SARS-CoV-2. The symptoms of COVID-19 infection can be seen after an average incubation period of 5-14 days. The time from the onset of the symptoms to fatality ranged from 6 to 41 days with a 14-day median period. This time depends on the patient's age and immune system status. This time was shorter for greater than 70-year-old patients relative to those under 70 years of age. Fever, cough, and fatigue are the most common symptoms at the onset of COVID-19. Other symptoms include sputum development, headaches, haemoptysis, diarrhoea, dyspnoea, and lymphopenia. Clinical characteristics were identified as pneumonia by a chest CT scan, however, there were irregular characteristics such as RNAaemia, acute spiral distress syndrome, acute cardiac injury, and the occurrence of opacity that led to death [5].

On January 20, 2020, it was acknowledged that the novel coronavirus should be classified under subgenus *Sarbecovirus* belonging to the *Betacoronavirus* genus; *Coronavirinae* subfamily, *Coronaviridae* family, and *Nidovirales* order. Thus, this virus was called SARS-CoV-2 since it is the sister of SARS [6]. Coronaviruses are pleomorphic RNA viruses with a diameter ranging from 150nm-160nm with a characteristic crown-shaped appearance. The main structural proteins are spike (S), membrane (M), envelope (E) and nucleocapsid (N). The nucleocapsid protein is bound to the RNA genome in a bead on a string fashion [5].

The genome of coronaviruses is the largest among the RNA viruses; its length is in the range of 27-32 kb. The genome of SARS-CoV-2 shows more similarity to the SARS-CoV (70%) than to the MERS-CoV. High homology was observed in the RNA binding domain of the SARS-CoV-2 and SARS-CoV. The occurrence of this contagious virus is like SARS-CoV in many ways. It was reported that both the viruses have the same mode of entry in the human cells, which is through the angiotensin-converting enzyme-2 (ACE2) receptor; thus it is expected that both the viruses have high clinical similarities [7]. It is also noted that the novel coronavirus Spike glycoprotein has modified itself through homologous recombination. The SARS-CoV-2 spike glycoprotein is a combination of the SARS-CoV bat and an unidentified Beta-CoV [8]. Another ground level similarity is that they both started at the spring festival in China. Billions of people travelled across the country, which also had a high number of tourist visitors from around the globe. This became favourable for the contagious disease to spread so rapidly throughout the world.

Reproduction number (R_0) is used to indicate the transmission capability of a virus. It indicates the number of new infections caused by an infected person in a non-experience population. Earlier WHO had given an estimated R_0 value of 1.4 – 2.5, but studies conducted in China using mathematical models indicated this value is an average of 3.28 [9]. This value is much higher than that of influenza, which has a value below 2 [10]. It is this high value of SARS-CoV-2, which makes it deadlier than many other viruses in terms of spreading. A research paper reported that the R^0 for India was lower, which was 1.82, than many highly infected countries. A few of the reasons could be the testing rate is lower than many countries and the high population of the country [11].

COVID-19 infection may lead to symptomatic and asymptomatic cases in infected individuals. The symptoms may be mild to life-threatening respiratory syndrome and multi-organ failure, some of which may lead to death. Certain predisposing factors are reported for the severe respiratory infection caused by SARS-CoV-2. The present chapter describes some of these risk factors encompassing age, gender, comorbid conditions, blood group and pre-natal transmission for severe COVID-19 disease. Assessment of these risk factors is essential for better patient management.

RISK FACTORS FOR SEVERE COVID-19 INFECTION

Numerous risk factors have been described for severe COVID-19 infection. These include age, gender, comorbid conditions (hypertension, diabetes, cardiovascular disease, and obesity), blood group and pre-natal transmission for severe COVID-19 disease (Fig. **1**).

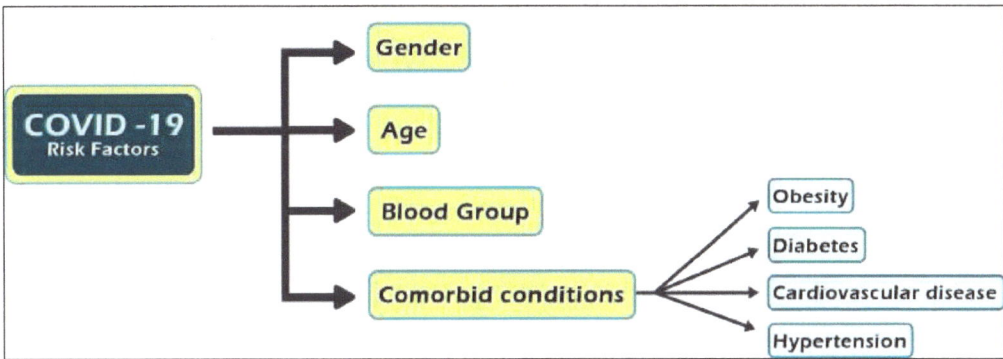

Fig. (1). Major risk factors influencing the severity of COVID-19 infection.

Age Distribution

There is a strong association between ageing and physiological changes. With these changes occurring in the body, there is a difference in tolerance level and response of the immune system. Thus, it can be expected that during an infection, the elderly population responds to it in a different manner as compared to the younger generation. A misconception had spread across countries in the initial stages that the infection of SARS-CoV-2 is confined to the elder age group and that too among those with comorbidities. The mortality due to the infection is there in all the age groups but is higher in the elder age groups [12].

In general, mortality increases exponentially with increasing age. Many diseases are age-related, such as hypertension, ischemic heart diseases, diabetes, chronic obstructive pulmonary diseases, *etc*. [13]. To be more precise with age, we would say that a biologically old person is more likely to have a higher chance of infection with SARS-CoV-2. A biologically old person may not necessarily be above 60 or 70 years old; 60 years old person may not have any of the above-stated diseases, but a 50 years old person may have. Therefore, this indicates that the 50 years old person is chronologically younger but biologically older as his body has one of the age-related diseases. The age-dependent risk of death is doubled with COVID-19 infection. This risk remains extremely low for children and young adults since there is a lower risk of age-related diseases. The vulnerability to COVID-19 and age-related diseases results from the same underlying cause, "ageing". Thus the correlation between the two is high; however, they are not directly related. Although all age-related diseases are not deadly such as osteoporosis, *etc.*, but they can create a complication in the body when COVID-19 infection is encountered [13].

In a study conducted on 2,449 patients, the maximum number of positive cases for COVID-19 was in the age group of 20-44 years with the positive percentage of 29% whereas, the minimum infections were observed in less than 20 years of age with 5% cases [14]. The second most positive cases were among 65-84 years of age (25%), followed by 18% in two age groups, including 45-54 and 55-64 years. On the contrary, the trend of hospitalization, ICU admission and deaths turned out to be different in the investigated age groups. Most cases for hospitalization were among the age group of 65-74 years old, followed by 20-44 years old, then 45-54 years, followed by 55-64 years in the same study. Further, a few people were hospitalized in other age groups, also including 75-84 years old, ≥85 years, and the least hospitalized age group was ≥19 years old. The ICU admissions trend was a little different; highest numbers were found in the age group of 65-84 years old, followed by 45-64 years old, then 20-44 years, then patients above or equal to 85 years. No ICU admissions were reported in the age group below or equal to 19 years. Among the known death cases in that study, the maximum deaths occurred in the age group of 65-84 years old; followed by the 85 and above age group, and to a lesser extent between the ages of 20-64 years [14]. In the earlier studies of this outbreak, it was reported that the elderly people had a severe infection as compared to the younger population. However, the same study depicted that the cases of infection among younger age groups were not negligible [15]. In a study conducted by CDC China, clinical data of around 72,000 COVID-19 patients from this region were collected [15]. Reports suggested that 86.6% of the infected population ranges from 30-79 years old. In this study, the highest cases were from the age group of 50-59 years old and the lowest number of patients was reported from the age group 90-99 years old individuals. Second highest among them were of ages groups 40-49 years old and 60-69 years old, both had 19.2% share of patients. Followed by these, the 30-39 years old age group had 17% patients, further 7.7% of patients were from 70-79 years age group, then 8.1% from 20-29 years old age group. The age group 80-89 years saw even lesser 2.9% of patients and 10-19 years old and 1-9 years old age group had 1.2% and 0.9% patients, respectively [15]. Italy has reported a high number of deaths during the pandemic since it has the second-highest elderly population in the world [16].

Surprisingly the statistics reported from India suggested that the maximum infections were in the age group of 30-39 years (21.7%) followed by 20-29 years (20.8%), then 40-49 years (17.4%), next 50-59 years (13.3%) and subsequently 60-69 years. Further, it may be noted that infections in the elderly age group (*i.e.*, >70 years) were below 5% and in the age group of 0-9 years and 10-19 years had 2.5% and 5% infections respectively [17]. The reason behind this could be that the people between the age group 20-50 years old have probably higher exposure to the virus since they are frequently coming out of their homes for work, to buy groceries or for any other reason. Another reason could be that the population being naïve and less literate, they do not take effective preventive measures, including social distancing and covering their faces with masks, consequently tend to get infected.

Gender

Previous investigations have suggested that the immune system is affected by the sex of an individual, which is a biological variable. Both innate and adaptive immune responses are dependent on gender variation and are maintained evolutionarily through different organisms [18]. Immune responses tend to change throughout life, depending on age and reproductive status. The sex chromosomes and hormonal regulation, including androgens, oestrogen and progesterone, play an important role in the differential regulation of immune responses among the sexes. The functionality of the immune system is also dependent on environmental factors such as nutritional level and microbiome in the body. Differential vulnerability and immune response of males and females to infectious diseases, autoimmune diseases and malignancies are also sex-dependent, and thus, the response to vaccinations is also affected accordingly [18]. The rate of mortality of males is higher than that of females at the same age. It is reported that at any given chronological age, males are biologically older than females. Hence, males are probably more vulnerable towards diseases than females. These diseases can either be age-related or infectious [13].

An important trend was observed when the contagious disease COVID-19 spread all over the world; it is that the infection was more prevalent in men than women. Before the outbreak reached American and European countries, China had already reported that men were more vulnerable to this virus than women [19]. But since the study was limited to China, it was not a very well accepted trend. However, when the outbreak was reported in other countries, trends were seen to be similar. Data analysis from Italy stated that the infected patients were around 65% males and 35% were females [20]. In addition, the early death ratio was 80:20 male to female. Even though these numbers are changing, the ratio of male to female infection rate and ratio of male to female deaths is still higher. Data from China also suggested a similar trend in which male to female infection ratio was about 60:40 and male to female death ratio was 70:30. Various theories have been given to justify these trends by scientists, but a firm conclusion is yet to be drawn [19, 20].

Another source revealed a similar trend that males have a higher percentage of infection in most geographical regions except in some European countries where the infections reported are higher among females than males [21]. It also articulates that in most countries, the proportion of COVID-19 related deaths is higher among males, with the ratio of deaths in males *versus* females is higher than 1. Some countries have reported a very high percentage of deaths in males, such as Thailand, which despite having 55.6% of the male infected population, the reported COVID-19 related deaths of males in the country are nearly 76% [21]. In some of the European countries, including Wales, Belgium, Netherlands, Sweden and Ukraine, the percentage of male infections is below 50%; nonetheless, the percentage of death of males is greater than 50% [21]. Scientists suggested that this could be due to various reasons such as smoking and drinking alcohol is more common among men than women in these regions. Another study reported on genetic predisposition suggested that ACE2 receptor works in an X-linked dominant pattern in severely affected patients. This might be one indication of why males have a high prevalence of the disease [22]. Previous demographic studies have suggested that males have higher health risks, including heart-related diseases [23]. WHO has done an analysis on the life expectancy of males and females based on various factors. It states that females tend to have higher life expectancy than males. Out of the top 40 causes of deaths, 33 are responsible for male deaths. In countries like China, Italy, South Korea, USA, *etc.* the maternal mortality rate is low as compared to South East Asian and central & West African countries [24]. Different factors have been reported to play a role in this; such as income level of a family, wealth of a country, diseases (hereditary and non-hereditary as well as communicable and non-communicable), reproductive and maternal health, and environmental factors [24]. Another report hypothesises that COVID-19 disease could have an immense effect on the male reproductive organs, specifically on testicles. It highlights that since ACE2 receptors are present in testicles, the virus could enter Sertoli cells and Leydig cell leading to inflammation. This could lead to fertility problems and could affect the production of sexual hormones. Similar problems in males were also reported during the SARS-CoV pandemic [25].

Blood Groups

Although blood type selection is genetically inherited, environmental factors also play an important role in which blood type will be passed on more frequently in a population. As seen in the geographical distribution of blood groups, most countries in the South American continent seem to have the highest population percentage of blood type O while most of the Asian countries have a majority population of blood type B [26]. Further, it has already been reported that some viruses have a preference for blood group type for susceptibility, such as the hepatitis B and Norwalk virus [27, 28]. While the blood group antigen A is called the primordial ancestral form, the blood group O (H) dominated as the most commonly occurring blood group worldwide under the selective pressure of life-threatening diseases [29]. Non-O(H) phenotypes display impaired development of adaptive and innate specificities of the immunoglobulin due to clonal selection and development of phenotypes in plasma proteins. People with blood group A have a substantially higher chance of developing certain forms of cancer and are also particularly prone to *Plasmodium falciparum* infection as compared to people with blood group O (H) [29]. The phenotype-determining blood group A glycotransferase(s), which affects the rates of anti-A/Tn cross-reactive immunoglobulins in phenotypic glycosidic accommodation, may also associate with the adhesion and entry of the parasite into host cells through the trans-species O-GalNAc glycosylation of abundant serine residues that occur during the life cycle of the parasite; except the likelihood of formation of antibody against the Tn antigen hybrid [29]. In comparison, the human blood group O (H), which lacks this enzyme, is considered to confer a survival advantage over the overall risk of developing cancer and people with this blood group seldom acquire life-threatening infections involving evolutionarily selective malaria strains [29].

It has been described that people with O blood group were probably less susceptible to SARS-CoV infection [30]. Further, lower blood group O susceptibility and higher blood group A susceptibility for SARS-CoV-2 may be correlated with the existence of natural anti-blood group antibodies, especially anti-A antibodies, in the blood [31]. This hypothesis still needs to be verified experimentally in large patient groups in future studies. Besides this, there might be some other ABO group based mechanism of susceptibility to COVID-19 infection.

Blood group distribution within countries could also be a reason why some countries are facing a smaller number of infections and deaths by the COVID-19. A major percentage of the world population has blood group O+, then A+ and then B+ type. USA currently being the most infected country in the world, has a population percentage of around 36% with blood group A+; this is second highest percent blood group type in the country [26]. Brazil currently having second-highest number of infected patients also has around 34% of the population with blood group A+. This high percentage of blood group type A could be one of the reasons why these countries have such high numbers of infected patients as well as high death rates. India, on the other hand, has the highest number of individuals with blood group B+ and second-highest numbers with O+ blood group, and China has about half of the population with O+ group type. It has also been postulated the selective blood group may also be related to good recovery rates in many countries [26]. We analysed the percent population of highly infected countries and the percentage of the population of blood group type A as indicated in Table **1**. We calculated the percent infection by the following formula and constructed a bar graph (Fig. **2**).

$$\text{Percent infection} = \frac{\text{number of infected patients in the stated country}}{\text{total number of infected patients in the world}} \times 100$$

The total number of infected people around the world as of 31st August 2020 were: 25,632,087.

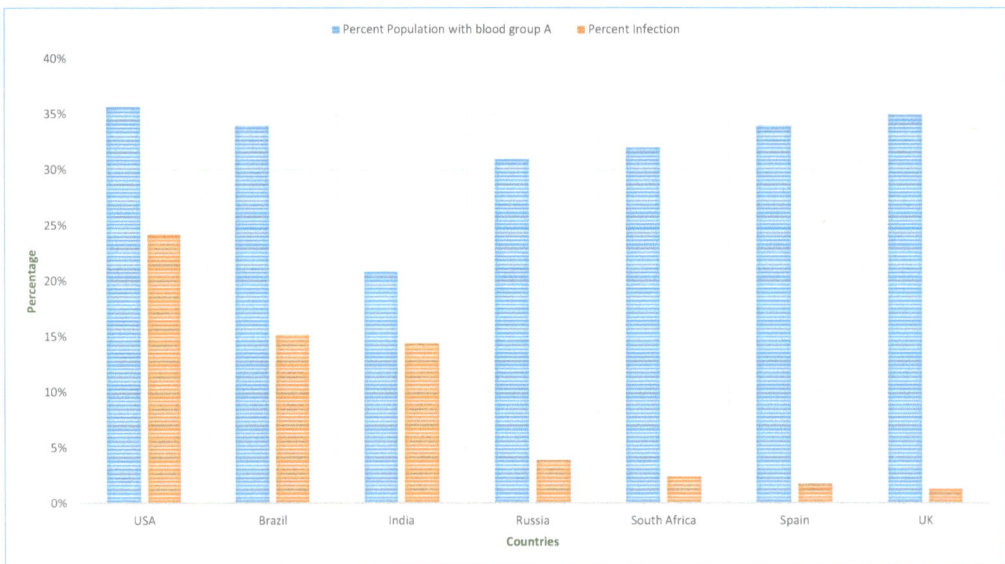

Fig. (2). Correlation of population infected with COVID-19 with the type A blood group. The data is updated until 31st of August 2020.

Table 1. Comparison of population infected with COVID-19 with the type A blood group.

Countries	Percent Population with Blood Group A	Infected Patients	Infection (%)
USA	35.7%	6207546	24.2%
Brazil	34%	3910901	15.2%
India	20.8%	3687939	14.4%
Russia	31%	995319	3.9%

(Table 1) cont.....

Countries	Percent Population with Blood Group A	Infected Patients	Infection (%)
South Africa	32%	627041	2.4%
Spain	34%	462858	1.8%
UK	35%	335813	1.3%

Note: The data for the table was taken from these references [2, 25, 32, 33, 34, 35]. The data is updated until 31st of August 2020.

We also analysed the percent population of those countries that have a good recovery rate, and we have tried to correlate it with the percentage of type O blood group population of that country as presented in Table **2**. Calculation of the recovered patients was done by the following formula and followed by the construction of a bar graph (Fig. **3**).

$$\text{Percent recovered} = \frac{\text{number of recovered patients in the stated country}}{\text{total number of infected people in the stated country}} \times 100$$

Total number of infected people around the world as on 31st August 2020 were: 25,632,087.

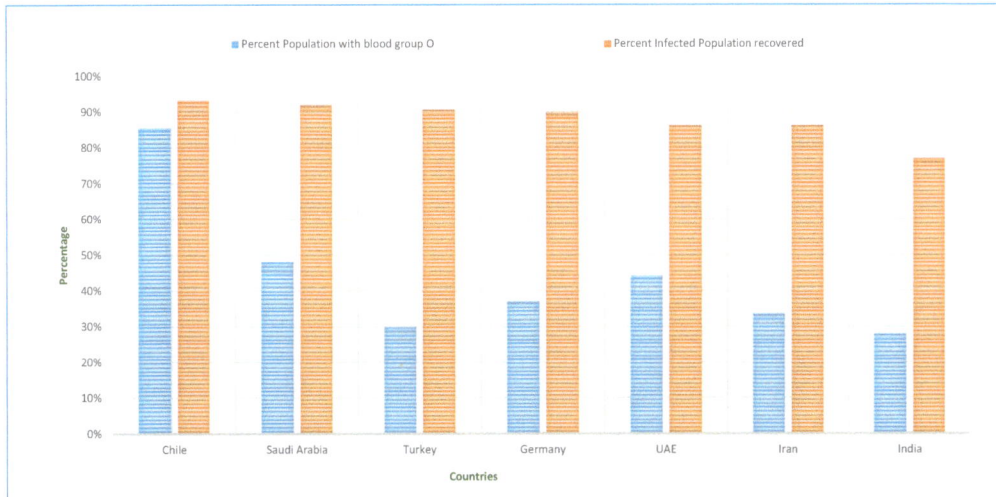

Fig. (3). Correlation of population recovered from COVID-19 with the type O blood group. The data is updated until 31st of August 2020.

Table 2. Comparison of population recovered from COVID-19 with the type O blood group.

Countries	Percent Population with Blood Group O	Infected Patients	Recovered Patients	Recovered Population (%)
Chile	85.5%	411726	383879	93.2%
Saudi Arabia	48.0%	315772	290796	92.0%

(Table 2) cont.....

Countries	Percent Population with Blood Group O	Infected Patients	Recovered Patients	Recovered Population (%)
Turkey	29.8%	270133	244926	90.6%
Germany	37.0%	244792	219900	89.8%
UAE	44.1%	70231	60931	86.1%
Iran	33.5%	375212	323233	86.1%
India	27.8%	3687939	287377	76.9%

Note: The data for the table was taken from these reference [2, 25, 32, 33, 34, 35]. The data is updated until 31st of August 2020.

The analysis revealed that the countries that had a good percentage of recovery from the disease were associated with the presence of a high percentage of blood group type O. The above graphs indicated that the countries with a high percentage population of blood group type A might be more susceptible to the infection of SARS-CoV-2. The most affected countries have nearly 30% or more of the blood group type A. This could be one of the reasons for the high percentage of COVID-19 cases in these countries. High recovery percentage was observed in the countries where people with blood type O are prevalent such as Chile, China, and Singapore, India having roughly 28% of the population with blood type O. Thus, people with group A are probably more susceptible to SARS-CoV-2 infection as compared to individuals with O group.

Comorbid Conditions

Earlier studies have reported that the existence of any comorbidity has about 3-4 times higher risk of developing respiratory diseases such as influenza, SARS and MERS [36 - 38]. Further, the studies have revealed that SARS-CoV-2 can be dangerous for people having comorbid conditions related to heart or lung disease, weak immunity, *etc*. A recent study has reported the effects of comorbid conditions in 1,590 infected patients from 575 different hospitals in China [39]. The authors examined the composite endpoints that consisted of admission to the intensive care unit or invasive ventilation or death. Out of the 1,590 cases studied, 25% had at least one co-morbidity, and among them, the highest number of patients had cardiovascular disease (53.7%), followed by hypertension (16.9%), diarrhoea (8.2%), cerebro-vascular disease (1.9%), chronic obstructive pulmonary disease (1.5%), chronic kidney disease (1.3%), malignancy (1.1%) and immunodeficiency (0.2%). Out of all the severe cases, 32.8% patients had at least one comorbidity and among non-severe cases, the percentage was 10.3%. The authors also reported that patients who had at least one comorbidity were older (mean age: 60.8) than those who did not have any comorbidity (mean age: 44.8). It was also concluded that more number of patients with comorbidity were more likely to have shortness of breath (41.4%) as compared to those without it (17.8%). A higher number of patients were reported for nausea (10.4% *vs.* 4.3%) and abnormal chest x-ray manifestation (29.2% *vs.* 15.1%) that had at least one comorbidity than those with none. Thus, it was concluded that circulatory and endocrine co-morbidities were prevalent among SARS-CoV-2 patients. Patients with at least one co-morbidity had poor clinical results and those with two or more comorbidities had worse results as compared to those who had none [39].

Hypertension is a condition that often develops with ageing and is not very common among the young population. An article published in "Hypertension Research" conducted a study on patients with COVID-19 [40]. In this study, the patients with hypertension were older and had a higher number of patients with diabetes as compared to non-hypertensive patients with COVID-19 infection. The requirement of the hypertensive patients for ICU and non-invasive mechanical ventilators was higher. Greater number of hypertensive patients reached case severity and the mortality ratio was also high as compared to non-hypertensive patients [40].

It has been reported that the SARS-CoV-2 binds to the angiotensin-converting enzymes 2 (ACE2) receptor to enter the target cell. Diabetes patients treated with ACE inhibitor and angiotensin II type-I receptor blocker leads to the up-regulation of ACE2 and will have markedly high expression of ACE2. Other than ARBs, angiotensin-converting enzyme inhibitors (ACEIs), which are antagonists of renin-angiotensin system, are used for the up-regulation of ACE2 as a treatment of hypertension, leading to higher chances of infection with SARS-CoV-2 [41, 42].

It has also been reported that diabetic patients have been linked to a longer stay in hospitals for treatment of COVID-19 [43]. Patients with diabetes were reportedly older than those without diabetes. Further, a higher number of diabetic and/or hyperglycaemic patients were hospitalized as compared to non-diabetic patients. The survival rate of the hospitalized patients with diabetes and/or uncontrolled hyperglycaemia were fourfold lower than those patients without diabetes and hyperglycaemia [43]. In another retrospective study, type 2 diabetes was reported to be more frequent among patients of COVID-19 infection as compared to type 1 diabetes [44].

Another study described that the case fatality rate of those COVID-19 patients who had cardiovascular disease was higher than other comorbid conditions, followed by chronic respiratory diseases, diabetes and hypertension, and fatality among patients with cancer were also notably high in critical cases [45].

The reports of a logarithmic increase in SARS-CoV-2 infections in the USA have become a worry for the country. Early reports from China, Italy and other European countries showed that body mass index (BMI) was rarely mentioned as a noteworthy clinical risk factor. Obesity is reported to be a common problem in the USA where about 36% of the total population is obese. The CDC has reported that individuals who are obese are highly susceptible to the SARS-CoV-2 infection [46]. Individuals with a BMI above 40 are required to be aware of this factor. For severe H1N1 pulmonary infections, obesity was also reported as an independent predisposition factor [47]. Additionally, impaired ventilation of the base of the lungs is associated with abdominal obesity, which results in lower oxygen saturation of blood. An immune response is impaired when there is an abnormal secretion of TNF-alpha and interferons that is characterised by chronic low-grade inflammation, a characteristic of abdominal obesity. A study reported that a higher number of obese patients with COVID-19 was admitted to intensive care units. Moderately obese and highly obese patients frequently required Intermittent Mandatory Ventilation (IMV) [48]. Multiple factors such as difference in immune response, chronic inflammatory status could be responsible for obese people to develop serious complications when a virus attacks their body. As stated above, ACE2 receptor is responsible for the entry of the virus. A recent study concluded that the expression of this receptor in the adipose tissue is more pronounced as compared to lung tissues. Thus, adipose tissue is more susceptible to viral infection. It is noteworthy that the expression level of the ACE2 protein was found to be same in both lungs and adipose tissues, but an obese person has a higher amount of adipose tissues, which makes them more vulnerable to COVID-19 [49]. Obesity has also been reported to be one of the subsequent consequences of having type 2 diabetes. Elevation in insulin levels during fasting as well as in postprandial state is one of the early signs related to obesity. After the failure of beta-cell compensation, type 2 diabetes is inclined due to insulin resistance [50].

We analysed the obesity conditions of the top-most infected countries of the world and tried to correlate this with the percentage of the COVID-19 infections (Table **3**). It was observed from the graph (Fig. **4**) that the countries with a high percentage of infection of the SARS-CoV-2 also have a high percentage of the obese population. A calculation of the percent infection was done using the following equation.

$$\text{Percent infection} = \frac{\text{number of infected in the stated country}}{\text{total number of infected people in the world}} \times 100$$

Table 3. Comparison of obesity and infection percentage of COVID-19.

Countries	Obesity (%)	Infected Patient	Infection (%)
USA	36.2%	3616827	24.2%
Brazil	22.1%	304574	14.4%
Russia	23.1%	173304	5.4%
Peru	19.7%	291911	2.5%
Columbia	22.3%	201252	2.4%
South Africa	28.3%	243506	2.4%
Mexico	28.9%	215940	2.3%

Note: The data for the table was taken from these reference [2, 51]. The data is updated until 31st of August 2020.

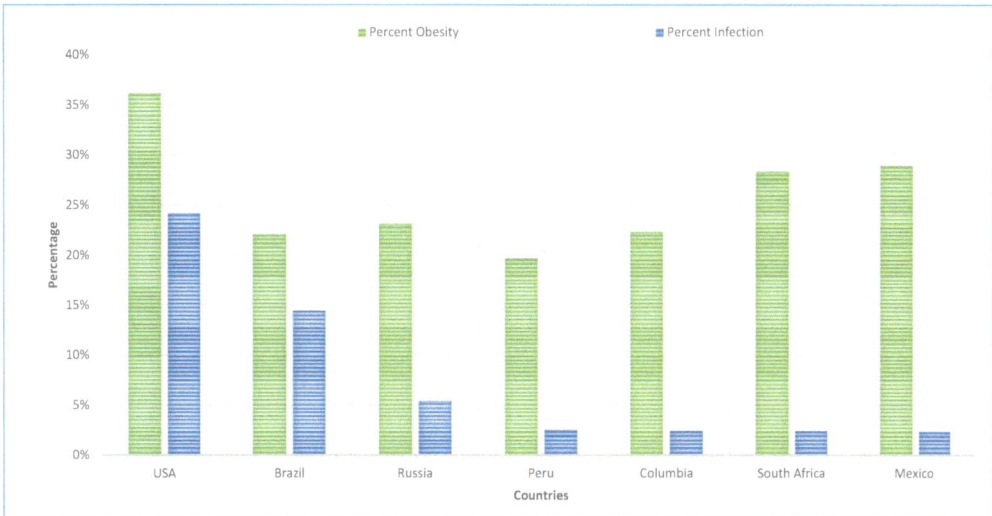

Fig. (4). Correlation of COVID-19 infection with obesity. The data is updated until 31st of August 2020.

Along with obesity, other cardiovascular conditions such as hypertension would drastically increase the chances of getting SARS-CoV-2. This condition commonly leads to breathing problems and has other pulmonary risks, which are very common symptoms of SARS-CoV-2. Thus, obesity can lead to unprecedented complications and lead to severe complications, sometimes even death.

Smoking has been associated with various diseases especially related to lungs, and it is one of the leading causes of deaths across the globe. According to WHO tobacco consumption claims around 8 million lives every year [52]. Contrasting results have been reported when tobacco consumption and COVID-19 are correlated. Studies conducted in France, USA and China suggested that the susceptibility of current smokers to COVID-19 infection might be less as compared to ex-smokers and non-smokers [53]. The interaction of ACE receptor and nicotine have been previously reported and it is indicated that nicotine has a role to play in the upregulation and downregulation of the ACE2 [54]. Thus, it is hypothesised that nicotine does have an influence on the interaction of the SARS-CoV-2 virus with the ACE2 receptor.

In an article reported in Nature, it was suggested that reduced kidney function had a direct impact on the case severity of the COVID-19 infection. Patients with lower glomerular filtration rates had a higher percentage of deaths with COVID-19 than those with normal or slightly low GFR [53].

Pre-natal Transmission

In many viral diseases, the pathogen present in the mother is passed on to the foetus *via* the placenta and causes the infection in the baby. The problem is particularly important in the context of the recent evidence of vertical maternal-foetal transmission of viral infections such as Zika, Ebola and Marburg that endanger the health and wellbeing of a diseased mother as well as the developing foetus. Trans-placental transmission of Zika virus leads to multiplication of the virus in human neural progenitor cells of the foetus that leads to modifications of the signaling pathways in host cells. This causes the death of developing neurons leading to microcephaly [55]. In this context, it may be noted that there might be a possibility that a SARS-CoV-2 infected pregnant female could pass it on to the foetus. From retrospective studies, it was reported that during the outbreak of SARS-CoV in 2002-03, there was no vertical transmission of the virus to infants. However, the same studies suggested that pregnant women with SARS infection had unfortunate clinical results as compared to non-pregnant women with infection [56]. During the MERS outbreak, the pregnant patients showed prenatal death, premature delivery, and maternal deaths but confirmed cases of vertical transfer of the virus were not reported [56].

It is still not clear if this viral infection can lead to higher risks of miscarriage, death, premature delivery, foetal tachycardia and foetal distress in pregnant females. But an important underlying question is whether the virus can be passed from a pregnant woman to her foetus. However, if it does get passed on, what would be the possible mechanism of its occurrence? This is not only a critical public health concern but also a topic of obstetric management in deciding the treatment provided to pregnant women. SARS-CoV-2 infection in pregnant females has been reported with maternal death, pneumonia, early pregnancy loss and several other problems [57]. Nevertheless, with almost all such cases, SARS-

CoV-2 has not been associated with vertical transmission. But with the cases where the babies were found to be positive, no evidence could be gathered to prove that the transmission was due to intrauterine vertical transmission rather, it was probably through droplet transmission by breastfeeding or while handling the baby [57].

CONCLUDING REMARKS

COVID-19 has spread across different parts of the globe in just a few months. Certain individuals are more susceptible to severe disease as compared to the rest of the population. These risk factors include age, gender, comorbidities, blood group and pre-natal transmission. A single factor cannot be the driving force for individuals' infection susceptibility; different permutation and combination of various factors might contribute towards the development of severity of COVID-19 infection. Future comprehensive investigations on different population groups should be designed to delineate the role of risk factors on severity of the viral infection. Assessment of these risk factors is essential for better management of COVID-19 patients.

CONSENT FOR PUBLICATION

Not Applicable.

CONFLICT OF INTEREST

The author declares no conflict of interest, financial or otherwise.

ACKNOWLEDGEMENTS

Zoya Shafat is supported by Research Fellowship by University Grant Commission (UGC), and Abu Hamza by Research Fellowship by Indian Council of Medical Research (ICMR), Government of India. The research in our laboratory is funded by Council of Scientific and Industrial Research (CSIR), India (37(1697)17/EMR-II) and Central Council for Research in Unani Medicine (CCRUM), Ministry of Ayurveda, Yoga and Naturopathy, Unani, Siddha and Homeopathy (AYUSH), India (F.No.3-63/2019-CCRUM/Tech).

REFERENCES

[1]   Jiang S, Shi Z, Shu Y, *et al.* A distinct name is needed for the new coronavirus. Lancet 2020; 395(10228): 949.
        [http://dx.doi.org/10.1016/S0140-6736(20)30419-0] [PMID: 32087125]

[2]   Coronavirus Update (Live): Cases and Deaths from COVID-19 Virus Pandemic - Worldometer [Internet]. Worldometers.info. 2020. Available from: https://www.worldometers.info/coronavirus/

[3]   Coronavirus disease 2019 (COVID-19) Situation Report – 59. Who.int. 2020. Available from:

https://www.who.int/docs/default-source/coronaviruse/situation-reports/20200319-sitrep-59--
ovid-19.pdf?sfvrsn=c3dcdef9_2

[4]   Ahmad T, Khan M, Haroon TH, *et al.* COVID-19: Zoonotic aspects. Travel Med Infect Di 2020; 36:
        p. 101607.
        [http://dx.doi.org/10.1016/j.tmaid.2020.101607] [PMID: 32112857]

[5]   Rothan HA, Byrareddy SN. The epidemiology and pathogenesis of coronavirus disease (COVID-19)
        outbreak. J Autoimmune 2020; p. 102433.
        [http://dx.doi.org/10.1016/j.jaut.2020.102433] [PMID: 32113704]

[6]   Islam A, Ahmed A, Naqvi IH, Parveen S. Emergence of deadly severe acute respiratory syndrome
        coronavirus-2 during 2019-2020. Virusdisease 2020; 1-9.
        [http://dx.doi.org/10.1007/s13337-020-00575-1] [PMID: 32292802]

[7]   Kannan S, Shaik Syed Ali P, Sheeza A, Hemalatha K. COVID-19 (Novel Coronavirus 2019) - recent
        trends. Eur Rev Med Pharmacol Sci 2020; 24(4): 2006-11.
        [http://dx.doi.org/10.26355/eurrev_202002_20378] [PMID: 32141569]

[8]   Shereen MA, Khan S, Kazmi A, Bashir N, Siddique R. COVID-19 infection: Origin, transmission, and
        characteristics of human coronaviruses. J Adv Res 2020; 24: 91-8.
        [http://dx.doi.org/10.1016/j.jare.2020.03.005] [PMID: 32257431]

[9]   Liu Y, Gayle AA, Wilder-Smith A, Rocklöv J. The reproductive number of COVID-19 is higher
        compared to SARS coronavirus. J Travel Med 2020; 27(2): taaa021.
        [http://dx.doi.org/10.1093/jtm/taaa021] [PMID: 32052846]

[10]   Inglesby TV. Public health measures and the reproduction number of SARS-CoV-2. JAMA 2020;
        323(21): 2186-7.
        [http://dx.doi.org/10.1001/jama.2020.7878] [PMID: 32356869]

[11]   Sinha S. Epidemiological dynamics of the COVID-19 pandemic in India: an interim assessment. Stat
        Appl 2020; 18: 333-50.

[12]   Le Couteur DG, Anderson RM, Newman AB. COVID-19 is a disease of older people. J Gerontol A
        Biol Sci Med Sci 2020; 10.

[13]   Blagosklonny MV. From causes of aging to death from COVID-19. Aging (Albany NY) 2020; 12(11):
        10004-21.
        [http://dx.doi.org/10.18632/aging.103493] [PMID: 32534452]

[14]   Covid CD, Team R. Severe outcomes among patients with coronavirus disease 2019 (COVID-
        19)—United States, February 12–March 16, 2020. MMWR Morb Mortal Wkly Rep 2020; 69(12):
        343-6.
        [http://dx.doi.org/10.15585/mmwr.mm6912e2] [PMID: 32214079]

[15]   Surveillances V. The epidemiological characteristics of an outbreak of 2019 novel coronavirus
        diseases (COVID-19)—China, 2020. China CDC Weekly 2020; 2(8): 113-22.
        [http://dx.doi.org/10.46234/ccdcw2020.032]

[16]   Which Country Has the Oldest Population? It Depends on How You Define 'Old.' – Population
        Reference Bureau. Prb.org. 2020. Available from: https://www.prb.org/which-country-has-the-ol-
        est-population/

[17]   Gupta N. Gupta N. 83% of India's coronavirus patients are below the age of 50: Health ministry data.
        India Today. 2020. Available from: https://www.indiatoday.in/india/story/83-of-india-s-coronav-
        rus-patients-are-below-the-age-of-50-health-ministry-data-1663314-2020-04-04

[18]   Klein SL, Flanagan KL. Sex differences in immune responses. Nat Rev Immunol 2016; 16(10): 626-
        38.
        [http://dx.doi.org/10.1038/nri.2016.90] [PMID: 27546235]

[19]   Jin JM, Bai P, He W, *et al.* Gender differences in patients with COVID-19: focus on severity and

mortality. Front Public Health 2020; 8: 152.
[http://dx.doi.org/10.3389/fpubh.2020.00152] [PMID: 32411652]

[20]   [Istituto superiore di Sanità] Coronavirus: in media 8 giorni tra ricovero e decesso, terapia antibiotica la più utilizzata. Regioni.it.. 2020. Available from: http://www.regioni.it/ sanita/2020/03/18/istituto-superiore-di-sanita-coronavirus-in-media-8-giorni-tra-ricovero-e-decesso-terapia-ant-biotica-la-piu-utilizzata-18-03-2020-607462/

[21]   COVID-19 sex-disaggregated data tracker – Global Health 50/50. Globalhealth5050.org. 2020. Available from: https://globalhealth5050.org/covid19/sex-disaggregated-data-tracker/

[22]   Darbeheshti F, Rezaei N. Genetic predisposition models to COVID-19 infection. Med Hypotheses 2020; 142: 109818.
[http://dx.doi.org/10.1016/j.mehy.2020.109818] [PMID: 32416414]

[23]   Albrektsen G, Heuch I, Løchen ML, *et al.* Lifelong gender gap in risk of incident myocardial infarction: the Tromsø Study. JAMA Intern Med 2016; 176(11): 1673-9.
[http://dx.doi.org/10.1001/jamainternmed.2016.5451] [PMID: 27617629]

[24]   World Health Organization. World health statistics overview 2019: monitoring health for the SDGs, sustainable development goals. World Health Organization 2019.

[25]   Illiano E, Trama F, Costantini E. Could COVID-19 have an impact on male fertility? Andrologia 2020; 52(6): e13654.
[http://dx.doi.org/10.1111/and.13654] [PMID: 32436229]

[26]   Blood Type Frequencies by Country including the Rh Factor - Rhesus Negative. Rhesusnegative.net. 2020. Available from: http://www.rhesusnegative.net/themission/bloodtypefrequencies/

[27]   Lindesmith L, Moe C, Marionneau S, *et al.* Human susceptibility and resistance to Norwalk virus infection. Nat Med 2003; 9(5): 548-53.
[http://dx.doi.org/10.1038/nm860] [PMID: 12692541]

[28]   Batool Z, Durrani SH, Tariq S. Association of ABO and Rh blood group types to hepatitis B, hepatitis C, HIV and Syphillis infection, a five year'experience in healthy blood donors in a tertiary care hospital. J Ayub Med Coll Abbottabad 2017; 29(1): 90-2.
[PMID: 28712183]

[29]   Arend P. Position of human blood group O(H) and phenotype-determining enzymes in growth and infectious disease. Ann N Y Acad Sci 2018; 1425(1): 5-18.
[http://dx.doi.org/10.1111/nyas.13694] [PMID: 29754430]

[30]   Cheng Y, Cheng G, Chui CH, *et al.* ABO blood group and susceptibility to severe acute respiratory syndrome. JAMA 2005; 293(12): 1450-1.
[http://dx.doi.org/10.1001/jama.293.12.1450-c] [PMID: 15784866]

[31]   Zhao J, Yang Y, Huang HP, *et al.* Relationship between the abo blood group and the COVID-19 susceptibility. medRxiv 2020.
[http://dx.doi.org/10.1101/2020.03.11.20031096]

[32]   Grünebaum A. Blood type and rh rhesus status by countries. 2020. Available from: https://www.babymed.com/pregnancy/blood-type-and-rh-rhesus-status-countries

[33]   What is the most common blood type? san diego blood bank. 2020. Available from: https://www.sandiegobloodbank.org/what-most-common-blood-type

[34]   Marian J. Blood type distribution by country in Europe 2020. https://jakubmarian.com/blood-typ--distribution-by-country-in-europe/

[35]   Dean L. Blood group antigens are surface markers on the red blood cell membrane. US: NCBI 2005.

[36]   Alqahtani FY, Aleanizy FS, Ali El Hadi Mohamed R, *et al.* Prevalence of comorbidities in cases of Middle East respiratory syndrome coronavirus: a retrospective study. Epidemiol Infect 2018; 1-5.
[http://dx.doi.org/10.1017/s0950268818002923] [PMID: 30394248]

[37]   Martínez A, Soldevila N, Romero-Tamarit A, *et al.* Risk factors associated with severe outcomes in adult hospitalized patients according to influenza type and subtype. PLoS One 2019; 14(1): e0210353. [http://dx.doi.org/10.1371/journal.pone.0210353] [PMID: 30633778]

[38]   Booth CM, Matukas LM, Tomlinson GA, *et al.* Clinical features and short-term outcomes of 144 patients with SARS in the greater Toronto area. JAMA 2003; 289(21): 2801-9. [http://dx.doi.org/10.1001/jama.289.21.JOC30885] [PMID: 12734147]

[39]   Guan WJ, Liang WH, Zhao Y, *et al.* Comorbidity and its impact on 1590 patients with covid-19 in china: a nationwide analysis. Eur Resp J 2020; 55(5): 2000547. [http://dx.doi.org/10.1183/13993003.00547-2020]

[40]   Huang S, Wang J, Liu F, *et al.* COVID-19 patients with hypertension have more severe disease: a multicenter retrospective observational study. Hypertens Res 2020; 43(8): 824-31. [http://dx.doi.org/10.1038/s41440-020-0485-2] [PMID: 32483311]

[41]   Fang L, Karakiulakis G, Roth M. Are patients with hypertension and diabetes mellitus at increased risk for COVID-19 infection? Lancet Respir Med 2020; 8(4): e21. [http://dx.doi.org/10.1016/S2213-2600(20)30116-8] [PMID: 32171062]

[42]   Brown JD. Antihypertensive drugs and risk of COVID-19? Lancet Respir Med 2020; 8(5): e28. [http://dx.doi.org/10.1016/S2213-2600(20)30158-2] [PMID: 32222168]

[43]   Bode B, Garrett V, Messler J, *et al.* Glycemic characteristics and clinical outcomes of COVID-19 patients hospitalized in the United States. J Diabetes Sci Technol 2020; 14(4): 813-21. [http://dx.doi.org/10.1177/1932296820924469] [PMID: 32389027]

[44]   Alkundi A, Mahmoud I, Musa A, Naveed S, Alshawaf M. Clinical characteristics and outcomes of COVID-19 hospitalized patients with diabetes in UK: A retrospective single centre study. Diabetes Res Clin 2020; Jul;165: p. 108263. [http://dx.doi.org/10.1016/j.diabres.2020.108263] [PMID: 32531325]

[45]   Wu Z, McGoogan JM. Characteristics of and important lessons from the coronavirus disease 2019 (COVID-19) outbreak in China. JAMA 2020. 323(13):1239-1242. [http://dx.doi.org/10.1001/jama.2020.2648]

[46]   People   of   Any   Age   with   Underlying   Medical   Conditions.   2020. https://www.cdc.gov/coronavirus/2019-ncov/need-extra-precautions/groups-at-higher-risk.html

[47]   Albashir AAD. The potential impacts of obesity on COVID-19. Clin Med (Lond) 2020; 20(4): e109-13. [http://dx.doi.org/10.7861/clinmed.2020-0239] [PMID: 32571783]

[48]   Kassir R. Risk of COVID-19 for patients with obesity. Obes Rev 2020; 21(6): e13034. [http://dx.doi.org/10.1111/obr.13034] [PMID: 32281287]

[49]   Malavazos AE, Corsi Romanelli MM, Bandera F, Iacobellis G. Targeting the adipose tissue in COVID-19. Obes 2020; 28(7): 1178-79. [http://dx.doi.org/10.1002/oby.22844]

[50]   Lockhart SM, O'Rahilly S. When two pandemics meet: Why is obesity associated with increased COVID-19 mortality? Med (N Y). 2020 Dec 18; 1(1): 33–42. [http://dx.doi.org/10.1016/j.medj.2020.06.005]

[51]   Global   Obesity   Levels   -   Obesity   -   ProCon.org.   Obesity.   2020.   Available   from: https://obesity.procon.org/global-obesity-levels/

[52]   Tobacco. Who.int. 2020. Available from: https://www.who.int/news-room/fact-sheets/detail/tobacco

[53]   Williamson EJ, Walker AJ, Bhaskaran K, *et al.* Factors associated with COVID-19-related death using OpenSAFELY. Nature 2020; 584(7821): 430-6. [http://dx.doi.org/10.1038/s41586-020-2521-4]

[54]   Oakes JM, Fuchs RM, Gardner JD, Lazartigues E, Yue X. Nicotine and the renin-angiotensin system. Am J Physiol Regul Integr Comp Physiol 2018; 315(5): R895-906.
[http://dx.doi.org/10.1152/ajpregu.00099.2018] [PMID: 30088946]

[55]   Faizan MI, Abdullah M, Ali S, Naqvi IH, Ahmed A, Parveen S. Zika virus-induced microcephaly and its possible molecular mechanism. Intervirology 2016; 59(3): 152-8.
[http://dx.doi.org/10.1159/000452950] [PMID: 28081529]

[56]   Schwartz DA, Graham AL. Potential maternal and infant outcomes from (Wuhan) coronavirus 2019-nCoV infecting pregnant women: lessons from SARS, MERS, and other human coronavirus infections. Viruses 2020; 12(2): 194.
[http://dx.doi.org/10.3390/v12020194] [PMID: 32050635]

[57]   Schwartz DA. An analysis of 38 pregnant women with COVID-19, their newborn infants, and maternal-fetal transmission of SARS-CoV-2: maternal coronavirus infections and pregnancy outcomes. Arch Pathol Lab Med 2020; 144(7): 799-805.
[http://dx.doi.org/10.5858/arpa.2020-0901-SA] [PMID: 32180426]

CHAPTER 7

Clinical Manifestations, Treatment, Immune Response and Pathogenesis of Covid-19

Irshad H. Naqvi[1],*, Md. Imam Faizan[2,3], Mohammad Islamuddin[2], Mohd Abdullah[1], Arpita Rai[4] and Shama Parveen[2],*

[1] *Dr. M. A. Ansari Health Centre, Jamia Millia Islamia, New Delhi, India*

[2] *Centre for Interdisciplinary Research in Basic Sciences, Jamia Millia Islamia, New Delhi, India*

[3] *Multidisciplinary Centre for Advanced Research and Studies, Jamia Millia Islamia, New Delhi, India*

[4] *Department of Oral Medicine and Radiology, Rajendra Institute of Medical Sciences, Ranchi, Jharkhand, India*

Abstract: The clinical symptoms of the Coronavirus Disease 2019 (COVID-19) may vary from asymptomatic to mild to severe to critical disease. The clinical symptoms include fever, body ache, severe weakness, cough, breathlessness, nausea/vomiting, diarrhoea, change in taste/smell, *etc.* The management of COVID-19 patients is in its evolutionary phase since the guidelines are being updated regularly due to the gradual addition of unique symptoms to the disease. A large number of asymptomatic cases, longer incubation periods, and high transmission rates are some of the concerns of the pandemic. The treatment is supportive in the absence of a specific therapeutic drug and a prophylactic vaccine. Numerous antipyretics, existing anti-viral drugs, antibiotics supplements, and other approaches are utilized for the management of COVID-19 patients. Though at early-stage (in the upper respiratory tract), the treatment of this infection is easier as compared to its advanced stage when the infection proceeds to the lower respiratory tract. Most of the severe cases may need hospitalization, regular monitoring, and oxygen supplementation. Patients with respiratory failure may need ventilator support. The SARS-CoV-2 mediated immune response has a significant impact on infection severity, which is represented as a cytokine storm and ultimately leads to acute respiratory distress syndrome (ARSD). The present chapter describes clinical manifestations and management of COVID-19 patients. Besides this, we have also discussed the host immune response and pathogenesis of the disease. Further comprehensive patient-based clinical studies will provide insight into the additional clinical manifestations, pathogenesis, and host immune response needed to clear the virus from the human body.

---

* **Corresponding authors Irshad H. Naqvi and Shama Parveen:** Dr. M. A. Ansari Health Centre, Jamia Millia Islamia, New Delhi, India and Centre for Interdisciplinary Research in Basic Sciences, Jamia Millia Islamia, New Delhi, India; E-mails: inaqvi@jmi.ac.in and sparveen2@jmi.ac.in, shamp25@yahoo.com

Keywords: Asymptomatic, COVID-19, Clinical manifestations, Critical illness, Cytokine storm, Management, Mild illness, Pathogenesis, SARS-CoV-2, Severe illness, Treatment.

INTRODUCTION

The initial outbreak of novel COVID-19, caused by severe acute respiratory syndrome coronavirus 2 (SARS-CoV-2), started in Wuhan, China, in late December 2019, which later took its position as a global pandemic [1]. Millions of confirmed cases and deaths have been reported worldwide due to this contagious infection and its severity. The symptoms of the initial cluster of this viral infection were reported to be like pneumonia, which then turned out to be more critical and severe in patients with comorbidities [1]. Though the virus is mainly transmitted from an infected individual to a healthy one *via* respiratory droplets, its asymptomatic scenario made its transmission more rapid [2]. Additionally, it becomes more challenging to handle the pandemic due to the exponential increase in the cases.

Clinically, COVID-19 patients have been found to show symptoms like fever, dry cough, breathing difficulties, arthralgia, diarrhea, *etc*. The immune response triggered through SARS-CoV-2 infection has an essential influence on the individuals' overall health condition. Some clinical findings suggested an abrupt rise in the activated cytokines in an advanced stage of its infection, termed as cytokine storm [3]. Interestingly, individuals with strong immunity were able to escape the harsh effect caused by this virus. Moreover, in multiple critical cases, patients were also shown to develop serious pneumonia-like symptoms together with acute respiratory distress syndrome (ARSD) and multi-organ collapse, which ultimately led to death [4]. In this chapter, we will elaborate mainly about COVID-19 patients' clinical manifestations and their management. An overview of the host immune response and viral pathogenesis will also be given in the latter part of the chapter.

CLINICAL MANIFESTATIONS

COVID-19 infection in humans may lead to symptomatic or asymptomatic cases. Individuals with COVID-19 infection show diverse symptoms ranging from mild to severe disease [5]. Commonly encountered initial symptoms mimic that of any other viral infection. Usually, the first symptoms to appear are the loss of smell (anosmia) and taste (ageusia: the tongue is not able to taste sweetness, saltiness, bitterness, and sourness), fever, cough, extreme weakness, and some experience shortness of breath. Other minor symptoms are headache, dizziness, runny nose, congestion, and nausea. Some patients may also develop gastrointestinal disturbances like diarrhea (Fig. **1**) [6 - 8].

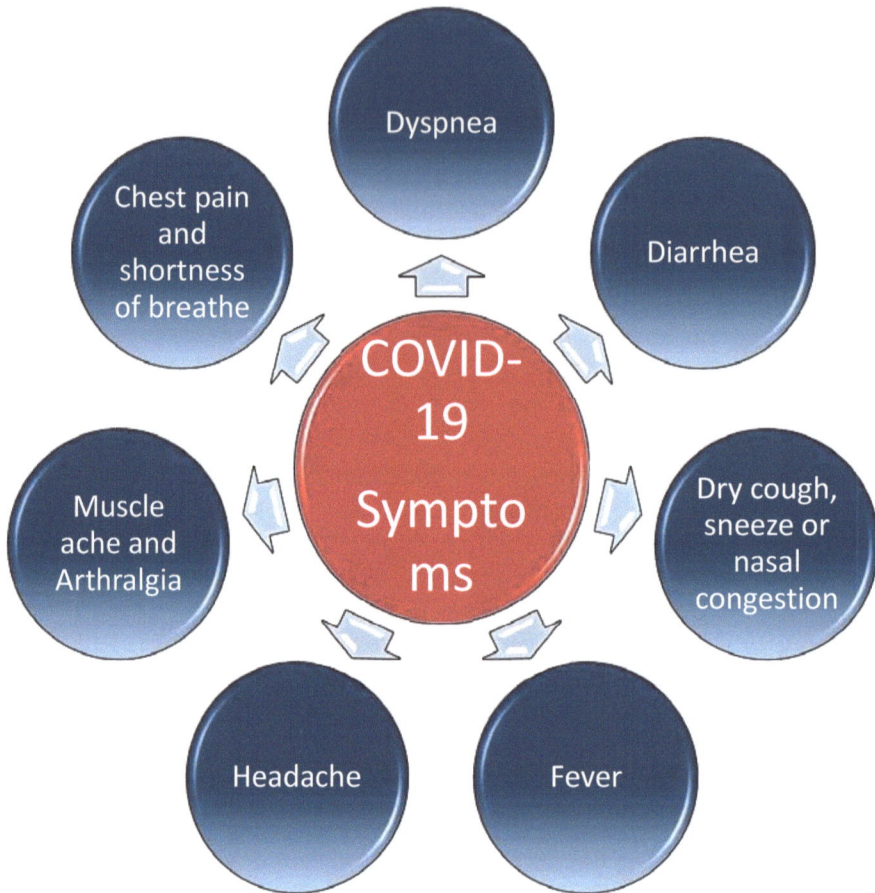

Fig. (1). Clinical manifestations of COVID-19.

Infection in most of the patients is mild or asymptomatic (80-90%). It is estimated that more than 40% people are wondering as asymptomatic COVID-19 individuals in society. It may also be noted that pre- and asymptomatic people are the most frequent source (almost 70-80%) of COVID-19 spread. It is estimated that around 10% of the cases are severe and around 5% of the cases develop a critical illness with respiratory failure, pneumonia, shock, ARSD, multi-organ failure, and ultimately death. Examination of CT scans of patients admitted to ICU revealed bilateral multiple lobular and subsegmental areas of consolidation. In addition, non-ICU patients bilateral ground-glass opacity and subsegmental areas of consolidation have also been documented. Laboratory investigations suggested that COVID-19 positive patients showed lymphocytopenia, leukocytopenia, an increase in lactic dehydrogenase enzyme, and an increase in C-reactive protein. Few immunocompromised or mid to older aged people may land onto a severe form of the disease called acute respiratory distress syndrome (ARDS). This severe form of the disease is represented with high-grade fever, drowsiness, confusion, cyanotic lips or face, hemoptysis, chest pain, oliguria or anuria, and respiratory failure, leading to a low level of oxygen saturation [9]. Occasionally, serious disease may present with a clinical feature of meningitis.

Incubation Period

The incubation period *i.e.*, time period of exposure to virus and development of first symptoms for COVID-19, is of usually 5 days. But this incubation period may vary up to 14 days also [10]. Patients are most contagious in the first 3 to 4 days after the development of symptoms, but may spread the disease before they become symptomatic (pre-symptomatic spread).

Transmission of Disease

The disease is usually transmitted to others by the 'droplets' arising from the sneeze or cough of an infected person. When an infected person is sneezing, coughing, simply talking, kissing, hugging, shouting or singing, droplets produced by him may be inhaled by the individual near him, causing the spread of the disease [11, 12]. Sharing taxis, public transport, washrooms or working in closed chambers for a long time may lead to transmission of the disease. This is the reason that the CDC has recommended social distancing of about six feet to prevent transmission of the infection [12]. The airborne spread of the infection theory is now gradually holding more weight for its transmission, which was not given importance earlier.

Contaminated droplets falling on the tabletops, chair handles, staircase railings, doorknobs, elevator buttons, *etc.*, may spread the disease when touched by the normal person, but it is less common as the virus gets destroyed as soon as the droplets get dry [10]. Therefore, surfaces do not become a common way of transmitting the disease. This is not an STD (sexually transmitted disease), but sputum and saliva contain a huge amount of virus, therefore, intimate contacts may transmit the virus easily. Aerosol transmission is reported in closed areas. Aerosol generated during flushing the toilets, medical procedures, *etc.*, may also transmit the disease easily. Breastfeeding may transmit the virus *via* milk as well as the baby coming in close contact with the mother [13].

Quarantine and Isolation

It has been demonstrated that this virus is transmitted from the droplets/aerosol produced during the sneeze or cough by the infected person. Therefore, keeping the infected person separate from others so that he is unable to further transmit the disease to healthy individuals is called **'isolation'** [14]. Implementation of aggressive isolation measures has led to a progressive reduction in COVID-19 cases. Keeping the non-symptomatic, apparently healthy individuals separately who had contact with the known positive patient is called as **'quarantine'** [14, 15]. This procedure is followed to observe whether he becomes symptomatic or not after the incubation period is completed. This is also done to save the healthy individuals who might have met them and unknowingly, the disease might have transmitted as an asymptomatic transmitter.

Treatment aimed at reducing transmission in the community is the best weapon. The purpose of both quarantine and isolation is to check the community transmission of the disease. **'Self-quarantine'** is widely practiced during an epidemic or pandemic when a suspected exposed person stays separately in his home in an isolated accommodation designed purposely and not leaving for the period he is required to quarantine. Only people who reside in the same household on the same premises may live with him and no visitors are permitted [16].

Peculiar Course of COVID-19

The patient manifests refractory fever, with a feeling of a state of malaise and dry cough. Within a week, elderly patients have impaired lung function and begin to experience symptoms of breathlessness. Sometimes dyspnea may be seen at the very onset of symptoms. While younger infected individuals are usually devoid of any respiratory ailment or other associated illnesses, but dyspnea may occasionally appear later. In such individuals, there may be a decrease in oxygen saturation (<93%), which is a crucial point for the rapid deterioration of respiratory functions. The first therapeutic approach is oxygen therapy that is usually effective in such cases. But in some cases, respiratory failure may occur. The next step is the NIV (non-invasive ventilation) that is quite effective. In a few cases, there is a sudden, unexpected worsening of clinical conditions. Patients require rapid intubation and invasive mechanical ventilation. However, after 24-48 hours, the patient usually shows marked improvement. Certain patients require continuous invasive therapy. In addition, mechanical ventilation is also recommended for 1-2 weeks.

CLINICAL MANAGEMENT

Oxygen Therapy: The First Step

There is no specific anti-viral drug against COVID-19, and no vaccine is currently available. The treatment is, thus, symptomatic, and **'oxygen therapy'** is the first step for effective management of respiratory damage in the patients. Non-invasive ventilation (NIV) and invasive mechanical ventilation (IMV) may be necessary for COVID-19 patients with respiratory failure. ICU admission is recommended to take care of such complications [17]. NIV is now recommended over IMV. Gattinoni and colleagues suggested that COVID-19-induced ARDS **(CARDS) is not a "Typical" ARDS.** In CARDS, good pulmonary compliance was demonstrated. NIV has shown to play a pivotal role in CARDS therapy in contrast to IMV [18].

Oxygen fast challenge: In COVID-19 patients with SpO_2 < 93-94% (< 88-90% if COPD) or a respiratory rate > 28-30 / min, or dyspnoea, oxygen administration by a 40% Venturi mask must be performed. After 5 to 10 minutes, if the patient shows some improvement, then the same treatment continues that is usually re-evaluated within the next 6 hours. In case of failure in improvement or worsening of conditions, the patient undergoes NIV treatment as per the requirement.

High nasal flow oxygen (HFNO) and non-invasive ventilation: It has been suggested that these approaches are usually performed by systems with good interface fitting that do not create widespread dispersion of exhaled air. This can be considered for the low risk of airborne transmission of COVID-19 [19]. High nasal flow cannula (HFNC) should be used in negative pressure rooms because of the risk of aerosol dispersal. It is used when the patient is not able to maintain saturation above 92% with usual oxygen support. HFNC can deliver a very high concentration of oxygen up to 50-60 liters per/mt. If saturation is not maintained with this HFNC, then the patient should be shifted to NIV.

Non-invasive ventilation and continuous positive airway pressure: This technique has a pivotal role in the management of COVID-19 associated respiratory failure. The continuous Positive Airway Pressure (CPAP) starts with 8-10 cmH_2O and FiO_2 60%. On the other hand, the NIV (*e.g.*, pressure support ventilation, PSV): starts with PEEP 5 cmH_2O after checking the tolerance of the patient.

Patients of COVID-19 may represent quite variable clinical manifestations with a wide range of presentations. These range from asymptomatic to mild to moderate symptoms to critical illness. The present chapter will discuss the clinical management of the disease according to the severity of the presentation. Many drugs are under clinical trials for the treatment of the disease across different parts of the globe. But no specific drug has been approved by the Food and Drug Administration (FDA) to date.

COVID patients are being classified under the following groups based on disease severity for management [20].

- Asymptomatic or pre-symptomatic infection: Covid positive but purely asymptomatic patients.
- Mild illness: Covid positive patients with a milder form of disease symptoms like a low-grade fever, cough, weakness, throat irritation, myalgia without any breathing difficulty or radiological abnormality.
- Moderate illness: Covid positive patients with oxygen saturation of approximately 94%, having clear-cut abnormality identified clinically and radiologically in the lungs.
- Severe illness: Covid positive patients with oxygen saturation less than 94% with tachypnea of more than 30 per minute or having more than 50% lung compromised with pneumonic infiltration.
- Critical illness: Covid positive patients with septic shock, multiple organ failure with respiratory failure.

It is estimated that around 70-80% of the infected individuals are asymptomatic or with very mild symptoms. The remaining 30% develop respiratory syndrome with the symptoms of high fever, and cough that further develops into severe respiratory failure, and many of them may require ICU admission.

Symptomatic or Pre-symptomatic Infection

Covid positive individuals without any symptoms should go for self-quarantine. If they are asymptomatic even after 10 days of positivity, they can discontinue their self-isolation. Current CDC guidelines are that a person with mild symptoms should isolate themselves for 10 days or till their febrile or breathing symptoms are gradually taken care of. No specific treatment is recommended for this category of COVID positive patients, but no further test is recommended for them [21].

Mild Illness

Patients with mild symptoms like fever, cough, myalgia, weakness, and throat irritation must be managed at home with proper regular telecommunication with medical staff. Individuals with risk factors should be closely monitored for any sudden deterioration. Otherwise, these individuals do not require any further investigational strategy. A detailed history of these patients must be recorded, including all the co-morbidities like sugar levels, blood pressure, *etc*. They must be monitored daily for temperature, oxygen saturation, and other vital statistics. The patients must be counseled regarding the signs and symptoms of complications arising due to severe respiratory disease.

Mild cases may be given simple antipyretics for fever and pain, as well as supplements, adequate nutrition, and rehydration. Patients with hypertension, diabetes mellitus, chronic kidney or lung disorder have to be monitored regularly. Limited data is available on the treatment of the mild symptomatic COVID positive patient with anti-virals or immunotherapy.

Moderate Illness

Obvious clinical respiratory difficulty rate, higher than 24 per/min with oxygen saturation approximately 94% in Covid positive cases, should be monitored closely. They should be isolated in Covid Care Centres since the conditions of such patients might suddenly deteriorate. Such patients should be monitored daily with complete blood count (CBC) along with other radiological investigations. Inflammatory markers like C-reactive protein (CRP), D-Dimer, serum ferritin must be evaluated as prognostic marker tools. Anxiety and fear are obvious with the patients and they should be supported by psychological counseling.

Personal Protective Equipment (PPE) use with single patient dedicated clinical instruments like a stethoscope, torch, hammer, blood pressure cuffs, thermometer, *etc.*, should be used to prevent transmission of infection. Limited entry in the room of patients of genuinely required individuals should be strictly followed. If possible, HEPA filter equipped room should be used to prevent the spread of aerosol generated infection.

Clinical Management of Moderate Disease

Patients with moderate disease must be closely monitored regularly. The oxygen supply for patients must be maintained so that the oxygen saturation increases from 92% to 96%. The patient should be maintained in a prone position and should be awake, that is good for saturation. The N95 masks should be used both by the health care workers and patients. ECG monitoring, CBC, liver function tests (LFT), kidney function test (KFT), absolute lymphocyte counts have to be monitored on daily basis. The D Dimer, CRP, and serum ferritin must be monitored every 72 hours. In addition, control of the co-morbid conditions must be strictly followed. Close monitoring of increasing breathing labor (use of accessory respiratory muscles), hemodynamic instability, and gradual increase in the oxygen requirement are indicators to shift the patient to a dedicated Covid care facility. Further, good provision of follow-up and transport facility should always be ready for these moderate cases.

Long-acting steroids, methyleprednisolone (0.5 to 1mg per kg), can be given intravenously for three days if the inflammatory markers are increased or the oxygen requirement is gradually increasing. Prophylactic use of anticoagulants is advocated (enoxapyrin 40m mg per day) [22]. The empirical antibiotics should not be started acquiring secondary infections unless pneumonia or sepsis is suspected. Other medications include antipyretics, supplements, *etc.*, as per the requirement of the patient.

SEVERE CASES MANAGEMENT

Urgent Supportive Therapy with Dedicated Monitoring

Oxygen supply should be provided for the patients as per the requirement to maintain oxygen saturation, while monitoring hemodynamic instability, renal and cardiac status, or patient landing into shock. Resuscitation facilities should always be ready.

Management of Respiratory Failure with Acute Respiratory Distress Syndrome (ARSD)

Respiratory failure with ARDS could be due to the intrapulmonary ventilation-perfusion mismatch or any cardiac shunt. This may shift the patient to mechanical ventilation. The standard oxygen management failure should be recognized as early as possible to prevent hypoxemic respiratory failure. High flow nasal cannula or non-invasive mechanical ventilation should be followed.

When the standard oxygen therapy starts failing, then the high flow oxygen nasal cannula or non-invasive mechanical ventilation (BIPAP/ CPAP) may be employed to prevent hypoxemic respiratory failure. This may reduce the risk of intubation. High flow nasal cannula (HFNO) is safe in mild to moderate and non-worsening hypercapnia. HFNO should be monitored by an experienced person so that, when required, he may be able to intubate the patient. Endotracheal intubation should be performed, keeping all the precautions, avoiding aerosol infection, and the patient should be deeply sedated.

The setting of the ventilator should be according to the guidelines for ARDS patients. Hyperventilation may be advocated to meet the pH range of blood gases from 7.30 to 7.45 as per the ventilator protocol. Prone position of the patient for 16 to 18 hours is recommended for the ARDS cases. Patients refractory to mechanical ventilation should be considered for extracorporeal life support (ECLS), if available. While transferring the patient, disconnection of the ET tube should be avoided to prevent atelectasis and failure of the ventilator setting.

Management of Extrapulmonary Manifestations and Systemic Complications

COVID-19 patients have reported the involvement of different organ systems leading to a complex situation. Kidney damage and Acute Kidney Injury are emerging as critical forms of associated manifestation of COVID-19. The clinical presentation of kidney damage ranges from mild proteinuria (more than 40% of the patients show abnormal proteinuria after hospital admission) to acute progressive renal injury (AKI). This renal injury is a marker of multi-organ dysfunction and severe disease that may need renal replacement therapy (RRT) along with the possibility of removal of cytokines. It is reported that up to 20% of COVID-19 admitted to ICU may need this RRT therapy [23].

Management of Septic Shock

Sepsis is a life-threatening situation during which the organs of the patients do not function properly. It is caused by a dysregulated host response to an infection [24]. COVID-19 patients with sepsis are in critical condition. They show a wide range of symptoms such as respiratory manifestations like severe dyspnea and hypoxemia, tachycardia, renal impairment with reduced urine output, altered mental status, *etc* [25]. Such patients should be started with vasopressors to maintain the mean arterial pressure and lactate once the patient is in a septic shock. Hypovolemia should be corrected quickly. The initiation of antimicrobial therapy with proper fluid management should be started immediately. Central venous catheter and the arterial catheter may be maintained depending upon the patient's requirement and available expert medical personnel [26].

Patients with septic shock should receive about 30 ml/kg of isotonic crystalloid in the first three hours. In children, it can be given up to 20 ml/kg as a bolus, then from 30 to 40 ml/ kg in about one hour. Crystalloids are normal saline or Ringer's lactate. The hypotonic solution, starch, gelatins should not be used in septic shock patients. The patients should be monitored for fluid overload while resuscitating. Intravenous vasopressors should be used when shock persists despite fluid resuscitation. Vasopressors may cause necrosis at the local site if given by a small vein or extravasated. If vasopressor and fluid resuscitation therapy are not able to maintain the signs of perfusion or cardiac instability, then inotropes like dobutamine may be utilized [26].

Other Therapeutic Measures

A low dose of methylprednisolone (1-2 mg per day) should be administered to patients who have shown gradually deteriorating oxygen saturation, worsening radiological pictures, and increased inflammatory response. High doses of glucocorticoid may further delay the removal of the virus from the body due to its immunosuppressive effect. Prophylactic use of anticoagulants should be used to avoid hypercoagulability [22, 27]. In addition, co-morbid conditions should be controlled effectively.

NEW INVESTIGATIONAL THERAPIES

The use of these therapies is with limited available documented evidence. It is expected with an evolving situation that more data will be available on these therapies in the future. Accordingly, their use recommendations will be incorporated and upgraded in future studies. Such drugs should be used in some defined situations and subgroups of cases.

Anti-Viral Drugs

Different permutation and combinations of existing anti-viral drugs are used for the treatment of COVID-19 patients. Lopinavir/ritonavir can be given (400/100 mg orally every 12 hours) [28]. But the use of this drug to treat COVID-19 patients is now debatable. Oseltamivir is anti-influenza drug that is also used in the treatment [29]. Favipiravir has also shown efficacy against SARS-CoV-2 in *in vitro* studies. In addition, alpha-interferon (*e.g.*, 5 million units by aerosol inhalation twice per day) is also prescribed. Remdesivir is an inhibitor of RNA polymerase with activity reported against many RNA viruses like Ebola. Only emergency use is permitted with this anti-viral drug in the following cases. This includes patients with moderate disease having raised liver enzymes (five times of upper limit). Other categories involve severe renal impairment requiring hemodialysis, pregnant and lactating mothers, and children more than twelve years of age. The recommended doses are 200 mg intravenous on day one and 100 mg daily for 5 days [30].

Tocilizumab

This inflammation inhibitor may be considered in moderately diseased persons demanding a gradual increase in oxygen supply in mechanically ventilated persons and patients on steroidal therapy [30]. The long term safety profile of the drug is still awaited. Some critical points should be considered before starting its use. Raised inflammatory markers like CRP, D-dimer, *etc.*, favors the recommendation of the drug. Strict monitoring is required for the possible development of neutropenia and secondary infections in patients. There should be no active bacterial or tubercular infection in the patients before initiation of the treatment. The recommended dose is 8 mg per kg, with a maximum of 800 mg may be given in dilution with normal saline in about one hour [31].

Hydroxychloroquine

This drug has shown *in vitro* activity against the SARS- CoV-2 and has some clinical benefits with limited evidence. While in other large observational studies, this drug has no role in preventing mortality and clinical outcome. This drug was initially used in the treatment of COVID-19 patients [30, 32]. But subsequent studies have shown that its role is a bit controversial.

Anticoagulant

COVID-19 patients showing thrombophilia or thrombosis are treated with certain anticoagulants like enoxaparin that is given 1 mg/kg twice daily. This thromboprophylaxis is associated with reduced mortality in such patients [33].

Convalescent Plasma

This treatment can be used in patients with moderate disease who are not responding to gradually increased oxygen despite steroidal therapy. Special prerequisites should be followed before the start of plasma therapy [34, 35]. This includes strict matching of blood groups. The donor should have a sufficient amount of antibodies developed to neutralize the antigen of the recipient. The recipients should be closely monitored for about 12 hours for any untoward reaction. The treatment should not be used in patients with IgA deficiency and immunoglobin allergy. The dose is variable between 4 to 13 ml /kg, and usually, 200 ml is given very slowly. This therapy has shown effectiveness in children infected with COVID-19.

Endogenous interferons are produced in response to viral infections and modulate the immune response by exerting anti-viral activity. In addition, other coronaviruses, namely MERS and SARS, have previously been shown to be highly susceptible to interferon treatment in *in vitro* conditions [36, 37].

Dexamethasone

This steroid is the first drug that has been authorized by the National Health Service (NHS), United Kingdom, and it reduces the risk of death in severe COVID-19 patients. It has been shown that this drug significantly reduces the risk of death of patients that are on ventilation by 35% and those on oxygen support by 20%. A recent study has shown that this drug reduces death by $1/3^{rd}$ among critically ill patients [38].

It may be noted that investigation of the long-term complications in the COVID-19 survivors is still in the preliminary stage. There are many unanswered questions in this category, like restoration of the normal respiratory, cardiovascular, renal, digestive functions in the individuals. In addition, the psychological behavior of the affected individuals has to be analyzed. Long term prospective studies on the patients are needed to answer these questions that will go a long way in the overall management of the affected individuals.

IMMUNE RESPONSE IN COVID-19

At present, inadequate data is available on SARS-CoV-2 and host immune response and is still under investigation. The SARS-CoV-2 infection triggers an innate and adaptive immune response, and hence assists the judgment of the infection. Although a very quick and systematized immune response exhibited an immediate and primary immune protection against the viral infection, disproportionate inflammatory innate immune response and uncontrolled adaptive immune defense of host may cause harm to the tissues at the point of virus entry as well as at an intrinsic level. Amplified proinflammatory host response was speculated to activate an immune pathology arising in the accelerated course of acute lung injury (ALI) and acute respiratory distress syndrome (ARDS) appearing in the infected patients [4, 20, 39]. For example, the extensive release of chemokine and cytokines, commonly named "cytokine storm", distinctly demonstrates an inconsistent host immune protection system (Fig. **2**).

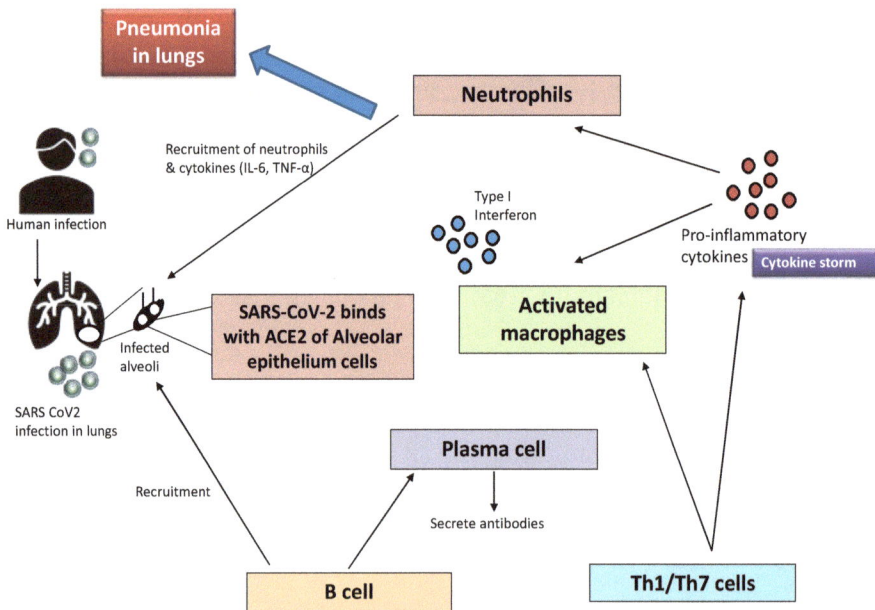

Fig. (2). Host immune responses to Covid-19 infection. SARS-CoV-2, with the help of their spike protein, infect the human cells expressing ACE2, such as alveolar epithelium cells. Cells infected by the virus can evade interferon type I (IFN-α/β). As a result, an inconsistent viral replication is initiated. The inflow of activated neutrophils and monocytes/macrophages developed an excessive production of pro-inflammatory cytokines. As a result of the "cytokine storms" wave the immunopathology of the lung developed. The inflammatory responses started due to the activation of specialized Th1/Th17 cells. Activated B cells differentiate into antibody-secreting plasma cells that generate neutralizing antibodies specific to SARS-CoV-2, which help in the clearance of viruses from the host.

Innate Immune Response

An innate immune response is the immediate and primary host's protection against a pathogen without previous exposure to it. It mainly dominates during the beginning hours to days of viral infection, which is represented by the activation of phagocytes and natural killer (NK) cells. Potential innate immune defense against viral infection depends massively upon type I interferon (IFN-α/β) responses and their downstream cascade, which supports inhibition of the viral replication as well as induction in the effective adaptive immune response. To escalate an anti-viral response, innate immune cells need to identify the virus intrusion with the help of pattern recognition receptor (PRR) through the pathogen-associated molecular patterns (PAMPs) presented by the pathogen. It may be noted that for RNA viruses like coronavirus, viral protein, and genomic RNA, as well as the intermediates produced at the time of viral replication, such as dsRNA, identified by the immune cells through their RNA receptors (TLR3 and TLR7) are present in endosomal and the RNA sensor (RIG-I/MDA5) in the cytoplasm [40]. It is also reported that the downstream signaling cascade activates to generate NF-κB, IRF3, and IRF7, followed by their nuclear translocation. Inside the nucleus, all these signaling transcription factors stimulate the synthesis of type I IFN and the pro-inflammatory cytokines like IL-6, TNF-α, IL-8, IL-1, and IL-12, and this primary response comprises the first wave of protection against infection at the site of viral entry [41]. The JAK-STAT pathway is initiated by the interaction of Type I IFN and interferon-α/β receptor (IFNAR). Here, the JAK1 and TYK2 kinases phosphorylate STAT1 and STAT2. This STAT1/2 and interferon regulatory factor 9 (IRF9) then forms a complex, and together, this complex moves inside the nucleus to trigger the initiation of transcription for anti-viral interferon-stimulated genes (ISGs).

Adaptive Immune Response

Generally, in viral infection, adaptive immunity, the major player is the Th1 type of cells and the generated Th1 type immune response plays an important role against virus infection. The antigen-presenting cells produce an atmosphere of cytokines that guides the direction to the T-cell responses. The overall adaptive host immune response is regulated by the T helper (Th) cells. At the same time, cytotoxic T (Tc) cells lead to the killing of cells infected with the virus. B-cells are the major players of the humoral immune response, and activated B cells give rise to plasma cells generating neutralizing antibodies specific to the virus. The antibodies neutralize the virus, and perform a protective role against virus infection at a later stage and prevent secondary infections in the future.

The T cell response was broadly investigated in SARS-CoV. It has been investigated that CD8+ T cell responses were more redundant with extensive size than the CD4+ T cell responses. In addition, virus-specific T cells from severe patients lead to a central memory phenotype along with a greater number of multi-functional CD4+ T cells (producing TNFα, IFNγ, and IL-2) as well as CD8+ T cells (generating IFNγ, TNFα and degranulated state), in comparison with the moderate and mild groups. Further, vigorous T cell activation correlates significantly with a greater number of neutralizing antibodies, at the same time, higher serum Th2 cytokines (IL-10, IL-4 and IL-5) has been discovered in the fatal group of patients [42]. Early increase in the number of CD8+ T cells correlates with disease severity in the case of coronavirus infection and effective Th1 type helper T cells are detected at the convalescent stage [43, 44]. As neutrophils have a harmful effect in almost all of the infections, in human coronavirus infection, the defensive or fatal role of Th17 remains unidentified.

Potential Immune Evasion

The current investigations demonstrate that the coronavirus inhibits host immune response. And, it is slightly elucidated why the incubation time is longer (2-11 days) in case of coronavirus infection compared to the influenza virus that is 1-4 days [45]. The longer incubation time is because of their immune avoidance features, as it skillfully evades human immune detection during the initial phase of infection. In short, most mechanisms basically depend on the suppression of innate immune reaction, particularly interferon type I (IFN-α/β) identification, and signaling. Structural proteins (*e.g.*, M and N), nonstructural (NS) proteins (*e.g.* NS4a, NS4b, NS15) and accessory protein of the coronaviruses are the essential and important factors in the modulation of host immune response [46].

PATHOGENESIS

The initial interaction of a healthy individual with the virus takes place through an infected person's exorcized respiratory droplets, which then find their way inside the body through mouth and nose. The inhaled viral particles are likely to fuse with the epithelial cells of the oral and nasal cavity, which are abundant in the receptor, ACE2 (angiotensin-converting enzyme 2). This receptor on the host cells acts as an anchor for the viral spike protein, using which viral particle binds and enters the host cell [47]. It has been reported that in about 80% of COVID-19 patients, the observed symptoms are mild and remain limited to the upper respiratory tract [8, 48]. As soon as the viral particles enter the cell, it takes over the host cell's metabolic system, consuming it and multiplying itself rapidly. Once the host cell's machinery is consumed, the newly synthesized viral particles bud off from the infected cell. At this stage, these newly viral particles are spread throughout the lower respiratory tract to infect the cells lining these tracts [49].

In the first week of the viral infection, the patient may not show any symptoms, but in some cases, due to an initial heavy load of viral particles, the patient starts to show fever, difficulty in breathing, arthralgia, diarrhea, sore throat, headache, *etc* [8]. In the case of COVID-19 progression, the individual's immune system plays an essential role. During its initial stage (infection in the upper respiratory tract), if the immune system is strong enough to fight back to the virus and stop its progression, then the person escapes from the severe stage of the disease. But if the patient has any underlying disease conditions, then the viral load is moved to the alveolar region of the lungs [50]. In healthy conditions, these alveoli help in the gaseous exchange. Interestingly, the cells in these alveoli regions are also abundant with ACE2 receptors, which gives the virus a suitable place for multiple infections [51]. In the phase where numerous viruses' attack the alveolar epithelial cells, a defense action of the host immune response takes place. This abnormal scenario not only evoked the immune cells but also alter the normal gaseous exchange. Clinically, this significant aspect of the disease is termed as a cytokine storm, which is a flood of immune cells inside the alveolar region, including activated inflammatory molecules (TNF-α, IL-1β, IL-8, IL-12, IP10, MIP1A, MCP1, IL-6) that fight against virus attack [52]. The effect of the cytokines storm is dysfunctional coagulation together with widespread damage of tissues. Among these multiple cytokines produced during the cytokine storm, the IL-6 acts as a protagonist, which is secreted by a wide range of cells, such as activated leukocytes, including some tissues. The role of IL-6 is well explained during inflammatory diseases, cancers, cardiovascular diseases, and autoimmune diseases. Interestingly, an essential role of IL-6 is also described during the progression of cytokine releasing syndrome (CRS) recently [53]. These immune cells later accumulate inside the alveolar region, forming a mixture of damaged and dead cells together with a sticky fluid collectively called an exudate. The advanced stage of COVID-19 that is diagnosed by X-ray images displays numerous white opacities in the lung cavity due to accumulation of these exudates. The COVID-19 patient symptoms resemble acute respiratory distress syndrome (ARDS) due to these accumulated exudates in which a patient strives for breathing [4]. Many of the patients die at this stage, but some of them also die due to the multi-organ failure followed by the ARSD (Fig. **3**) [54].

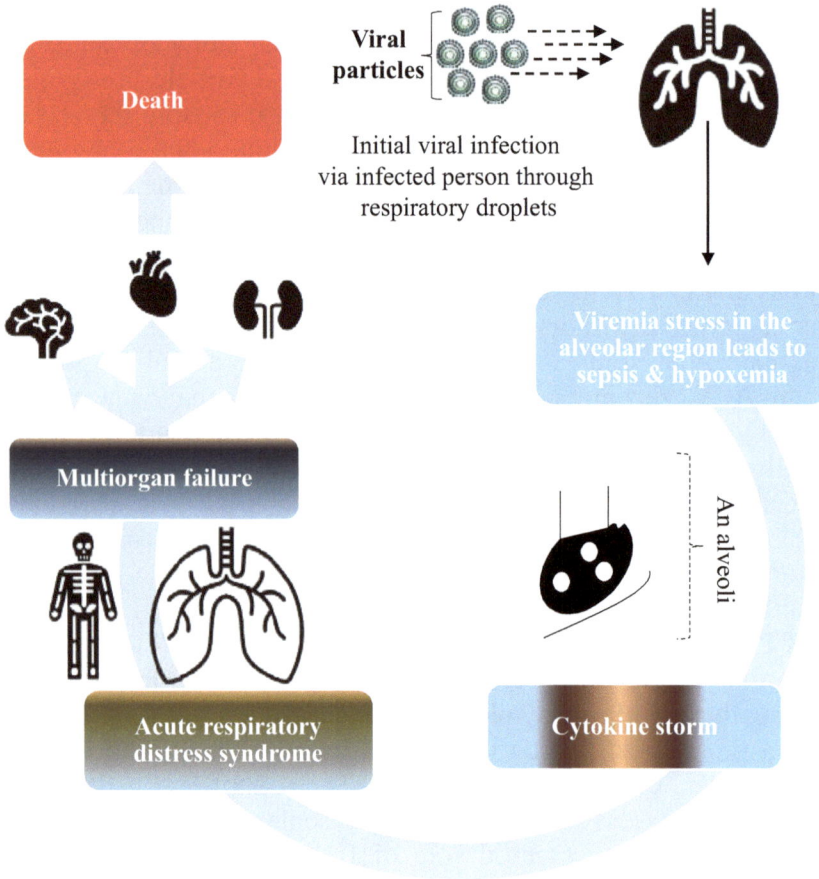

Mechanism of COVID-19

Fig. (3). A schematic representation of the pathogenesis of COVID-19.

CONCLUDING REMARKS

Numerous symptoms have been added to the list of existing COVID-19 clinical signs. Therefore, the treatment guidelines of COVID-19 patients are updated regularly by the WHO. Usually, the treatment is symptomatic since anti-viral agents are not available against SARS-CoV-2. Treatment of mild cases is manageable mostly at home since the symptoms resemble the regular viral infection. Severe cases need hospitalization and oxygen support. Patients with existing co-morbid conditions must be monitored on a regular basis for severe disease. In addition, treatment of the high-risk individuals encompassing health care workers, immunocompromised individuals, and persons with co-morbidities should be prioritized for their effective treatment. The ongoing accelerated drug trials in different parts of the globe will contribute towards the formulation of anti-viral agents against SARS-CoV-2.

Despite numerous publications on the viral pathophysiology, the SARS-CoV-2 mediated host immune response is still poorly understood. The viral infection mediated cytokine storm is a predominant phenomenon of host defense against the viral infection. This elevated level of cytokines not only has a significant impact on the disease progression, but it also provides the essential cellular workforce to fight against the infection in healthy individuals. Collaborative efforts of pathologists, immunologists, and clinicians are the need of the hour to delineate the attributes of the pathogenesis of this emerging viral pathogen.

CONSENT FOR PUBLICATION

Not Applicable.

CONFLICT OF INTEREST

The author declares no conflict of interest, financial or otherwise.

ACKNOWLEDGEMENTS

Md Imam Faizan is supported by Research Fellowship by the Indian Council of Medical Research (ICMR), Government of India. Mohammad Islamuddin is supported by Fellowship from University Grants Commission (UGC), Government of India. The research in our laboratory is funded by the Council of Scientific and Industrial Research (CSIR), India (37(1697)17/EMR-II) and Central Council for Research in Unani Medicine (CCRUM), Ministry of Ayurveda, Yoga and Naturopathy, Unani, Siddha and Homeopathy (AYUSH), India (F.No.3-63/2019-CCRUM/Tech).

REFERENCES

[1]   Shi H, Han X, Jiang N, *et al.* Radiological findings from 81 patients with COVID-19 pneumonia in Wuhan, China: a descriptive study. Lancet Infect Dis 2020; 20(4): 425-34.
      [http://dx.doi.org/10.1016/S1473-3099(20)30086-4] [PMID: 32105637]

[2]   Liu X, Zhang S. COVID-19: Face masks and human-to-human transmission. Influenza Other Respi Viruses 2020; 14(4): 472-3.
      [http://dx.doi.org/10.1111/irv.12740]

[3]   Jose RJ, Manuel A. COVID-19 cytokine storm: the interplay between inflammation and coagulation.

Lancet Respir Med 2020; 8(6): e46-7.
[http://dx.doi.org/10.1016/S2213-2600(20)30216-2] [PMID: 32353251]

[4]   Xu Z, Shi L, Wang Y, *et al.* Pathological findings of COVID-19 associated with acute respiratory distress syndrome. Lancet Respir Med 2020; 8(4): 420-2.
[http://dx.doi.org/10.1016/S2213-2600(20)30076-X] [PMID: 32085846]

[5]   Kim GU, Kim M-J, Ra SH, *et al.* Clinical characteristics of asymptomatic and symptomatic patients with mild COVID-19. Clin Microbiol Infect 2020; 26(7): 948.e1-3.
[http://dx.doi.org/10.1016/j.cmi.2020.04.040] [PMID: 32360780]

[6]   Arons MM, Hatfield KM, Reddy SC, *et al.* Presymptomatic SARS-CoV-2 infections and transmission in a skilled nursing facility. N Engl J Med 2020; 382(22): 2081-90.
[http://dx.doi.org/10.1056/NEJMoa2008457] [PMID: 32329971]

[7]   Menni C, Valdes A, Freydin MB, *et al.* Loss of smell and taste in combination with other symptoms is a strong predictor of COVID-19 infection. MedRxiv 2020.
[http://dx.doi.org/10.1101/2020.04.05.20048421]

[8]   Zhou F, Yu T, Du R, *et al.* Clinical course and risk factors for mortality of adult inpatients with COVID-19 in Wuhan, China: a retrospective cohort study. Lancet 2020; 395(10229): 1054-62.
[http://dx.doi.org/10.1016/S0140-6736(20)30566-3] [PMID: 32171076]

[9]   (CDC). USCfDCaP. "Coronavirus Disease 2019 (COVID-19)—Symptoms" 2020. https://www.cdc.gov/coronavirus/2019-ncov/symptoms-testing/symptoms.html

[10]   WHO QAocC Q&A on coronaviruses (COVID-19). 2020. https://www.who.int/emergencies/diseases/novel-coronavirus-2019/question-and-answers-hub/q-a-detail/q-a-coronaviruses2020.

[11]   Hamner L, Dubbel P, Capron I, *et al.* High SARS-CoV-2 attack rate following exposure at a choir practice—Skagit County, Washington, March 2020. MMWR Morb Mortal Wkly Rep 2020; 69(19): 606-10.
[http://dx.doi.org/10.15585/mmwr.mm6919e6] [PMID: 32407303]

[12]   https://www.ecdc.europa.eu/en/covid-19/questions-answersQAoC-ECfDPaCRA. European Centre for Disease Prevention and Control. Retrieved 30 April 2020. 2020

[13]   Groß R, Conzelmann C, Müller JA, *et al.* Detection of SARS-CoV-2 in human breastmilk. Lancet 2020; 395(10239): 1757-8.
[http://dx.doi.org/10.1016/S0140-6736(20)31181-8] [PMID: 32446324]

[14]   Lawrence JMD. Infection control in the community. Elsevier Health Sciences 2003; p. 136.

[15]   Quarantine and Isolation. Centers for Disease Control and Prevention 2018.

[16]   GOV.UK. Advice for home isolation https://www.gov.uk/government/publications/wuhan-nove--coronavirus-self-isolation-for-patients-undergoing-testing/advice-sheet-home-isolation2020.

[17]   Cascella M, Rajnik M, Cuomo A, Dulebohn SC, Di Napoli R. Features, Evaluation, and Treatment of Coronavirus. StatPearls Publishing 2020; LLC: 2020.

[18]   Gattinoni L, Coppola S, Cressoni M, Busana M, Rossi S, Chiumello D. Covid-19 does not lead to a "typical" acute respiratory distress syndrome. Am J Respir Crit Care Med 2020; 201(10): 1299-300.
[http://dx.doi.org/10.1164/rccm.202003-0817LE] [PMID: 32228035]

[19]   Hui DS, Chow BK, Lo T, *et al.* Exhaled air dispersion during high-flow nasal cannula therapy *versus* CPAP *via* different masks. Eur Respir J 2019; 53(4): 1802339.
[http://dx.doi.org/10.1183/13993003.02339-2018] [PMID: 30705129]

[20]   Huang C, Wang Y, Li X, *et al.* Clinical features of patients infected with 2019 novel coronavirus in Wuhan, China. Lancet 2020; 395(10223): 497-506.
[http://dx.doi.org/10.1016/S0140-6736(20)30183-5] [PMID: 31986264]

[21]   Kimball A, Hatfield KM, Arons M, *et al.* Asymptomatic and presymptomatic SARS-CoV-2 infections

in residents of a long-term care skilled nursing facility—King County, Washington, March 2020. MMWR Morb Mortal Wkly Rep 2020; 69(13): 377-81.
[http://dx.doi.org/10.15585/mmwr.mm6913e1] [PMID: 32240128]

[22]   Bikdeli B, Madhavan MV, Jimenez D, *et al.* Endorsed by the ISTH, NATF, ESVM, and the IUA, Supported by the ESC Working Group on Pulmonary Circulation and Right Ventricular Function COVID-19 and thrombotic or thromboembolic disease: Implications for prevention, antithrombotic therapy, and follow-up: JACC state-of-the-art review. J Am Coll Cardiol 2020; 75(23): 2950-73.
[http://dx.doi.org/10.1016/j.jacc.2020.04.031] [PMID: 32311448]

[23]   Cheng Y, Luo R, Wang K, *et al.* Kidney disease is associated with in-hospital death of patients with COVID-19. Kidney Int 2020; 97(5): 829-38.
[http://dx.doi.org/10.1016/j.kint.2020.03.005] [PMID: 32247631]

[24]   Singer M, Deutschman CS, Seymour CW, *et al.* The third international consensus definitions for sepsis and septic shock (Sepsis-3). JAMA 2016; 315(8): 801-10.
[http://dx.doi.org/10.1001/jama.2016.0287] [PMID: 26903338]

[25]   Seymour CW, Kennedy JN, Wang S, *et al.* Derivation, validation, and potential treatment implications of novel clinical phenotypes for sepsis. JAMA 2019; 321(20): 2003-17.
[http://dx.doi.org/10.1001/jama.2019.5791] [PMID: 31104070]

[26]   Alhazzani W, Møller MH, Arabi YM, *et al.* Surviving Sepsis Campaign: guidelines on the management of critically ill adults with Coronavirus Disease 2019 (COVID-19). Intensive Care Med 2020; 46(5): 854-87.
[http://dx.doi.org/10.1007/s00134-020-06022-5] [PMID: 32222812]

[27]   Arachchillage DRJ, Laffan M. Abnormal coagulation parameters are associated with poor prognosis in patients with novel coronavirus pneumonia. J Thromb Haemost 2020; 18(5): 1233-4.
[http://dx.doi.org/10.1111/jth.14820] [PMID: 32291954]

[28]   Bimonte S, Crispo A, Amore A, Celentano E, Cuomo A, Cascella M. Potential antiviral drugs for SARS-Cov-2 treatment: preclinical findings and ongoing clinical research. *In Vivo* 2020; 34(3)(Suppl.): 1597-602.
[http://dx.doi.org/10.21873/invivo.11949] [PMID: 32503817]

[29]   Chen N, Zhou M, Dong X, *et al.* Epidemiological and clinical characteristics of 99 cases of 2019 novel coronavirus pneumonia in Wuhan, China: a descriptive study. Lancet 2020; 395(10223): 507-13.
[http://dx.doi.org/10.1016/S0140-6736(20)30211-7] [PMID: 32007143]

[30]   WHO; "Solidarity" clinical trial for COVID-19 treatments. https://www.who.int/emergencies/ diseases/novel-coronavirus-2019/global-research-on-novel-coronavirus-2019-ncov/so-idarity-clinical-trial-for-covid-19-treatments2020.

[31]   Pharmacopoeia B, Commission BP. Medicines and healthcare products regulatory agency. London 2010; 3(6): 1844.

[32]   WHO. Q&A : Hydroxychloroquine and COVID-19. https://www.who.int/news-room/q-a-detail-q-a-hydroxychloroquine-and-covid-19

[33]   Kollias A, Kyriakoulis KG, Dimakakos E, Poulakou G, Stergiou GS, Syrigos K. Thromboembolic risk and anticoagulant therapy in COVID-19 patients: emerging evidence and call for action. Br J Haematol 2020; 189(5): 846-7.
[http://dx.doi.org/10.1111/bjh.16727] [PMID: 32304577]

[34]   Teixeira da Silva JA. Convalescent plasma: A possible treatment of COVID-19 in India. Med J Armed Forces India 2020; 76(2): 236-7.
[http://dx.doi.org/10.1016/j.mjafi.2020.04.006] [PMID: 32296259]

[35]   Shen C, Wang Z, Zhao F, *et al.* March 2020, posting date. Treatment of 5 critically ill patients with COVID19 with convalescent plasma. JAMA 2020; 323(16): 1582-9.
[http://dx.doi.org/10.1001/jama.2020.4783]

[36]   Gralinski LE, Baric RS. Molecular pathology of emerging coronavirus infections. J Pathol 2015; 235(2): 185-95.
[http://dx.doi.org/10.1002/path.4454] [PMID: 25270030]

[37]   Arabi YM, Shalhoub S, Mandourah Y, *et al.* Ribavirin and interferon therapy for critically ill patients with middle east respiratory syndrome: a multicenter observational study. Clin Infect Dis 2020; 70(9): 1837-44.
[http://dx.doi.org/10.1093/cid/ciz544] [PMID: 31925415]

[38]   Ledford H. Coronavirus breakthrough: dexamethasone is first drug shown to save lives. Nature 2020; 582(7813): 469.
[http://dx.doi.org/10.1038/d41586-020-01824-5] [PMID: 32546811]

[39]   Wu F, Zhao S, Yu B, *et al.* A new coronavirus associated with human respiratory disease in China. Nature 2020; 579(7798): 265-9.
[http://dx.doi.org/10.1038/s41586-020-2008-3] [PMID: 32015508]

[40]   García LF. Immune response, inflammation, and the clinical spectrum of COVID-19. Front Immunol 2020; 11: 1441.
[http://dx.doi.org/10.3389/fimmu.2020.01441] [PMID: 32612615]

[41]   de Wit E, van Doremalen N, Falzarano D, Munster VJ. SARS and MERS: recent insights into emerging coronaviruses. Nat Rev Microbiol 2016; 14(8): 523-34.
[http://dx.doi.org/10.1038/nrmicro.2016.81] [PMID: 27344959]

[42]   Li CK, Wu H, Yan H, *et al.* T cell responses to whole SARS coronavirus in humans. J Immunol 2008; 181(8): 5490-500.
[http://dx.doi.org/10.4049/jimmunol.181.8.5490] [PMID: 18832706]

[43]   Shin H-S, Kim Y, Kim G, *et al.* Immune responses to Middle East respiratory syndrome coronavirus during the acute and convalescent phases of human infection. Clin Infect Dis 2019; 68(6): 984-92.
[http://dx.doi.org/10.1093/cid/ciy595] [PMID: 30060038]

[44]   Prompetchara E, Ketloy C, Palaga T. Immune responses in COVID-19 and potential vaccines: Lessons learned from SARS and MERS epidemic. Asian Pac J Allergy Immunol 2020; 38(1): 1-9.
[PMID: 32105090]

[45]   Lessler J, Reich NG, Brookmeyer R, Perl TM, Nelson KE, Cummings DA. Incubation periods of acute respiratory viral infections: a systematic review. Lancet Infect Dis 2009; 9(5): 291-300.
[http://dx.doi.org/10.1016/S1473-3099(09)70069-6] [PMID: 19393959]

[46]   Faure E, Poissy J, Goffard A, *et al.* Distinct immune response in two MERS-CoV-infected patients: can we go from bench to bedside? PLoS One 2014; 9(2): e88716.
[http://dx.doi.org/10.1371/journal.pone.0088716] [PMID: 24551142]

[47]   Zhang H, Penninger JM, Li Y, Zhong N, Slutsky AS. Angiotensin-converting enzyme 2 (ACE2) as a SARS-CoV-2 receptor: molecular mechanisms and potential therapeutic target. Intensive Care Med 2020; 46(4): 586-90.
[http://dx.doi.org/10.1007/s00134-020-05985-9] [PMID: 32125455]

[48]   Wu Z, McGoogan JM. Characteristics of and important lessons from the coronavirus disease 2019 (COVID-19) outbreak in China: summary of a report of 72 314 cases from the Chinese Center for Disease Control and Prevention. JAMA 2020; 323(13): 1239-42.
[http://dx.doi.org/10.1001/jama.2020.2648] [PMID: 32091533]

[49]   Lui G, Ling L, Lai CK, *et al.* Viral dynamics of SARS-CoV-2 across a spectrum of disease severity in COVID-19. J Infect 2020; 81(2): 318-56.
[http://dx.doi.org/10.1016/j.jinf.2020.04.014] [PMID: 32315724]

[50]   Shi Y, Wang Y, Shao C, Huang J, Gan J, Huang X, *et al.* COVID-19 infection: the perspectives on immune responses. Cell Death Differ 2020; 27: 1451-4.
[http://dx.doi.org/10.1038/s41418-020-0530-3]

[51]   Jia HP, Look DC, Shi L, *et al.* ACE2 receptor expression and severe acute respiratory syndrome coronavirus infection depend on differentiation of human airway epithelia. J Virol 2005; 79(23): 14614-21.
[http://dx.doi.org/10.1128/JVI.79.23.14614-14621.2005] [PMID: 16282461]

[52]   Azkur AK, Akdis M, Azkur D, *et al.* Immune response to SARS-CoV-2 and mechanisms of immunopathological changes in COVID-19. Allergy 2020; 75(7): 1564-81.
[http://dx.doi.org/10.1111/all.14364] [PMID: 32396996]

[53]   Moore JB, June CH. Cytokine release syndrome in severe COVID-19. Science 2020; 368(6490): 473-4.
[http://dx.doi.org/10.1126/science.abb8925] [PMID: 32303591]

[54]   Wang T, Du Z, Zhu F, *et al.* Comorbidities and multi-organ injuries in the treatment of COVID-19. Lancet 2020; 395(10228): e52.
[http://dx.doi.org/10.1016/S0140-6736(20)30558-4] [PMID: 32171074]

CHAPTER 8

COVID-19: Current Diagnostic Approaches

Anwar Ahmed[1,2,*], **Fahad N. Almajhdi**[1,5], **Md. Imam Faizan**[3,4], **Tanveer Ahmad**[3] and **Shama Parveen**[4,*]

[1] *Centre of Excellence in Biotechnology Research, College of Science, King Saud University, Riyadh, Saudi Arabia*

[2] *Department of Biochemistry, College of Science, King Saud University, Riyadh, Saudi Arabia*

[3] *Multidisciplinary Centre for Advanced Research and Studies, Jamia Millia Islamia, New Delhi, India*

[4] *Centre for Interdisciplinary Research in Basic Sciences, Jamia Millia Islamia, New Delhi, India*

[5] *Department of Botany & Microbiology, College of Science, King Saud University, Riyadh, Saudi Arabia*

Abstract: Coronavirus Disease 2019 (COVID-19) has spread rapidly across the world, leading to a pandemic. The diagnostic methods for COVID-19 are still in the evolutionary phase since scientists are continuously trying to implement the latest technologies to achieve this objective. The infection is difficult to diagnose in the early stage as patients can stay asymptomatic from 2 to 14 days or more. A rapid, sensitive, and specific reverse transcription real-time PCR (rRT-PCR) detects viral RNA and is used to detect early infections to prevent disease spread. Although the gold standard in diagnosis, this method cannot be implemented in remote areas because of the requirements of expensive setup and trained staff. Therefore, a relatively economical method known as loop-mediated isothermal amplification (LAMP), which also detects viral RNA, is designed for use at point-of-care and remote settings. The non-nucleic acid based rapid antigen detection method detects viral antigen on nasal/pharyngeal specimen and implies current viral infection. The serological diagnostic methods detect early serological markers (IgM/IgG) in the serum of patients after a week of infection. Antigen detection and serological diagnostic methods are rapid, specific, and sensitive, with the potential to screen a large number of people during a pandemic. Thus, the genome and antigen-based diagnostic assay can detect the virus in the early stages of infection, while serological methods can be used to diagnose infections at later stages. The combination of nucleic acid and non-nucleic acid laboratory detection methods can assist in a timely and accurate diagnosis of COVID-19 that will be a step towards better patient management and containment of the pandemic.

* **Corresponding author Anwar Ahmed and Shama Parveen:** Centre of Excellence in Biotechnology Research, College of Science, King Saud University, Riyadh, Saudi Arabia and Centre for Interdisciplinary Research in Basic Sciences, Jamia Millia Islamia, New Delhi, India; E-mails: anahmed@ksu.edu.sa and sparveen2@jmi.ac.in, shamp25@ yahoo.com

Keywords: Asymptomatic, Antigen detection, COVID-19, Diagnosis, ELISA, SARS-CoV-2, LAMP, Rapid diagnostic test, Real-time PCR, Serology.

INTRODUCTION

China encountered cases of pneumonia of unknown etiology in Wuhan City of Hubei Province during December 2019. The causative agent was found to be a previously unknown coronavirus and was named severe acute respiratory syndrome coronavirus 2 (SARS-CoV-2) [1, 2], and the disease was called COVID-19. The SARS-CoV-2 threat emerged in China and later rapidly spread to other countries and was declared a pandemic on 11th March, 2020 by the WHO [3]. Rapid spreading patterns of SARS-CoV-2 suggested that its human-to-human transmission was quite efficient as compared to SARS-CoV [4, 5]. More than 24 million global cases and 0.83 million deaths till 31st August 2020, have been attributed to the virus.

Clinical characteristics alone cannot establish COVID-19 in patients as the early symptoms often overlap with that of flu, including fever, cough, or shortness of breath, weakness, body ache, *etc*. The infection spreads rapidly and is difficult to diagnose clinically in the early stages as patients can stay asymptomatic from 2 to 14 days or more. The initial diagnosis of COVID-19 was based on imaging, but this was not feasible for the diagnosis of a large part of the population and has health hazards associated with it [6, 7].

Since early laboratory diagnosis of COVID-19 is crucial for the prevention and control of this pandemic, the rapid, reliable, and quick nucleic acid-based detection approaches like rRT-PCR are currently used in the diagnosis. It is a robust, sensitive, and accurate diagnostic method and was developed to identify patients in the early stages of infection [8]. Although successfully implemented, rRT-PCR is expensive and requires costly instrumentation and trained staff; therefore, it cannot be implemented at point-of-care and remote settings. Therefore, another relatively cheap method of target DNA or RNA sequence amplification, known as loop-mediated isothermal amplification (LAMP), has been designed. LAMP has some advantages of being cheap, sensitive, and specific and can be applied at point-of-care and remote testing [9, 10]. Various LAMP assays have been developed for SARS-CoV-2 detection [11, 15].

RNA viruses (SARS-CoV-2) have an error-prone replication system that may affect the binding potential of the oligos in rRT-PCR and LAMP and result in misdiagnosis or false negatives. Therefore, non-nucleic acid based serological diagnostic tools are used wherein the earliest serological marker (IgM or IgG) in the serum of the person are detected after 5 or 6 days of infection to know the person's exposure to the particular pathogen. Various serological diagnostic (SD) methods like Rapid diagnostic tests (RDTs), Enzyme-linked immunosorbent assay (ELISA), Neutralization assay (NA), and Chemiluminescent immunoassay (CLIA) detect serum antibodies against highly immunogenic spike (S) or nucleocapsid (N) protein. Serological diagnostic tests are rapid and can be used for point-of-care testing to detect qualitatively the presence or absence of antibodies against a pathogen. Another non-nucleic acid based antigen detection test detects viral antigen in nasal/pharyngeal specimens of the patient. It is rapid, specific, and implies current infection. The present review summarizes all the molecular, serological, and antigen detection tests that are available for the diagnosis of SARS-CoV-2 infection. Early and accurate diagnosis of the infection will assist in timely management of clinical cases that will be a step towards containment of the ongoing pandemic.

SAMPLE COLLECTION

The preferred samples include nasopharyngeal (NP) swabs/aspirates or other upper respiratory tract specimens, such as throat swabs and saliva, for initial screening for SARS-CoV-2. Samples are taken with a flocked swab, preferably with aluminum or plastic shaft, to collect maximum quantity with minimum PCR inhibitors. The NP swabs are preferred due to the ease of collection by the healthcare worker and are comfortable for the patient as well. The samples (swabs) should be collected in a viral transport medium and transported to the laboratory immediately in an icebox to prevent degradation of viral nucleic acid. Improper sample collection and inadequate processing may lead to false results.

The lower respiratory tract sample collection includes bronchoalveolar lavage from the patients showing severe pneumonia. Further, stool samples were also positive for some patients showing severe pneumonia. The healthcare worker collecting the sample should take appropriate precautions, including the use of full Personal Protective Equipment (PPE) kit. The processing of the samples in the laboratory should be done in BSL2/3 facilities using the WHO guidelines and appropriate precautions.

REAL-TIME REVERSE TRANSCRIPTASE-PCR (RT-PCR)

The complete genome sequencing of the SARS-CoV-2 was a fundamental requirement for designing and development of nucleic acid based diagnostic tests. The genome sequence of the SARS-CoV-2 (WH-Human_1) was revealed and it had 14 ORFs that encode 27 proteins like the SARS-like bat coronaviruses [16 - 18]. The genome sequence analysis also identified some specific sequences associated with only the SARS-CoV-2 genome [19]. The primers and probes are designed from these specific sequences and are the backbone of the polymerase chain reaction (PCR) based diagnostics. The PCR based detection methods are rapid, sensitive, and specific and, therefore, considered as the gold standard for the detection of viruses and other microorganisms. The modified form of PCR, the real-time reverse transcriptase-PCR (rRT-PCR), is considered the most effective and reliable test for the detection of SARS-CoV-2 since it quantitates the nucleic acid present in the sample [20 - 22].

The rRT-PCR is performed with genetic material obtained from clinical samples. SARS-CoV-2 genomic RNA extraction is carried out, followed by its conversion to cDNA by reverse transcription. PCR amplification of the target regions in the genomic cDNA is carried out in multiple cycles. With each cycle, DNA is synthesized and a complementary fluorescence probe or fluorescent dye binds to the newly synthesized DNA, thus emitting radiations to be recorded. This cyclic process keeps repeating until sufficient fluorescent signals are generated to be detected by the system. The cycle number at which the sufficient signals are observed is called the cycle threshold (Ct). The fluorescence is monitored in real-time throughout the reaction and is displayed as an amplification plot for each reaction (Fig. **1**) [23].

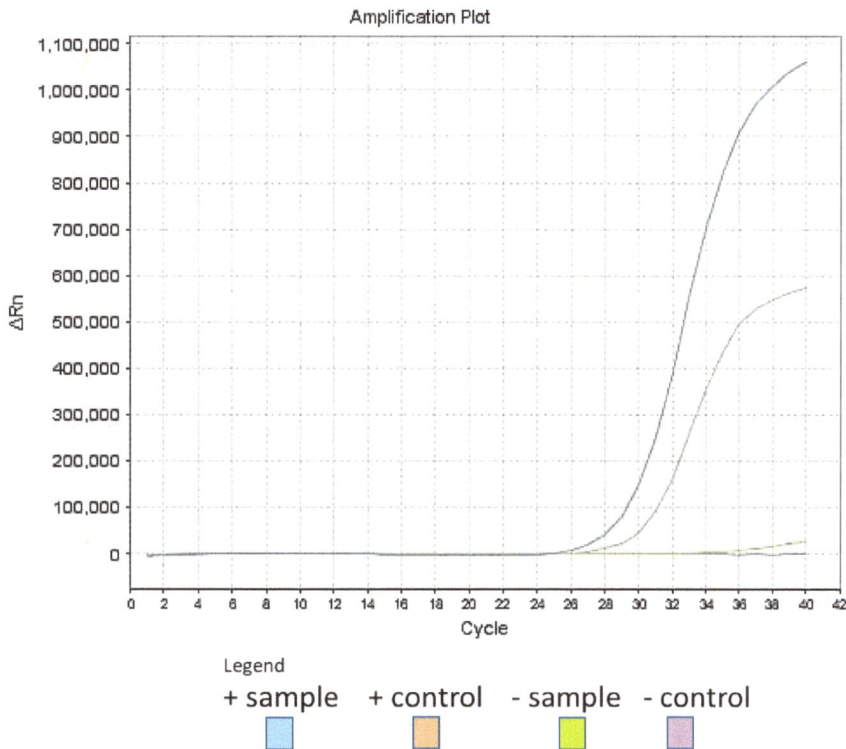

Fig. (1). Amplification plot of real-time rRT-PCR assay. The positive sample and positive control show amplification while the negative control and negative sample did not show any amplification.

The lower the Ct value, the higher is the viral RNA load and vice versa. It may be noted that Ct values of patients with severe pneumonia are lower than individuals with mild symptoms of COVID-19. The real-time PCR can give a positive result on the first day of the appearance of COVID-19 symptoms and the peak is usually observed within the first week itself. The PCR positivity in the infected patients usually starts declining by the end of 3 weeks, and later, it becomes undetectable. However, some patients have shown PCR positivity after 6 weeks of initial confirmation of the infection of COVID-19.

The target genes for RT-PCR based diagnostic for SARS-CoV-2 are RNA dependent RNA polymerase (RdRp), envelope gene (E), ORF1ab fragment, nucleocapsid protein gene (N), S gene, and the non-structural polyprotein pp1ab [19, 24 - 28]. Some diagnostic kits target more than one gene or one region in the viral genome to improve the specificity of the detection [17, 19, 29]. The infection is confirmed in the patients when the amplification of both the genes or both target regions in the genome is positive [26]. Some of the single gene and double gene target-based RT-PCR diagnostic kits for SARS-CoV-2 are commercially available (Table **1**).

Table 1. Commercially available RT-PCR kits for the detection of SARS-CoV-2.

Country of Origin	Commercial Kit Name	Target Genes	Company
Germany	RealStar® SARS-CoV-2 RT-PCR Kit	E, S	Altona Diagnostics
China	Real-Time Fluorescent RT-PCR Kit for Detecting SARS-CoV-2	ORF1ab	BGI
Korea	RADI COVID-19 Detection kit	RdRp, S	KH Medical
Germany	RIDA®GENE SARS-CoV-2 Real-time PCR test kit	E	R-Biopharm AG
Spain	VIASURE SARS-CoV-2 S gene Real-Time PCR Detection Kit	ORF1ab, N	CerTest Biotec
Korea	Allplex™ 2019-nCoV Assay	RdRp, N, Ea	Seegene
England	Primerdesign Ltd COVID-19 genesig® Real-Time PCR assay	RdRp	PrimerDesign
USA	CDC 2019-Novel Coronavirus (2019-nCoV) Real-Time RT-PCR Diagnostic Panel	RNase P, N	Centers for Disease Control and Prevention (CDC), USA
USA	LabCorp COVID-19 RT-PCR test	RNase P	Laboratory Corporation of America
Korea	2019 Novel Coronavirus Real-time PCR Kit	N gene, E gene, and RdRp gene	Kogene Biotech

(Table 1) cont.....

Country of Origin	Commercial Kit Name	Target Genes	Company
Korea	AccuPower ® SARS-CoV-2 Real-Time RT-PCR Kit	E and RdRp gene	Bioneer
USA	Cobas SARS-CoV-2 test	ORF1 and E genes	Roche Molecular Systems
Hungary	GSD NovaPrime® SARS-CoV-2 (COVID-19) Real-Time PCR	N gene	Eurofins Technologies
USA	Abbott RealTime SARSCoV-2 Amplification Reagent Kit	RdRp and N-genes	Abbott Molecular Division Inc.
USA	QIAstat-Dx Respiratory 2019-nCoV Panel	Orf1ab and E genes	Qiagen
Turkey	Bio-Speedy Covid-19 QPCR detection kit	RdRp gene	Bioeksen, Buyukdere
France	ARGENE® SARS-COV-2 R-GENE®	RdRp and N-genes	BIOMERIEUX S.A
USA	BD SARS-CoV-2 Reagents for BD MAX System	N gene (N1 and N2 region)	Becton Dickinson and Company
USA	TaqPath COVID-19 CE-IVD RT-PCR Kit	Orf-1ab, N Protein, S Protein, MS2	Life Technologies Corporation
USA	Lyra SARS-CoV-2 Assay	non-structural Polyprotein (pp1ab)	Quidel

Although rRT-PCR is extremely sensitive and specific and, therefore, a gold-standard for the detection of various pathogens, it still has some limitations. A positive test result indicates the presence of viral genetic material but does not suggest the viability and, thus, the transmissibility of the virus. False negatives are often encountered during COVID-19 rRT-PCR tests; therefore, the internal control, the positive control, and negative control are involved in the experimental setup. The requirement of sophisticated instrumentation, constant and regular electric supply and trained staff to accurately run the rRT-PCR tests make this technology less feasible in remote areas and for various point-of-care settings [30].

LOOP-MEDIATED ISOTHERMAL AMPLIFICATION (LAMP)

Scientists have developed another relatively cheap method of isothermal one-step amplification of target DNA or RNA sequence known as loop-mediated isothermal amplification (LAMP) [9, 31]. LAMP has many advantages of being cheap, sensitive, and specific and can be used in remote areas and for various point-of-care testings with minimum facilities since the procedure does not require a thermal cycler and can be performed in a heating block or water bath [9].

LAMP requires the selection of the regions of the viral genome that are highly conserved. The published full-length genome sequences of SARS-CoV-2 available at different genome databases can be retrieved and aligned using MEGA and BioEdit software [32 - 34]. The entropy plot, which shows variability at individual nucleotide positions in the alignment [35 - 37], can reveal low entropy sites (highly conserved sites) that can be considered for primer designing for LAMP reaction [38].

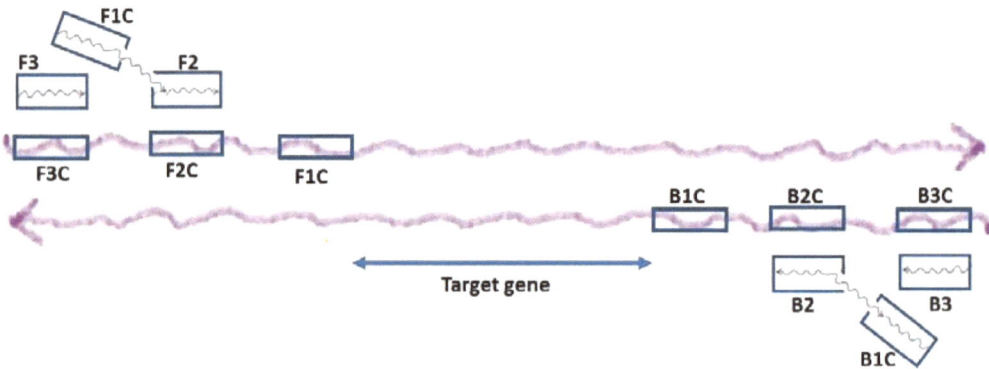

Fig. (2). Primers used and target region selected for LAMP assay. Initially, the FIP (F1C+F2) and BIP (B1C+B2) primers anneal to the complementary regions F2C and B2C in the target region and synthesis takes place. This is followed by annealing of outer primers (F3 or B3) to complementary regions F3C and B3C and results in the formation of self-hybridizing loop structures. Subsequent reactions result in the formation of huge number of different cauliflower shaped DNA structures with multiple loops and different stem lengths.

LAMP is performed at constant temperature and makes use of single strand-displacing DNA polymerase to generate a huge amount of double-stranded concatemeric amplicons within an hour that can be detected by naked eyes [9]. The technique makes use of single strand-displacing Bst DNA polymerase and a set of 4 primers (FIP [F1C+F2], BIP [B1C+B2], F3, and B3) that are specific to 6 target regions (B3, B2, B1, F1c, F2c and F3c) to generate millions of DNA or RNA target copies within an hour [9] (Fig. **2**). In LAMP reaction, initially, the inner primers *i.e.*, FIP or BIP, anneal to complementary sequences F2c or B2c in the target region. In a subsequent reaction, invasion by inner primer takes place that displaces the strand with the help of modified DNA polymerase and separates the target dsDNA. The F3 or B3 outer primers then anneal to F3c and B3c in the target DNA and invade again and to form a self-hybridizing loop structure. This results in dumbbell-shaped DNA structure formation and is the starting structure for exponential amplification. This results in the amplification of different sized

DNA structures with stem-loop of different lengths and different cauliflower resembling structures with numerous loops.

LAMP assay can be extremely sensitive compared to PCR and can even detect 10 gene copies in a reaction [10]. A modified form of LAMP can use intercalating fluorescent dyes for real-time observation of amplification [39]. Large quantities of DNA are amplified in LAMP reactions and it is, therefore, possible to detect the product colorimetrically with the naked eye [40 - 42]. Moreover, no purification of the starting material is required for LAMP and the sample can be used directly in the reaction [43 - 45]. These features make LAMP a possible technique to conduct high throughput tests with a non-purified sample without any sophisticated instrument for detection in remote areas and for various point-of-care settings. LAMP has been in use to detect SARS [46], Dengue [47], influenza [48], HSV [49], CMV [50], HPV [51] and many other viruses. Although LAMP assays for SARS-CoV-2 detection are also available [11 - 14, 52, 53], they are yet to be commercialized (Table **2**).

Table 2. LAMP protocols reported for the detection of SARS-CoV-2.

Target Region	Detection Method	References
orf1ab, S gene and N gene	Colorimetric change	[13]
orf1ab and *S* genes	Turbidity monitoring and visual observation	[54]
Nucleocapsid gene	Colorimetric change	[52]
Nsp3, Spike, and Orf8	Colorimetric detection	[11]
N gene	Colorimetric change	[55]
orf1ab and N gene	Colorimetric change	[56]
The 2941-3420 nt of the COVID-19 Wuhan-H--1 complete genome (MN908947)	SYBR Green I by eye, fluorescence, or gel electrophoresis	[12]
Orf 1a, S, Orf 8, and N	Fluorescence	[57]
RdRP and E genes	Hydroxynaphthol violet to blue color	[58]

LAMP-based diagnosis also has some limitations. Like rRT-PCR, this test also indicates the presence of viral genetic material but does not suggest the viability and, thus, transmissibility of the virus. The negative LAMP tests for COVID-19 do not give information about the patient's previous infection or the immunity status. The technology is emerging and is likely to improve in the future to accommodate more efficient detection of emerging viral pathogens.

SEROLOGICAL DIAGNOSIS

RNA viruses have an error-prone replication system due to which mutations are introduced into its genome. The error rate is high, and therefore, intra-host variants of SARS-CoV-2 can be observed. These variations may be an adaptation of the virus to the new environment or a mechanism to evade the host immune response. This is also a step towards higher rates of sustained human-to-human transmission, which is a potential threat to public health. This error-prone replication system of the virus may result in the emergence of mutations at the targeted sites, which affect the binding potential of the oligos and/or probes in rRT-PCR and LAMP assays and may result in misdiagnosis or false negatives. To overcome this issue in diagnosis, the serological diagnostics are used wherein the earliest serological marker (IgM or IgG) in the serum of the patients is detected.

Serological methods are the indirect measurements of the host immune response to an infection. These are serum-based tests that give an idea about the person's exposure to a pathogen by detecting serological markers against it. These tests are generally performed in patients with mild to moderate illness and assist in the identification of patients with a good immune system that are being protected from becoming seriously ill. Serological diagnosis of SARS-CoV-2 has become essential in the community to assess the extent of COVID-19 spread by quantification of the number of infections, including asymptomatic or recovered individuals. This contrasts with the rRT-PCR and LAMP tests which only indicate the presence of pathogen genetic material and do not specify person's past infection. Serological tests, therefore, provide details of the prevalence of a disease in a population by diagnosing individuals for antibodies against the virus proteins.

The antibodies are the earliest serological markers against the infective agent that begin to develop in the early stages of infection. Total antibodies to SARS-CoV-2 are observed by the fifth day of infection, but a higher level can be seen in the second and third week of infection [59]. IgM are the earliest markers observed after infection and reach its peak level in the third week post-infection. During week four, almost equal levels of IgM and IgG are observed. But during the fifth week, the level of IgM declines and by the seventh week, it is almost non-traceable [60, 61]. Whereas the level of IgG has been observed to be static after four weeks and is also observed till the seventh week [62]. IgM and IgG antibodies are generated against the abundant protein like nucleocapsid protein (N) and the spike or attachment (S) protein's receptor-binding domain (RBD) of SARS-CoV-2.

The S protein is found on the surface of the virus and its receptor-binding domain (RBD-S) helps in the attachment of the virus to host cells through interaction with angiotensin-converting enzyme 2 (ACE2) receptor [63]. Whereas the N protein is an abundant protein and is involved in the transcription, replication, and packaging of the viral genome [64, 65]. Both the S and N proteins have been reported to be highly immunogenic [66 - 68] and, therefore, are potential antigenic targets for serological diagnosis of COVID-19 infection. The antibodies against RBD are neutralizing and are, therefore, specific, while the antibodies generated against N are abundant. Therefore, including the antibodies generated against both the antigens (N and RBD) would result in specificity and sensitivity [60]. A study conducted on the sensitivities of the rRT-PCR and ELISA (IgM against nucleocapsid protein) showed that during the first 5.5 days of infection, the sensitivity of rRT-PCR is maximum, whereas after 5.5 days, the sensitivity of ELISA is higher [69]. Therefore, testing the patient first with rRT-PCR and later in the second week by ELISA can increase the accuracy of the diagnosis.

Serological diagnostic tests are rapid and can be used for point of care testing to detect the presence or absence of antibodies against N or RBD-S of SARS-CoV-2. However, the serological tests have disadvantages due to cross-reactivity with SARS and perhaps other Coronaviruses. Serological tests like RDT and CLIA are rapid tests, whereas ELISA may take 3-6 hours for completion of the reaction. Neutralization assay (NA) is a culture-based diagnosis, therefore, it takes 3-5 days to complete. RDT is a qualitative test that reveals the presence or absence of antibodies against viruses whereas ELISA and CLIA are quantitative in nature. NA detects virus inhibitory antibodies present in patient serum and takes many days before the result is displayed. These serological tests are summarized below:

RAPID DIAGNOSTIC TEST (RDT)

Rapid diagnostic tests (RDTs) are qualitative (positive or negative) tests and detect the presence or absence of antibodies against the pathogen present in patient serum by utilizing lateral flow strip technology (Fig. **3A**). The RDT kits are portable and can be used with minimum resources available and for various point-of-care testings. They require no special training and are easy to perform without the use of any sophisticated and costly instrument. The assay can provide results within 15 minutes and reduce the burden of repeated visits of the patient/relatives to the diagnostic center or hospitals, thus also reducing their risk of exposure to the disease. The RDTs also assist in providing the correct treatment regimen to the patient by avoiding presumptive treatment.

These assays use blood, saliva, or nasal swab fluid samples as diagnostic material. The samples are applied to the marked well on the strip followed by drops of the buffer. The fluid is allowed to move through the strip to the other end. Within minutes the colored lines develop at the indicated sites suggesting positive or negative results (Fig. **3B**). In COVID-19 patients, RDTs measure for patient early-stage antibodies (IgM) and late-stage antibodies (IgG) against N or S proteins.

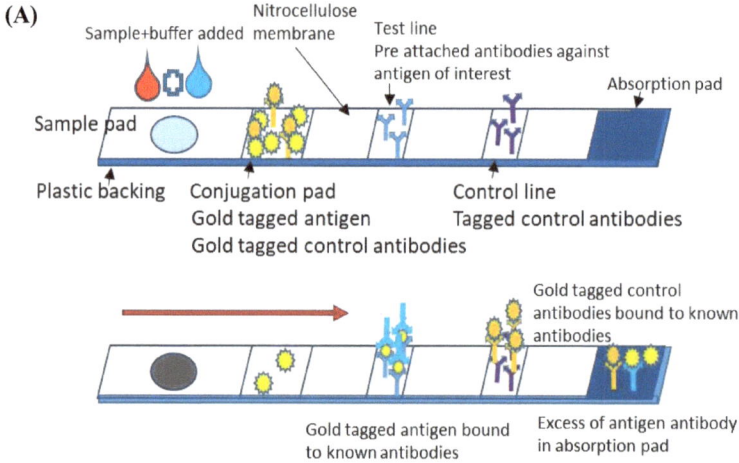

(A)

Fig. (3A). Schematic diagram for RDT. At one end of the strip on the conjugation pad, indicator-labeled antibodies (control antibodies) and indicator labeled target antigen are placed. A second antibody specific to the different epitope of the target antigens is bound to the test line. Another antibody specific for the control antibody is bound at the control line. Blood, serum, or saliva mixed with buffer are added to the sample pad. A capillary flow draws the fluid to the other end of the strip. If antibodies are present in the sample, they bind to the labeled antigen in a conjugation pad and are trapped on the test line and become visible. Tagged control antibodies are trapped on the control line and become visible.

(B)

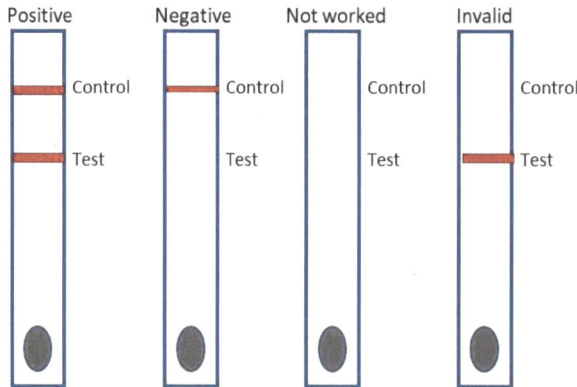

Fig. (3B). Interpretation of results: Positive: Two distinct colored lines appear, one in the control region and another in the test region. **Negative:** Only one colored line appears in the control region. **No Line:** Test has not worked. Repeat the test with a new test device. If the problem persists, discontinue using the test kit. **Invalid:** No control line appears. Reason may be the insufficient specimen volume or incorrect procedural technique.

ENZYME-LINKED IMMUNOSORBENT ASSAY (ELISA)

It is a plate-based qualitative or quantitative immunological assay technique designed to measure antibodies, antigens, and proteins in biological samples (whole blood, plasma, or serum samples). ELISA can be performed in a large number of samples at a time; thus, it produces rapid results. ELISA has limitations as the tests require time for standardization and its commercialization needs approval from concerned authorities. ELISA is a well established, quick, and cost-effective laboratory technique and produces results in 1 to 3 hours of sample collection.

ELISA for COVID-19 includes a plate with an antigen (N or S protein) immobilized on it. Patient samples are incubated with the immobilized protein to bind to antibodies (IgG or IgM) present in the patient sample. After washing, the bound antibody-antigen complex is incubated with another antibody that is linked to an enzyme. Detection is based on the production of a color or fluorescent signal by the activity of the conjugated enzyme on incubation with a substrate (Fig. **4**).

CHEMILUMINESCENT IMMUNOASSAY (CLIA)

This is a laboratory technique used to detect immune response (antibodies) against the virus or its specific protein (N and S protein of SARS-CoV-2) in combination with the luminescence detection system (Fig. **4**). CLIA is a quantitative, highly specific, and sensitive test and is conducted in a laboratory using patients' whole blood, plasma, or serum sample [70]. The test makes use of enzyme-labeled antibodies, which generate luminescent signals to be identified by a detector. The reaction proceeds with the mixing of patient's sample with known viral fixed protein followed by enzyme-labeled antibodies. The viral protein reacting antibodies (primary IgG, IgM, and IgA) in the patient sample (if present) will form a complex with the protein. The complex is detected by the addition of enzyme-labeled secondary antibodies that are specific to the primary antibody. On the addition of substrate to the complex, the enzymatic reaction occurs that produces light. The intensity of the light emitted is proportional to the number of antibodies present in a patient sample.

Another modified form of test is chemiluminescent microparticle immunoassay that makes use of protein-coated microparticles known as chemiluminescent microparticle instead of simple protein. For SARS-CoV-2 antibodies detection, various methods, including colloidal gold and chemiluminescence immunoassay, are available [71].

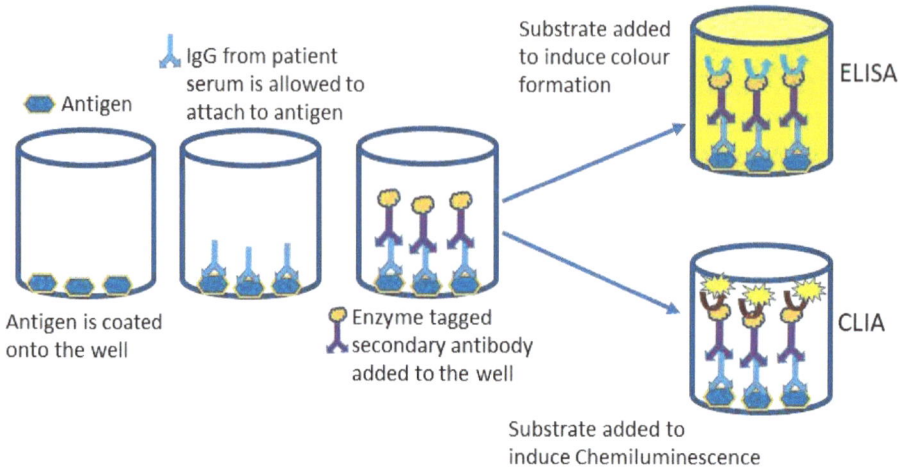

Fig. (4). The basic setup in ELISA and CLIA assay. The antigen (target S or N protein) is immobilized on the surface of microplate wells. Serum antibodies (the primary antibody, if present) against the target protein bind to the antigen of interest. The primary antibodies are then recognized by anti-primary (secondary antibody) antibodies conjugated to an enzyme. In ELISA, the conjugated enzyme gives color on the addition of substrate, while in CLIA, luminescence is observed.

NEUTRALIZATION ASSAY (NA)

This assay is used to identify the neutralizing antibodies (NAbs) that are induced either by infection or vaccination against virus. Neutralization assays use patient's antibodies (from whole blood, serum, or plasma) to prevent viral infection of cells in a laboratory setting. The assay detects active and effective antibodies that can block virus replication through binding to some vital protein on the virus. These NAbs thus provide protection against the viral infection or are used for the treatment of the infection by blocking viral replication. Vaccines against smallpox, polio, and influenza viruses have been developed based on higher levels of NAbs generated against their respective targets [72].

Plasma fusion, which is also known as plasma therapy, is a passive immune therapy that has been effectively used to treat some viral infections. The success of the therapy lies with the higher amount of NAbs in the plasma of the recovered patient as a donor [73]. Plasma fusion therapy has been successfully used to treat patients with viral infections such as SARS-CoV [74], influenza [75], and Ebola viruses [73]. Although the NAbs data in COVID-19 is still in the preliminary stages of research, the therapy was considered for its treatment by transfusion of plasma from COVID-19 recovered patients and has shown some promising results as therapy for its prophylaxis and treatment [76]. The commercially available diagnostic kits for detection of SARS-CoV-2 based on serology are summarized in Table **3**.

Table 3. Commercially available serological kits for the diagnosis of COVID-19.

Commercial Kit Name	Target	Technology	Company
Alinity i SARS-CoV-2 IgG	Nucleocapsid	Chemiluminescent Microparticle Immuno Assay (CMIA)	Abbott
Architect SARS-CoV-2 IgG	Nucleocapsid	CMIA	Abbott
Anti-SARS-CoV-2 Rapid Test	Spike	Lateral Flow (RDT)	Autobio
Platelia SARS-CoV-2 Total Ab	Nucleocapsid	ELISA	Bio-Rad Laboratories, Inc
qSARS-CoV-2 IgG/IgM Rapid Test	Spike and Nucleocapsid	Lateral Flow (RDT)	Cellex, Inc.
LIAISON SARS-CoV-2 S1/S2 IgG	Spike	CMIA	DiaSorin
SARS-CoV-2 RBD IgG test	Spike	ELISA	Emory Medical Laboratories
SARS-COV-2 ELISA (IgG)	Spike	ELISA	EUROIMMUN
RightSign COVID-19 IgG/IgM Rapid Test Cassette	Spike	Lateral Flow (RDT)	Hangzhou Biotest Biotech
COVID-19 IgG/IgM Rapid Test Cassette	Spike	Lateral Flow (RDT)	Healgen
SCoV-2 Detect IgG ELISA	Spike	ELISA	InBios
Mt. Sinai Laboratory COVID-19 ELISA Antibody Test	Spike	ELISA	Mount Sinai Hospital Clinical Laboratory
VITROS Anti-SARS-CoV-2 IgG test	Spike	Chemiluminescence immune assay (CLIA)	Ortho-Clinical Diagnostics, Inc.
VITROS Immunodiagnostic Products Anti-SARS-CoV-2 Total Reagent Pack and Calibrator	Spike	CLIA	Ortho-Clinical Diagnostics, Inc.
Elecsys Anti-SARS-CoV-2	Nucleocapsid	Electro-chemiluminescence immunoassay (ECLIA)	Roche
ADVIA Centaur SARS-CoV-2 Total (COV2T)	Spike	CMIA	Siemens Healthcare Diagnostics
Vibrant COVID-19 Ab Assay	Spike and Nucleocapsid	CLIA	Vibrant America Clinical Labs
New York SARS-CoV Microsphere Immunoassay for Antibody Detection	Nucleocapsid	Microsphere Immunoassay (MIA)	Wadsworth Center, New York State Department of Health
Atellica IM SARS-CoV-2 Total (COV2T)	Spike	CMIA	Siemens Healthcare Diagnostics

(Table 3) cont.....

Commercial Kit Name	Target	Technology	Company
Dimension EXL SARS-CoV-2 Total antibody assay (CV2T)	Spike	ELISA	Siemens Healthcare Diagnostics
Dimension Vista SARS-CoV-2 Total antibody assay (COV2T)	Spike	ELISA	Siemens Healthcare Diagnostics

RAPID ANTIGEN DETECTION TEST (RADT)

During the initial stages of the pandemic, there have been two types of diagnostic tests approved for SARS-CoV-2 detection, the polymerase chain reaction (PCR) tests and serological tests, thus, identifying an active COVID-19 infection and late infection, respectively. The latest approved test is a rapid antigen detection test (RADT) for use in the detection of SARS-CoV-2 antigens in an ongoing pandemic. They are non-nucleic acid strip based rapid detection test utilizing nasal/nasopharyngeal swab as a testing material to directly detect viral antigen (nucleocapsid protein) in the specimen (Table **4**). RADTs are primarily lateral flow immuno-assays utilizing colloid gold conjugate pad together with the membrane strip that is pre-coated on a test line with antibodies against the antigen of SARS-CoV-2. The test is similar to CLIA shown above in serology with minor alterations. In serology (CLIA), antibodies against the SARS-CoV-2 antigens are detected in the serum of the patient, while in RADT, an antigen is detected in the specimen from the patient. If the specimen withdrawn from a nasopharyngeal swab has SARS-CoV-2 antigens, a colored band appears on the test line due to the formation of antigen–antibody gold conjugate complex. The N protein of SARS-CoV-2 is an abundant antigen that can be identified in the patients. Therefore, antibodies are used against nucleocapsid to detect SARS-CoV-2 presence in the specimen. Antigen detection tests are rapid and provide results within minutes. The sensitivity of the RADT is lower than that of RT-PCR, as shown in earlier studies where enzyme-linked immunosorbent assays (ELISA) developed for SARS-CoV have limits of detection of 50 pg/ ml [77, 78]. The false-negative are also major concerns with RADT and are due to low viral load and inconsistency in sampling or sample processing [79]. A recent study showed that RADT for N protein of SARS-CoV-2 has been shown to be effective with a higher viral load specimen (Ct value of $\leq$30 in qRT-PCR) while the specimen with Ct value of $\leq$40 has shown less sensitivity of detection [80]. Therefore, RADT assay can be useful in excluding patients with high viral loads. The specificity of RADT for SARS-CoV-2 is also a concern due to the potential cross-reactivity of SARS-CoV-2 antigens with the other human CoV. Efforts are going on to increase the sensitivity of the RADT by using monoclonal antibodies against the SARS-CoV-2 antigens and utilizing more sensitive colloidal gold-labeled immunoglobulins [81, 82]. Furthermore, RADT can be improved for clinical utilization by somehow increasing the concentration of the antigen to be detected and by amplifying the detection phase [82-83].

Table 4. Commercially available rapid antigen diagnosis tests (RADT) for COVID-19.

Commercial Kit Name	Target	Technology	Company
BinaxNOW COVID-19 Ag Card	Nucleocapsid	CLIA	Abbott Diagnostics Scarborough, Inc
LumiraDx SARS-CoV-2 Ag Test	Nucleocapsid	CLIA	LumiraDx UK Ltd.
BD Veritor System for Rapid Detection of SARS-CoV-2	Nucleocapsid	CLIA	Becton, Dickinson and Company (BD)
Sofia SARS Antigen FIA	Nucleocapsid	CLIA	Quidel Corporation

Despite many limitations, the use of RADT has advantages of rapid detection of antigen (15–30 min compared to hours for RT-PCR), easy interpretation of results, and low technical skill requirement. Together with minimum infrastructure requirement compared to nucleic acid based diagnostics, the RADT is worth pursuing.

CONCLUDING REMARKS

Viral diagnostics is the emerging field of research and must incorporate newer technologies to increase the sensitivity and specificity of detection of the pathogens. We have reviewed different approaches that are available for laboratory diagnosis of SARS-CoV-2 infection. The nucleic acid-based molecular diagnostics (rRT-PCR and LAMP) are rapid and sensitive and can detect the virus in the early stages of infections, while serological diagnostics can be used to detect infection in late stages in patients with mild to moderate illness (Fig. **5**). Recently introduced antigen detection tests (RADT) are rapid, specific but less sensitive than nucleic acid based tests. RADT can be used to sort out the high viral load of patients from asymptomatic or low viral load patients due to its high throughput potential. Serological diagnosis can be used for high throughput mass screening during a pandemic and, therefore, can determine the extent of the spread of infections in the community. Thus, testing the patient first with molecular diagnostics or RADT and later in the second week by serological tests can increase the accuracy of the diagnosis of COVID-19.

A major concern is the screening of asymptomatic individuals using a random testing approach in a community. However, one of the major unanswered questions includes the exact duration of the immune response in asymptomatic and symptomatic individuals and its correlation to disease severity. The serological tests are based on this immune response, it is likely that the guidelines for these tests can be modified in the near future. Therefore, the forthcoming months will add to the existing data of screening of the suspected COVID-19 patients using molecular, antigenic, or serological approaches. However, the timely detection of SARS-CoV-2 is likely to decrease the community transmission of the infection that will assist in saving mankind from the menace of COVID-19.

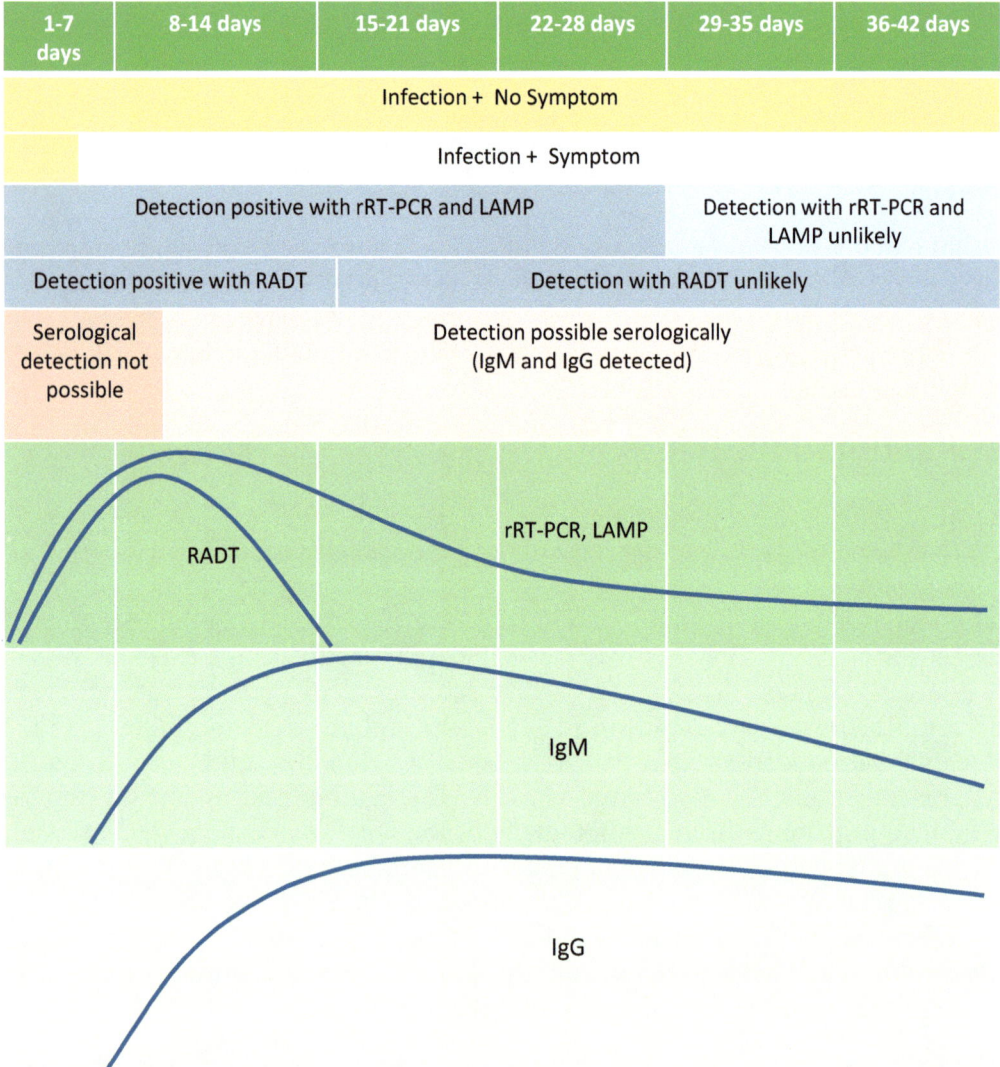

Fig. (5). Timings for successful detection of SARS-CoV-2 by nucleic acid based (rRT-PCR and LAMP), antigen (RADT) and serology based diagnostic tests post-infection.

CONSENT FOR PUBLICATION

Not Applicable.

CONFLICT OF INTEREST

The author declares no conflict of interest, financial or otherwise.

ACKNOWLEDGEMENTS

We extend appreciation to the Centre of Excellence in Biotechnology Research, Deanship of Scientific Research, King Saud University, Riyadh, Saudi Arabia, for support. The research in our laboratory is funded by the Council of Scientific and Industrial Research (CSIR), India (37(1697)17/EMR-II) and Central Council for Research in Unani Medicine (CCRUM), Ministry of Ayurveda, Yoga and Naturopathy, Unani, Siddha and Homeopathy (AYUSH) (F.No.3-63/2019-CCRUM/Tech).

REFERENCES

[1]   Zhu N, Zhang D, Wang W, *et al.* China novel coronavirus investigating and research team. A novel coronavirus from patients with pneumonia in China, 2019. N Engl J Med 2020; 382(8): 727-33.
      [http://dx.doi.org/10.1056/NEJMoa2001017] [PMID: 31978945]

[2]   The species Severe acute respiratory syndrome-related coronavirus: classifying 2019-nCoV and naming it SARS-CoV-2. Nat Microbiol 2020; 5(4): 536-44.
      [http://dx.doi.org/10.1038/s41564-020-0695-z] [PMID: 32123347]

[3]   Mahase E. Covid-19: WHO declares pandemic because of "alarming levels" of spread, severity, and inaction. BMJ 2020; 368: m1036.
      [http://dx.doi.org/10.1136/bmj.m1036] [PMID: 32165426]

[4]   Chen N, Zhou M, Dong X, *et al.* Epidemiological and clinical characteristics of 99 cases of 2019 novel coronavirus pneumonia in Wuhan, China: a descriptive study. Lancet 2020; 395(10223): 507-13.
      [http://dx.doi.org/10.1016/S0140-6736(20)30211-7] [PMID: 32007143]

[5]   Chan JF, Yuan S, Kok KH, *et al.* A familial cluster of pneumonia associated with the 2019 novel coronavirus indicating person-to-person transmission: a study of a family cluster. Lancet 2020; 395(10223): 514-23.
      [http://dx.doi.org/10.1016/S0140-6736(20)30154-9] [PMID: 31986261]

[6]   Chung M, Bernheim A, Mei X, *et al.* CT imaging features of 2019 novel coronavirus (2019-nCoV). Radiology 2020; 295(1): 202-7.
      [http://dx.doi.org/10.1148/radiol.2020200230] [PMID: 32017661]

[7]   Pan Y, Guan H. Imaging changes in patients with 2019-nCov. Eur Radiol 2020; 30(7): 3612-3.
      [http://dx.doi.org/10.1007/s00330-020-06713-z] [PMID: 32025790]

[8]   Corman VM, Drosten C. Authors' response: SARS-CoV-2 detection by real-time RT-PCR. Euro Surveill 2020; 25(21): 2001035.
      [http://dx.doi.org/10.2807/1560-7917.ES.2020.25.21.2001035] [PMID: 32489177]

[9]   Notomi T, Okayama H, Masubuchi H, *et al.* Loop-mediated isothermal amplification of DNA. Nucleic Acids Res 2000; 28(12): E63.
      [http://dx.doi.org/10.1093/nar/28.12.e63] [PMID: 10871386]

[10]   Shirato K, Yano T, Senba S, *et al.* Detection of Middle East respiratory syndrome coronavirus using reverse transcription loop-mediated isothermal amplification (RT-LAMP). Virol J 2014; 11: 139.
[http://dx.doi.org/10.1186/1743-422X-11-139] [PMID: 25103205]

[11]   Park GS, Ku K, Baek SH, *et al.* Development of reverse transcription loop-mediated isothermal amplification assays targeting severe acute respiratory syndrome coronavirus 2 (SARS-CoV-2). J Mol Diagn 2020; 22(6): 729-35.
[http://dx.doi.org/10.1016/j.jmoldx.2020.03.006] [PMID: 32276051]

[12]   Lamb LE, Bartolone SN, Ward E, Chancellor MB. Rapid detection of novel coronavirus/Severe Acute Respiratory Syndrome Coronavirus 2 (SARS-CoV-2) by reverse transcription-loop-mediated isothermal amplification. PLoS One 2020; 15(6): e0234682.
[http://dx.doi.org/10.1371/journal.pone.0234682] [PMID: 32530929]

[13]   Huang WE, Lim B, Hsu CC, *et al.* RT-LAMP for rapid diagnosis of coronavirus SARS-CoV-2. Microb Biotechnol 2020; 13(4): 950-61.
[http://dx.doi.org/10.1111/1751-7915.13586] [PMID: 32333644]

[14]   James AS, Alawneh JI. COVID-19 infection diagnosis: potential impact of isothermal amplification technology to reduce community transmission of SARS-CoV-2. Diagnostics (Basel) 2020; 10(6): E399.
[http://dx.doi.org/10.3390/diagnostics10060399] [PMID: 32545412]

[15]   Kashir J, Yaqinuddin A. Loop mediated isothermal amplification (LAMP) assays as a rapid diagnostic for COVID-19. Med Hypotheses 2020; 141: 109786.
[http://dx.doi.org/10.1016/j.mehy.2020.109786] [PMID: 32361529]

[16]   Wu A, Peng Y, Huang B, *et al.* Genome composition and divergence of the novel coronavirus (2019-nCoV) originating in China. Cell Host Microbe 2020; 27(3): 325-8.
[http://dx.doi.org/10.1016/j.chom.2020.02.001] [PMID: 32035028]

[17]   Wang H, Li X, Li T, *et al.* The genetic sequence, origin, and diagnosis of SARS-CoV-2. Eur J Clin Microbiol Infect Dis 2020; 39(9): 1629-35.
[http://dx.doi.org/10.1007/s10096-020-03899-4] [PMID: 32333222]

[18]   Khailany RA, Safdar M, Ozaslan M. Genomic characterization of a novel SARS-CoV-2. Gene Rep 2020; 19: 100682.
[http://dx.doi.org/10.1016/j.genrep.2020.100682] [PMID: 32300673]

[19]   Sethuraman N, Jeremiah SS, Ryo A. Interpreting diagnostic tests for SARS-CoV-2. JAMA 2020; 323(22): 2249-51.
[http://dx.doi.org/10.1001/jama.2020.8259] [PMID: 32374370]

[20]   Shen M, Zhou Y, Ye J, *et al.* Recent advances and perspectives of nucleic acid detection for coronavirus. J Pharm Anal 2020; 10(2): 97-101.
[http://dx.doi.org/10.1016/j.jpha.2020.02.010] [PMID: 32292623]

[21]   Wan Z, Zhang Y, He Z, *et al.* A melting curve-based multiplex RT-qPCR assay for simultaneous detection of four human coronaviruses. Int J Mol Sci 2016; 17(11): E1880.
[http://dx.doi.org/10.3390/ijms17111880] [PMID: 27886052]

[22]   Noh JY, Yoon SW, Kim DJ, *et al.* Simultaneous detection of severe acute respiratory syndrome, Middle East respiratory syndrome, and related bat coronaviruses by real-time reverse transcription PCR. Arch Virol 2017; 162(6): 1617-23.
[http://dx.doi.org/10.1007/s00705-017-3281-9] [PMID: 28220326]

[23]   Higuchi R, Fockler C, Dollinger G, Watson R. Kinetic PCR analysis: real-time monitoring of DNA amplification reactions. Biotechnology (N Y) 1993; 11(9): 1026-30.
[PMID: 7764001]

[24]   Lorusso A, Calistri P, Mercante MT, *et al.* A "One-health" approach for diagnosis and molecular characterization of SARS-CoV-2 in Italy. One Health 2020; 10: 100135.

[http://dx.doi.org/10.1016/j.onehlt.2020.100135] [PMID: 32313828]

[25]   Lv DF, Ying QM, Weng YS, *et al.* Dynamic change process of target genes by RT-PCR testing of SARS-Cov-2 during the course of a Coronavirus Disease 2019 patient. Clin Chim Acta 2020; 506: 172-5.
[http://dx.doi.org/10.1016/j.cca.2020.03.032] [PMID: 32229107]

[26]   Wang M, Zhou Y, Zong Z, *et al.* A precision medicine approach to managing 2019 novel coronavirus pneumonia. Precis Clin Med 2020; 3(1): 14-21.
[http://dx.doi.org/10.1093/pcmedi/pbaa002] [PMID: 32330209]

[27]   Xiao AT, Tong YX, Gao C, Zhu L, Zhang YJ, Zhang S. Dynamic profile of RT-PCR findings from 301 COVID-19 patients in Wuhan, China: A descriptive study. J Clin Virol 2020; 127: 104346.
[http://dx.doi.org/10.1016/j.jcv.2020.104346] [PMID: 32361324]

[28]   Hogan CA, Sahoo MK, Huang C, *et al.* Comparison of the panther fusion and a laboratory-developed test targeting the envelope gene for detection of SARS-CoV-2. J Clin Virol 2020; 127: 104383.
[http://dx.doi.org/10.1016/j.jcv.2020.104383] [PMID: 32353760]

[29]   Ishige T, Murata S, Taniguchi T, *et al.* Highly sensitive detection of SARS-CoV-2 RNA by multiplex rRT-PCR for molecular diagnosis of COVID-19 by clinical laboratories. Clin Chim Acta 2020; 507: 139-42.
[http://dx.doi.org/10.1016/j.cca.2020.04.023] [PMID: 32335089]

[30]   Nayak S, Blumenfeld NR, Laksanasopin T, Sia SK. Point-of-care diagnostics: recent developments in a connected age. Anal Chem 2017; 89(1): 102-23.
[http://dx.doi.org/10.1021/acs.analchem.6b04630] [PMID: 27958710]

[31]   Niemz A, Ferguson TM, Boyle DS. Point-of-care nucleic acid testing for infectious diseases. Trends Biotechnol 2011; 29(5): 240-50.
[http://dx.doi.org/10.1016/j.tibtech.2011.01.007] [PMID: 21377748]

[32]   Tamura K, Stecher G, Peterson D, Filipski A, Kumar S. MEGA6: molecular evolutionary genetics analysis version 6.0. Mol Biol Evol 2013; 30(12): 2725-9.
[http://dx.doi.org/10.1093/molbev/mst197] [PMID: 24132122]

[33]   Shannon CE. The mathematical theory of communication. 1963. MD Comput 1997; 14(4): 306-17.
[PMID: 9230594]

[34]   Hall TA. BioEdit: a user-friendly biologicalsequence alignment editor and analysis programfor Windows 95/98/NT. Nucleic Acids Symp Ser 1999; 41: 95-8.

[35]   Ahmed A, Haider SH, Parveen S, *et al.* Co-circulation of 72bp duplication group a and 60bp duplication group b respiratory syncytial virus (RSV) strains in Riyadh, Saudi Arabia during 2014. PLoS One 2016; 11(11): e0166145.
[http://dx.doi.org/10.1371/journal.pone.0166145] [PMID: 27835664]

[36]   Malasao R, Okamoto M, Chaimongkol N, *et al.* Molecular characterization of human respiratory syncytial virus in the Philippines, 2012-2013. PLoS One 2015; 10(11): e0142192.
[http://dx.doi.org/10.1371/journal.pone.0142192] [PMID: 26540236]

[37]   Al-Hassinah S, Parveen S, Somily AM, *et al.* Evolutionary analysis of the ON1 genotype of subtype a respiratory syncytial virus in Riyadh during 2008-16. Infect Genet Evol 2020; 79: 104153.
[http://dx.doi.org/10.1016/j.meegid.2019.104153] [PMID: 31881360]

[38]   Silva SJRD, Pardee K, Pena L. Loop-mediated isothermal amplification (LAMP) for the diagnosis of zika virus: a review. Viruses 2019; 12(1): E19.
[http://dx.doi.org/10.3390/v12010019] [PMID: 31877989]

[39]   Oscorbin IP, Belousova EA, Zakabunin AI, Boyarskikh UA, Filipenko ML. Comparison of fluorescent intercalating dyes for quantitative loop-mediated isothermal amplification (qLAMP). Biotechniques 2016; 61(1): 20-5.
[http://dx.doi.org/10.2144/000114432] [PMID: 27401670]

[40]   Goto M, Honda E, Ogura A, Nomoto A, Hanaki K. Colorimetric detection of loop-mediated isothermal amplification reaction by using hydroxy naphthol blue. Biotechniques 2009; 46(3): 167-72. [http://dx.doi.org/10.2144/000113072] [PMID: 19317660]

[41]   Miyamoto S, Sano S, Takahashi K, Jikihara T. Method for colorimetric detection of double-stranded nucleic acid using leuco triphenylmethane dyes. Anal Biochem 2015; 473: 28-33. [http://dx.doi.org/10.1016/j.ab.2014.12.016] [PMID: 25575759]

[42]   Tanner NA, Zhang Y, Evans TC Jr. Visual detection of isothermal nucleic acid amplification using pH-sensitive dyes. Biotechniques 2015; 58(2): 59-68. [http://dx.doi.org/10.2144/000114253] [PMID: 25652028]

[43]   Nie K, Qi SX, Zhang Y, *et al.* Evaluation of a direct reverse transcription loop-mediated isothermal amplification method without RNA extraction for the detection of human enterovirus 71 subgenotype C4 in nasopharyngeal swab specimens. PLoS One 2012; 7(12): e52486. [http://dx.doi.org/10.1371/journal.pone.0052486] [PMID: 23272248]

[44]   Nyan DC, Ulitzky LE, Cehan N, *et al.* Rapid detection of hepatitis B virus in blood plasma by a specific and sensitive loop-mediated isothermal amplification assay. Clin Infect Dis 2014; 59(1): 16-23. [http://dx.doi.org/10.1093/cid/ciu210] [PMID: 24704724]

[45]   Lee D, Shin Y, Chung S, Hwang KS, Yoon DS, Lee JH. Simple and highly sensitive molecular diagnosis of zika virus by lateral flow assays. Anal Chem 2016; 88(24): 12272-8. [http://dx.doi.org/10.1021/acs.analchem.6b03460] [PMID: 28193014]

[46]   Hong TC, Mai QL, Cuong DV, *et al.* Development and evaluation of a novel loop-mediated isothermal amplification method for rapid detection of severe acute respiratory syndrome coronavirus. J Clin Microbiol 2004; 42(5): 1956-61. [http://dx.doi.org/10.1128/JCM.42.5.1956-1961.2004] [PMID: 15131154]

[47]   Parida M, Horioke K, Ishida H, *et al.* Rapid detection and differentiation of dengue virus serotypes by a real-time reverse transcription-loop-mediated isothermal amplification assay. J Clin Microbiol 2005; 43(6): 2895-903. [http://dx.doi.org/10.1128/JCM.43.6.2895-2903.2005] [PMID: 15956414]

[48]   Ito M, Watanabe M, Nakagawa N, Ihara T, Okuno Y. Rapid detection and typing of influenza A and B by loop-mediated isothermal amplification: comparison with immunochromatography and virus isolation. J Virol Methods 2006; 135(2): 272-5. [http://dx.doi.org/10.1016/j.jviromet.2006.03.003] [PMID: 16616961]

[49]   Enomoto Y, Yoshikawa T, Ihira M, *et al.* Rapid diagnosis of herpes simplex virus infection by a loop-mediated isothermal amplification method. J Clin Microbiol 2005; 43(2): 951-5. [http://dx.doi.org/10.1128/JCM.43.2.951-955.2005] [PMID: 15695716]

[50]   Suzuki R, Yoshikawa T, Ihira M, *et al.* Development of the loop-mediated isothermal amplification method for rapid detection of cytomegalovirus DNA. J Virol Methods 2006; 132(1-2): 216-21. [http://dx.doi.org/10.1016/j.jviromet.2005.09.008] [PMID: 16289345]

[51]   Hagiwara M, Sasaki H, Matsuo K, Honda M, Kawase M, Nakagawa H. Loop-mediated isothermal amplification method for detection of human papillomavirus type 6, 11, 16, and 18. J Med Virol 2007; 79(5): 605-15. [http://dx.doi.org/10.1002/jmv.20858] [PMID: 17385684]

[52]   Baek YH, Um J, Antigua KJC, *et al.* Development of a reverse transcription-loop-mediated isothermal amplification as a rapid early-detection method for novel SARS-CoV-2. Emerg Microbes Infect 2020; 9(1): 998-1007. [http://dx.doi.org/10.1080/22221751.2020.1756698] [PMID: 32306853]

[53]   Kitagawa Y, Orihara Y, Kawamura R, *et al.* Evaluation of rapid diagnosis of novel coronavirus disease (COVID-19) using loop-mediated isothermal amplification. J Clin Virol 2020; 129: 104446.

[http://dx.doi.org/10.1016/j.jcv.2020.104446] [PMID: 32512376]

[54]   Yan C, Cui J, Huang L, *et al*. Rapid and visual detection of 2019 novel coronavirus (SARS-CoV-2) by a reverse transcription loop-mediated isothermal amplification assay. Clin Microbiol Infect 2020; 26(6): 773-9.
[http://dx.doi.org/10.1016/j.cmi.2020.04.001] [PMID: 32276116]

[55]   Lu R, Wu X, Wan Z, Li Y, Jin X, Zhang C. A novel reverse transcription loop-mediated isothermal amplification method for rapid detection of SARS-CoV-2. Int J Mol Sci 2020; 21(8): E2826.
[http://dx.doi.org/10.3390/ijms21082826] [PMID: 32325642]

[56]   Lalli MA, Chen X, Langmade SJ, Fronick CC, Sawyer CS, Burcea LC, *et al*. Rapid and extraction-free detection of SARS-CoV-2 from saliva with colorimetric LAMP. medRxiv 2020.
[http://dx.doi.org/10.1101/2020.05.07.20093542]

[57]   Ganguli A, Mostafa A, Berger J, *et al*. Rapid isothermal amplification and portable detection system for SARS-CoV-2. BioRxiv 2020; 2020.05.21.108381.
[http://dx.doi.org/10.1073/pnas.2014739117] [PMID: 32511358]

[58]   Lau YL, Ismail I, Mustapa NI, *et al*. Real-time reverse transcription loop-mediated isothermal amplification for rapid detection of SARS-CoV-2. PeerJ 2020; 8: e9278.
[http://dx.doi.org/10.7717/peerj.9278] [PMID: 32547882]

[59]   Lou B, Li TD, Zheng SF, *et al*. Serology characteristics of SARS-CoV-2 infection after exposure and post-symptom onset. Eur Respir J 2020; 56(2): 2000763.
[http://dx.doi.org/10.1183/13993003.00763-2020] [PMID: 32430429]

[60]   To KK, Tsang OT, Leung WS, *et al*. Temporal profiles of viral load in posterior oropharyngeal saliva samples and serum antibody responses during infection by SARS-CoV-2: an observational cohort study. Lancet Infect Dis 2020; 20(5): 565-74.
[http://dx.doi.org/10.1016/S1473-3099(20)30196-1] [PMID: 32213337]

[61]   Xiang F, Wang X, He X, Peng Z, Yang B, Zhang J, *et al*. Antibody detection and dynamic characteristics in patients with COVID-19. Clin Infect Dis 2020; Nov 5;71(8): 1930-4.
[http://dx.doi.org/10.1093/cid/ciaa461] [PMID: 32306047]

[62]   Xiao AT, Gao C, Zhang S. Profile of specific antibodies to SARS-CoV-2: The first report. J Infect 2020; 81(1): 147-78.
[http://dx.doi.org/10.1016/j.jinf.2020.03.012] [PMID: 32209385]

[63]   Zhou P, Yang XL, Wang XG, *et al*. A pneumonia outbreak associated with a new coronavirus of probable bat origin. Nature 2020; 579(7798): 270-3.
[http://dx.doi.org/10.1038/s41586-020-2012-7] [PMID: 32015507]

[64]   Chang CK, Sue SC, Yu TH, *et al*. Modular organization of SARS coronavirus nucleocapsid protein. J Biomed Sci 2006; 13(1): 59-72.
[http://dx.doi.org/10.1007/s11373-005-9035-9] [PMID: 16228284]

[65]   Hurst KR, Koetzner CA, Masters PS. Identification of *in vivo* interacting domains of the murine coronavirus nucleocapsid protein. J Virol 2009; 83(14): 7221-34.
[http://dx.doi.org/10.1128/JVI.00440-09] [PMID: 19420077]

[66]   Woo PC, Lau SK, Wong BH, *et al*. Differential sensitivities of severe acute respiratory syndrome (SARS) coronavirus spike polypeptide enzyme-linked immunosorbent assay (ELISA) and SARS coronavirus nucleocapsid protein ELISA for serodiagnosis of SARS coronavirus pneumonia. J Clin Microbiol 2005; 43(7): 3054-8.
[http://dx.doi.org/10.1128/JCM.43.7.3054-3058.2005] [PMID: 16000415]

[67]   Adams ER, Ainsworth M, Anand R, Andersson MI, Auckland K, Baillie JK, *et al*. Antibody testing for COVID-19: A report from the National COVID scientific advisory panel. MedRxiv 2020.
[http://dx.doi.org/10.1101/2020.04.15.20066407]

[68]   Chen S, Lu D, Zhang M, *et al*. Double-antigen sandwich ELISA for detection of antibodies to SARS-

associated coronavirus in human serum. Eur J Clin Microbiol Infect Dis 2005; 24(8): 549-53.
[http://dx.doi.org/10.1007/s10096-005-1378-7] [PMID: 16133409]

[69]   Guo L, Ren L, Yang S, *et al.* Profiling early humoral response to diagnose novel coronavirus disease
       (COVID-19). Clin Infect Dis 2020; 71(15): 778-85.
       [http://dx.doi.org/10.1093/cid/ciaa310] [PMID: 32198501]

[70]   Wang Q, Du Q, Guo B, *et al.* A method to prevent sars-cov-2 igm false positives in gold
       immunochromatography and enzyme-linked immunosorbent assays. J Clin Microbiol 2020; 58(6):
       e00375-20.
       [http://dx.doi.org/10.1128/JCM.00375-20] [PMID: 32277023]

[71]   Zhong L, Chuan J, Gong B, *et al.* Detection of serum IgM and IgG for COVID-19 diagnosis. Sci
       China Life Sci 2020; 63(5): 777-80.
       [http://dx.doi.org/10.1007/s11427-020-1688-9] [PMID: 32270436]

[72]   Zinkernagel RM. On natural and artificial vaccinations. Annu Rev Immunol 2003; 21: 515-46.
       [http://dx.doi.org/10.1146/annurev.immunol.21.120601.141045] [PMID: 12500980]

[73]   van Griensven J, Edwards T, de Lamballerie X, *et al.* Ebola-Tx Consortium. Evaluation of
       convalescent plasma for ebola virus disease in guinea. N Engl J Med 2016; 374(1): 33-42.
       [http://dx.doi.org/10.1056/NEJMoa1511812] [PMID: 26735992]

[74]   Wong VW, Dai D, Wu AK, Sung JJ. Treatment of severe acute respiratory syndrome with
       convalescent plasma. Hong Kong Med J 2003; 9(3): 199-201.
       [PMID: 12777656]

[75]   Zhou B, Zhong N, Guan Y. Treatment with convalescent plasma for influenza A (H5N1) infection. N
       Engl J Med 2007; 357(14): 1450-1.
       [http://dx.doi.org/10.1056/NEJMc070359] [PMID: 17914053]

[76]   Casadevall A, Pirofski LA. The convalescent sera option for containing COVID-19. J Clin Invest
       2020; 130(4): 1545-8.
       [http://dx.doi.org/10.1172/JCI138003] [PMID: 32167489]

[77]   Che XY, Qiu LW, Pan YX, *et al.* Sensitive and specific monoclonal antibody-based capture enzyme
       immunoassay for detection of nucleocapsid antigen in sera from patients with severe acute respiratory
       syndrome. J Clin Microbiol 2004; 42(6): 2629-35.
       [http://dx.doi.org/10.1128/JCM.42.6.2629-2635.2004] [PMID: 15184444]

[78]   Di B, Hao W, Gao Y, *et al.* Monoclonal antibody-based antigen capture enzyme-linked
       immunosorbent assay reveals high sensitivity of the nucleocapsid protein in acute-phase sera of severe
       acute respiratory syndrome patients. Clin Diagn Lab Immunol 2005; 12(1): 135-40.
       [http://dx.doi.org/10.1128/CDLI.12.1.135-140.2005] [PMID: 15642998]

[79]   Tang YW, Schmitz JE, Persing DH, Stratton CW. Laboratory diagnosis of COVID-19: current issues
       and challenges. J Clin Microbiol 2020; 58(6): e00512-20.
       [http://dx.doi.org/10.1128/JCM.00512-20] [PMID: 32245835]

[80]   Diao B, Wen K, Chen J, *et al.* Diagnosis of acute respiratory syndrome coronavirus 2 infection by
       detection of nucleocapsid protein. MedRxiv 2020.
       [http://dx.doi.org/10.1101/2020.03.07.20032524]

[81]   Li Z, Yi Y, Luo X, *et al.* Development and clinical application of a rapid IgM-IgG combined antibody
       test for SARS-CoV-2 infection diagnosis. J Med Virol 2020; 92(9): 1518-24.
       [http://dx.doi.org/10.1002/jmv.25727] [PMID: 32104917]

[82]   La Marca A, Capuzzo M, Paglia T, Roli L, Trenti T, Nelson SM. Testing for SARS-CoV-2 (COVID-
       19): a systematic review and clinical guide to molecular and serological *in-vitro* diagnostic assays.
       Reprod Biomed Online 2020; 41(3): 483-99.
       [http://dx.doi.org/10.1016/j.rbmo.2020.06.001] [PMID: 32651106]

CHAPTER 9

Natural Compounds as Potential Therapeutic Agents against COVID-19

Ayesha Tazeen[1], Farah Deeba[1], Zoya Shafat[1], Md. Imam Faizan[1,2], Maryam Sarwat[3], Mohammad Khalid Parvez[4] and Shama Parveen[1,*]

[1] *Centre for Interdisciplinary Research in Basic Sciences, Jamia Millia Islamia, New Delhi, India*

[2] *Multidisciplinary Centre for Advanced Research and Studies, Jamia Millia Islamia, New Delhi, India*

[3] *Amity Institute of Pharmacy, Amity University, Noida, Uttar Pradesh, India*

[4] *Department of Pharmacognosy, College of Pharmacy, King Saud University, Riyadh, Saudi Arabia*

Abstract: Research scientists across the globe are attempting to unearth the possible therapeutic agents against Coronavirus disease 2019 (COVID-19). The natural compounds from plant sources constitute a rich source of potential antiviral, antibacterial, antioxidant, anticancer, immune enhancer and other activities with minimal side effects. Approximately 25% of the European Medical Agency (EMA) or Food and Drug Administration (FDA) approved drugs are based on plant products highlighting their importance in the medical field. In recent years, *in-silico* methods have provided fast and cost-efficient approaches for designing potential inhibitors. Several virtual screening, molecular simulation, pharmacokinetics and druggability studies have been carried out to identify potential inhibitors against structural (spike, envelope, and membrane) and non-structural (Protease, RdRp, endoribonucleoase) proteins of SARS-CoV-2. In the present chapter, we have reviewed all such studies that recommended naturally occurring bioactive compounds (flavonoids, terpenes, curcuminoids, tannins, essential oil *etc.*) of plant origin as potential inhibitors of COVID-19. We have listed 100 such potential compounds and have analyzed significance of some of these (Myricitrin, Baicalin, Hesperidin, Theaflavin, Apigenin, Isothymol, Saikosaponin U, Curcumin, Tannin *etc.*) in detail based on computational studies. Furthermore, we have also studied several medicinal plants (*Curcuma longa, Vitis vinifera, Glycyrrhiza glabra, Malus domestica, Azadirachta indica, Camellia sinensis and Nigella sativa*). These plants are part of normal human diet and can also be considered as potential herbs with immune system enhancing effects. In addition, these phytoconstituents should be further analyzed in detail for toxicity, pharmacokinetics, antiviral and therapeutic potential in cell culture and animal models against SARS-CoV-2.

* **Corresponding author Shama Parveen:** Centre for Interdisciplinary Research in Basic Sciences, Jamia Millia Islamia, New Delhi, India; E-mails: sparveen2@jmi.ac.in and shamp25@yahoo.com

Keywords: Curcuminoids, Flavonoids, Natural compounds, Plants, SARS-CoV-2, Terpenes, Therapeutics.

INTRODUCTION

Plants have been used by the human beings as health resource for millions of years before the evolution of science. During the course of history, the medicinal plants have played a significant role in the therapeutic approach for different diseases. The ancient civilizations utilized the medicinal plants by consuming them in raw form. After learning that many diseases can be cured using plants, the ancient civilizations started to collect evidence to assess their therapeutic values. Initially, it was mainly dependent on the trial and error method; however, after extensive exploration and discovery of important effects of specific plants for treating the diseases, it became clearer. Eventually, they developed the understanding that harvesting the herbs at the right time, followed by their preservation in specific preparations, may increase their efficacy and availability for a long duration.

The Egyptians described several plant-based preparations around 1500 BC [1, 2]. Later on, the Romans and Greeks further developed and refined these plant-based extracts and preparations [3]. By the early 17th century, several plants were documented and majority of them can be found in the first official drug book from Great Britain, the *Pharmacopeia Londonensis* [1, 4]. The herbal preparations still receive universal attention, with a considerable increase in their use in the developed countries with its market expansion in the United States and European countries [5]. Several ointments, tea, alcoholic extracts and salves were often recommended for treating many diseases ranging from wounds of war to menstrual complications [1, 2]. Furthermore, several other countries have their own traditional system of medicine with official transcripts and books such as India, China, Korea, Japan, Africa and many others. The traditional Chinese medicine (TCM) and Indian traditional medicinal system are one of the oldest systems, presently under the jurisdiction of the National Health Commission and Ministry of AYUSH, respectively. The Indian traditional medicinal system has unique characteristics with different well-acknowledged traditional systems of medicine, such as Unani, Ayurveda, Siddha, Naturopathy and with some classical transcripts including Unani Pharmacopeia of India, Rigveda, and Sushruta Samhita.

SIGNIFICANCE OF PLANTS DERIVED COMPOUNDS AS ANTIVIRALS

Nature is a silent companion to human world which provides a reliable source of different phytochemicals. In recent times, a lot of efforts have been made to identify antiviral compounds from various plants and other natural resources as they are a rich source of phytochemicals like flavonoids, polyphenols, alkaloids, saponins, anthocyanins, tannins, including others. These purified natural compounds offer a rich supply for novel antiviral drug development, as evident by several ancient practices and recent research works. These phytochemicals also exhibit several therapeutic properties and novel scaffolds for designing new medications. Around 40% of the available drugs in the market are directly or indirectly derived from the plants [6]. Notably, while mono or poly-herbal preparations are complex products containing multiple pharmacologically active secondary metabolites, isolated bioactive compounds frequently perform better and in a specific way. Furthermore, even for a plant species, the nature and relative quantities of the active phytoconstituents may vary due to its geographical origin, cultivar, environmental conditions, plant parts used, storage condition, preparation method, contamination, and adulteration.

Nonetheless, herbal compounds, by the virtue of their structural diversity, provide a great opportunity to screen compounds against SARS-CoV-2 with a distinct mechanism of action and novel structure. Identifying the antiviral mechanisms of the natural compounds helps in exploring their activities and exactly at which stage (entry, replication, assembly, release, and virus–host interactions) they may interrupt the life cycle of the virus. Improved understanding of the mode of action of natural antiviral compounds may prove to be helpful in providing a new insight for developing novel antiviral drugs for efficacious viral control.

Considering the present scenario of COVID-19, this chapter summarizes some notable natural compounds studied against the SARS-CoV-2 since its outbreak. Several *in-silico* but very few *in vitro* studies have been done to identify the antiviral and immuno-modulatory properties of these compounds against SARS-CoV-2. Several of these have been suggested for the prevention and treatment of mild COVID-19 symptoms in addition to the routine therapeutic approaches against this infection. It may be noted that scientific evidence of their recommendations against SARS-CoV-2 is still currently under study. Thus, the option to use these natural compounds as accepted antivirals is yet to be established.

ANTIVIRAL ACTIVITY OF SELECTED NATURAL COMPOUNDS AGAINST SARS-COV-2

The plant produces a wide range of secondary metabolites or other phytochemicals such as lignans, flavonoids, tannins, phytoalexins, saponins, terpenes and several other polyphenols which plays a vital role in plant's growth, metabolism and development. The flavonoids comprise a major group of secondary metabolites found in seeds, stem, leaves, fruits, vegetables, nuts, spices, bark and tea [7]. These compounds are synthesized in response to abiotic stress environments and play a significant role in defending the plants against insects and pathogens. Due to virtue of their previously known properties (antiviral, anti-inflammatory, antioxidant, *etc.*) and significant interactions against different RNA-dependent RNA polymerase (RdRp), main protease/ 3-chymotrypsin-like cysteine protease (M^{Pro}/ $3CL^{pro}$), spike and other proteins of SARS-CoV-2, they can be used for further experimental validations in cell culture and animal models. Since some of the compounds have already shown significant antiviral activities against the *Coronaviruses* (SARS-CoV and MERS), it makes them more noteworthy. In addition, some of the identified compounds are known to have good ADMET properties (absorption, distribution, metabolism, excretion, and toxicity of a drug molecule), therefore, these may be directly used for clinical studies as natural compounds are known to exhibit very low to no toxicity.

In this review, we have listed 100 natural compounds from different plant sources which showed most significant antiviral activities against SARS-CoV-2. Also, we have described in detail some of the most potential antiviral compounds and plants which can be used as prophylaxis for COVID-19 on the basis of their interaction with target proteins, binding affinity, previously known antiviral activities and also ease of availability (Fig. **1**).

FLAVONOIDS

The flavonoids consist of flavan nucleus and a 15 carbon skeleton consisting of 2 benzene rings connected *via* heterocyclic pyrene ring. The flavonoids are categorized into several classes, including biflavanoids, isoflavanoids, flavones, flavonols, anthocyanidins, flavanones, flavans, *etc*. Several flavonoids were identified as potential antiviral agents against SARS-CoV-2; some of which are listed in Table **1**. These flavonoids can be used for experimental studies in animal models due to the virtue of their properties and significant interactions against several proteins of SARS-CoV-2.

Myricitrin

Myricitrin is a flavonol and a glycosylated analog of myricetin, found in *Myrica esculenta, Myrica Cerifera, Nelumbo nucifera, Nymphaea odorata* and several other plant species. Myricitrin is an anti-tussive (helps to relieve or prevent cough) molecule. It exhibits antiviral activity against Ebola virus, human immune deficiency virus (HIV), herpes simplex virus (HSV) as reported by several previous studies [8, 9]. Two different significant studies by Joshi and colleagues, and Qamar and co-workers found that Myricitrin exhibits a strong binding affinity with the active site residue of M^{Pro} of SARS-CoV-2 with a binding energy of -8.9 and -15.64 kcal/mol, respectively [8, 9]. Joshi and colleagues also showed that it exhibited a strong interaction with human ACE-2 (hACE-2) and RdRp with a binding energy of -7.5 and -7.9 kcal/mol, respectively [9].

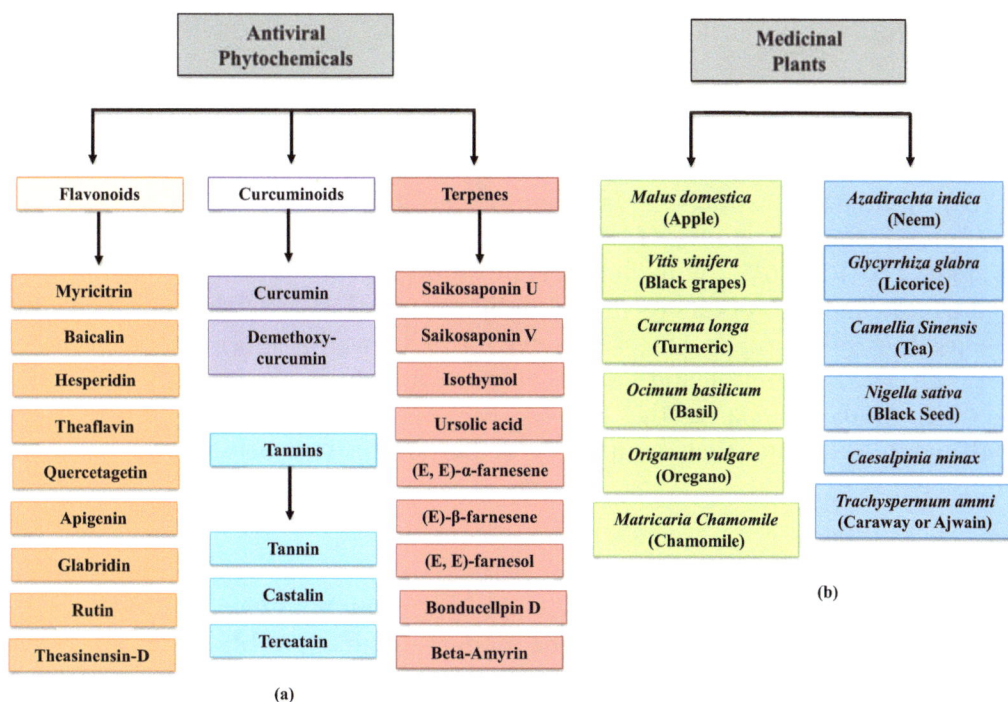

```
          Antiviral                                    Medicinal
        Phytochemicals                                   Plants

   Flavonoids   Curcuminoids   Terpenes        Malus domestica      Azadirachta indica
                                                   (Apple)               (Neem)

   Myricitrin     Curcumin     Saikosaponin U    Vitis vinifera      Glycyrrhiza glabra
                                                 (Black grapes)        (Licorice)
    Baicalin      Demethoxy-   Saikosaponin V
                   curcumin                       Curcuma longa       Camellia Sinensis
   Hesperidin                    Isothymol         (Turmeric)              (Tea)

   Theaflavin     Tannins       Ursolic acid     Ocimum basilicum     Nigella sativa
                                                    (Basil)            (Black Seed)
  Quercetagetin               (E, E)-α-farnesene
                                                 Origanum vulgare     Caesalpinia minax
    Apigenin       Tannin     (E)-β-farnesene       (Oregano)
                                                                     Trachyspermum ammi
    Glabridin      Castalin   (E, E)-farnesol   Matricaria Chamomile (Caraway or Ajwain)
                                                   (Chamomile)
     Rutin        Tercatain   Bonducellpin D
                                                              (b)
  Theasinensin-D               Beta-Amyrin

                      (a)
```

Fig. (1). (a) Potential antiviral phytochemicals against SARS-CoV-2 **(b)** Some significant plants with therapeutic properties and potential antiviral phytochemicals.

Baicalin

Baicalin, a glycosyloxyflavone, a monosaccharide derivative, is a prodrug, non-steroidal and anti-inflammatory drug. It exhibits antiviral activity against several viruses, including SARS-CoV, Chikungunya virus, H1N1-pdm09 influenza strain, which has experimentally been proved. It is found mainly in different species of *Scutellaria,* including *S. lateriflora, S.baicalensis* and *S. galericulata.* Significantly, Baicalin is a component of an important and widely used prescription drug or herbal supplement "**Sho-Saiko-To**", also known as "Xiǎocháihútāng (XCHT)" in Chinese. Its formula is listed in China in Pharmacopoeia of the People's Republic of China and in Japan as a Kampo medicine (Adaptation of Traditional Chinese Medicine). The active ingredients of Sho-Saiko-To discovered so far include Baicalin, Saikosaponins, Gingerol, Glycyrrhizin, Baicalein, Wogonin and Ginsenosides. Islam and colleagues found that Baicalin has a strong affinity with the residues of protease of SARS-CoV-2 with a binding energy of -8.1 kcal/mole. Joshi and co-workers have also reported significant interaction of Baicalin with protease, hACE-2 and RdRp [9, 10]. Significantly, Baicalin has the structural similarity with the apo-form of protease.

Hesperidin

Hesperidin is a disaccharide derivative and a major flavanone glycoside in citrus peel. It is found in many citrus fruits *(Citrus spp.), Mentha spp., Yellow Toadflax, Linaria vulgaris,* and several others. It exhibits antiviral (influenza and hepatitis virus), antioxidant, anticancer and antibacterial activities. Many authors have performed docking studies for Hesperidin against protease RdRp and spike protein of SARS-CoV-2 with significant results [9, 11 - 13]. Tallei and colleagues and Utomo and co-workers reported binding energies of -10.4 and -9.61 kcal/mol against the spike protein [11, 12]. Hesperidin showed a strong binding affinity between -13.5 kcal/mol and -8.3 kcal/mol for M^{Pro} in three different studies. Another study compared the affinity of several compounds with the drug Nelfinavir and found that the affinity of hesperidin was better as compared to Nelfinavir [11].

Theaflavin

Theaflavin is a type of natural biflavonoid found mainly in *Camellia sinensis* (tea plant) and other related plants. It is the main red pigment of black tea with strong antioxidant properties. It has well-known antiviral (SARS-CoV, HSV, tobacco mosaic virus), antibacterial and anticancer activities. A recent investigation studied several compounds used in Chinese traditional medicines against RdRp and identified Theaflavin as a potential inhibitor of SARS-CoV-2. Interestingly, tea is one of the most basic drinks consumed universally, and thus, Theaflavin can be considered as a significant anti-SARS dietary polyphenol [14].

Quercetagetin

Quercetagetin is a type of hexahydroxyflavone which is derived from quercetin (a well-known antiviral flavonoid). It is found mainly in the genus *Eriocaulon.* Singh and colleagues found that Quercetagetin has a strong binding affinity with the active site residues in the catalytic pocket of RdRp of SARS-CoV-2 with binding energy as -7.0 kcal/mol. The authors also compared their findings with RdRp of SARS-CoV-1 and found the affinity to be nearly consistent (-7.8 Kcal/mol) for both the viruses suggesting that it may inhibit the activities of RdRp, resulting in blocking of replication and viral transcription. The author also showed that Quercetagetin also has favorable pharmacokinetics properties (Toxicity, ADMET and druggability) [15].

Apigenin

Apigenin is a type of flavone, a tri-hydroxyflavone. It is found abundantly in several fruits and vegetables such as *Malus domestica, Thymus vulgaris, Capsicum annuum, Allium sativum, Apium graveolens,etc*. It is also an important component of *Matricaria chamomilla* (Chamomile) in the form of essential oil (Chamomile oil). It exhibits antiviral (HIV, HSV, foot-and-mouth disease virus, Epstein-Barr virus, enterovirus-71), antibacterial, antioxidant, anti-inflammatory, anti-metastatic, anticancer and other activities. A recent report compared the binding affinities of RdRp of both SARS-CoV and SARS-CoV-2 and concluded that Apigenin has a significant binding energy of -7.0 kcal/mol and -6.5 kcal/mol with residues of RdRp. Ramaiah and colleagues showed that Apigenin also exhibits a strong interaction with protease of SARS-CoV-2 with binding affinities of -7.8 and 7.0 kcal/mol [15, 16].

Glabridin

Glabridin is a type of hydroxyl-isoflavans. It is found majorly in *Glycyrrhiza glabra* (Licorice), which is a well-known medicinal plant. It exhibits antiviral, anti-inflammatory, antioxidant, antibacterial, antifungal activities. Two recent investigations reported binding energy of Glabridin as –8.0 kcal/mol and -8.1 kcal/mol with the residues of protease of SARS-CoV-2 [10, 16].

Table 1. Potential antiviral flavonoids against SARS-CoV-2 studied using *in-silico* approaches.

S.No.	Compound	Plant	Reported Activities of the Compound	Studied Protein	Reference
1	Baicalin	*Scutellaria baicalensis, S. lateriflora, S. galericulata*	Antiviral, Anticancer, Anti-inflammatory, Antibacterial	Protease, Spike, RdRp	[9, 10]
2	Hesperidin	*Citrus fruit (Citrus spp.), Mentha spp., Linaria vulgaris*	Antiviral, Anticancer, Antibacterial, Antioxidant	Spike, Protease, RdRp	[9, 11 - 13]
3	Glabridin	*Glycyrrhiza glabra*	Antiviral, Antioxidant Antibacterial, Anti-inflammatory, Antifungal	Protease	[9, 16]

S.No.	Compound	Plant	Reported Activities of the Compound	Studied Protein	Reference
4	Rhoifolin	*Rhus succedanea, Citrus aurantium, Bergamot, Citrus paradisi, Citrus limon, Lablab purpureus, Lycopersicon esculentum, Cynara scolymus, Musa spp., Vitis vinifera*	Antiviral, Anticancer	Protease, Spike	[11]
5	Pectolinarin	*Cirsium spp., Linaria vulgaris*	Anti-inflammatory, Antihemorrhagic, Antiproliferative, Anticancer	Spike, Protease	[11]
6	Galangin	*Alpinia galangal, Helichrysum aureonitens*	Anticancer, Antiviral, Antimicrobial	Protease	[12]
7	Theaflavin	*Camellia Sinensis*	Antiviral (SARS-CoV), Antimicrobial, Antioxidant, Anticancer	RdRp	[14]
8	Quercetagetin	*Genus Eriocaulon*	Antiviral	RdRp	[15]
9	Apigenin	*Camellia Sinensis, Malus domestica, Thymus vulgaris, Matricaria chamomilla, Capsicum annuum, Allium sativum var, Apium graveolen*	Antiviral, Anticancer Antibacterial, Anti-Inflammatory, Antioxidant, Antimetastatic	Protease, RdRp	[15, 16]
10	Glycoumarin	*Glycyrrhiza glabra*	Antibacterial	Protease	[16]
11	Liquiritigenin	*Glycyrrhiza glabra, Glycyrrhiza uralensis*	Antiviral, Anti-inflammatory, Antimicrobial, Anticancer	Protease	[16]
12	5,7-dimethoxyflavaN-4'-O-β-dglucopyranoside	*Caesalpinia minax*	Antiviral	Protease	[20]
13	Myricitrin	*Vitis vinifera, Myrica Cerifera, Myrica esculenta, Nelumbo nucifera, Nymphaea odorata*	Anti-tussive, Antiviral, Antioxidant, Anti-inflammatory, Protein kinase C inhibitor	Protease, Spike, RdRp	[9, 24]

(Table 1) cont.....

S.No.	Compound	Plant	Reported Activities of the Compound	Studied Protein	Reference
14	3,5,7,30,40,50-hexahydroxy flavanone-3-Obeta-Dglucopyranoside	*Phaseolus vulgaris*	Anticancer	Protease	[24]
15	(2S)-Eriodictyol 7-O-(6"-O-galloyl)-beta-D-glucopyranoside	*Phyllanthus emblica*	-	Protease	[24]
16	Myricetin 3-Obeta-Dglucopyranoside	*Camellia sinensis*	Anti-inflammatory, Antioxidant, Antiviral	Protease	[24]
17	Licoleafol	*Glycyrrhiza uralensis*	Antioxidant	Protease	[24]
18	Cyanidin 3-Glucoside	*Blackberry*	Antiviral, Antioxidant Anti-inflammatory	Protease	[25]
19	5,7,3',4'-Tetrahydroxy-2'-(3,3-dimethylallyl) isoflavone	*Psorothamnus arborescens*	Anti-leishmanial	Protease	[24]
20	Myricetin	*Petroselinum crispum, Foeniculum vulgare, Lycium barbarum,Vaccinium subg. Oxycoccus*	Antiviral, Anticancer, Anti-Inflammatory, Antioxidant, Anti-Carcinogen	RdRp	[15]
21	Theasinensin-D	*Camellia sinensis*	Antioxidant, Antiviral	Protease	[26]
22	Crysophanic acid	*Aloe vera, Citri Reticulatae Pericarpium,*	Anti-Inflammatory, Antiviral	Protease	[22]
23	Avicularin	*Psidium guyava, Lespedeza cuneata, Polygonum aviculare*	Antiviral, Antioxidant, Anti-Inflammatory, Hepatoprotective Activity	Spike, NSP9, Protease	[27]
24	Guajaverin	*Psidium guyava*	Antiviral	Spike, NSP9, Protease	[27]
25	Isoxanthohumol	*Sophora flavescens, Humulus lupulus*	Antiviral (SARS-Cov), Anti-Carcinogenic, Antioxidant, Anti-Inflammatory, Anti-Angiogenic	Protease	[28]
26	Chrysanthemin	*Vitis vinifera, Hibiscus sabdariffa*	Antibacterial, Anti-tussive	Spike, RdRp, Protease	[9]

(Table 1) cont.....

S.No.	Compound	Plant	Reported Activities of the Compound	Studied Protein	Reference
27	Taiwanhomoflavone A	*Cephalotaxus wilsoniana*	Anticarcinogenic, Anti-Inflammatory, Anti-Neoplastic	Spike, RdRp, Protease	[9]
28	Afzelin	*Nymphaea odorata*	Antiviral, Anticancer Antioxidant, Anti-Inflammatory, Antibacterial	Spike, RdRp, Protease	[9]
29	Biorobin	*Ficus benjamina, Cassia occidentalis, Medicago species, Trigonella species*	Antiviral, Anti-Inflammatory	Spike, RdRp, Protease	[9]
30	Nympholide-A	*Nymphaea lotus*	Antiviral (Influenza), Analgesic, Anti-Cancer	Spike, RdRp, Protease	[9]
31	Morin	*Morus alba, Vaccinium myrtillus*	Anti-inflammatory, Antioxidant, Antiviral	Protease, Spike	[11]
32	Rutin	*Nigella sativa*	Antiviral (SARS-CoV), Antioxidant, Anti-inflammatory	Protease, Spike	[13]
33	Kaempferol	*Citrus paradise, Hamamelis*	Antioxidant, Antiviral	Protease, Spike	[11]

TERPENES AND TERPENOIDS

Terpenes and terpenoids are the biggest and diverse classes of organic compounds or secondary metabolites. Terpenes contain 5 carbon isoprene units assembled with each other in different ways. These terpenoids are the modified class of terpenes having different functional groups and oxidized methyl group arranged at various positions. On the basis of carbon units, terpenoids are categorized as sesterpenes, sesquiterpenes, monoterpenes, diterpenes and triterpenes. Terpenoids are biologically active and used worldwide for treating several diseases. Terpenes and terpenoids are the main components of several types of essential oils, flowers and many other plants such as conifers. Some of the studied significant terpenoids are listed in Table **2**.

Saikosaponin U and Saikosaponin V: Saikosaponin U and Saikosaponin V are triterpene saponin glycosides. They exhibit a wide range of pharmacological activities. These are the major bioactive components of traditional oriental medicinal plants, especially the traditional Chinese medicine plants such as *Scrophularia scorodonia, Bupleuri Radix,* and different species of *Bupleurum and Heteromorpha.* These are known for antiviral (human CoV, RSV, influenza virus, hepatitis virus *etc*), antioxidant, anti-inflammatory, antipyretic, anti-tumor, antimalaria, anticancer and immunomodulatory effects. The study by Sinha and colleagues found that Saikosaponin U and Saikosaponin V had the best affinity with NSP15 endoribonuclease of SARS-CoV-2 with a binding energy of -8.3 kcal/mol and -7.2 kcal/mol, respectively [17]. Furthermore, Saikosaponin U and Saikosaponin V also interacted with residues of spike glycoprotein with a binding energy of -8.4 kcal/mol and -8.2 kcal/mol, respectively [17].

Isothymol: Isothymol or carvacol is a natural monoterpene derived from cymene and is commonly used as a food additive. It is found in many important medicinal plants and seeds, including *Ammoides verticillata, Trachyspermum ammi, Nigella sativa, Origanum vulgare, and Lippia graveolens.* It exhibits antiviral (murine norovirus, HSV, RSV, bovine viral diarrhoea virus), antibacterial, and antifungal activities. Abdelli and co-workers studied several compounds and found this compound as a top potential inhibitor with good drug-like property and was tested negative for toxicity. The study showed that isothymol also exhibited good interaction with the ACE2 receptor of SARS-CoV-2 with binding affinity as -5.7 kcal/mol [18].

Ursolic acid: Ursolic acid or Urson is one of the most ubiquitous types of pentacyclic triterpenoid of medicinal herbs. It is an integral part of the human diet as it is present in many fruits, vegetables and herbs. It is found abundantly in *Malus domestica, Ocimum basilicum, Vaccinium myrtillus, Vaccinium oxycoccos, Rosmarinus officinalis, Thymus vulgaris, Mentha piperita, Prunus domestica* and several other common herbs and plants. Numerous extensive studies have been done on Ursolic acid to recognize its properties, which reflects the tremendous interest in this compound. It is known for its antiviral (human papillomavirus, HSV, HIV, hepatitis, dengue and influenza viruses), anticancer, antioxidative, anti-inflammatory, anti-carcinogenic and anti-tumor activities. Ramaiah and co-workers have reported significant interaction of Ursolic acid with residues of different models of protease with a binding affinity of -8.2 kcal/mol and -7.6 kcal/mol, which may hinder the viral replication [16].

(E, E)-α-farnesene, (E)-β-farnesene, (E, E)-farnesol: The (E,E)-farnesol is a farnesane sesquiterpenoid, the (E,E)-α-farnesene is 1,3,6,10-tetraene and the (E)-β-farnesene is 11-Dimethyl-3-methylenedodeca-1, 6, 10-triene, and these are members of Sesquiterpenoids. These are components of many essential oils, and plants such as *Malus domestica, Matricaria recutita, Zingiber ocinale Roscoe,etc.* These are known for their antiviral, anti-inflammatory and antimicrobial activities. Silva and colleagues studied around 170 compounds found in essential oils. They concluded that three compounds, namely E,E)-α-farnesene, (E)-β-farnesene and (E,E)-farnesol showed significant interactions with NS15 protein (endoribonuclease) of SARS-CoV-2. The binding energies (using Molegro Virtual Docker) were found to be 115.0, 115.4 and 112.0 KJ/mol for E,E)-α-farnesene, (E)-β-farnesene and (E,E)-farnesol, respectively [19].

Bonducellpin D: Bonducellpin D is a cassane furano-diterpenes. It is mainly isolated from traditional Chinese medicinal plant *Caesalpinia minax* seeds. It is known to exhibit antiviral (parainfluenza-3 virus) activity. Gurung and colleagues found that this compound is the best-ranked lead molecule which interacted with M^{Pro} of SARS-CoV-2 with a high binding affinity of −9.28 kcal/mol as compared to the control antiviral drug, Saquinavir. It also showed high inhibition constant of -156.75 nM. The study also found that Bonducellpin D exhibited broad-spectrum inhibition potential as it showed inhibitory activity against the same enzyme of SARS and MERS [20].

Beta-Amyrin: Beta-Amyrin is a type of pentacyclic tri-terpenol found in higher plants. It is found in the medicinal plants *Azadirachta Indica, Aspergillus nidulans, Guiera senegalensis* and *Guiera senegalensis*. It is commonly known as "cure all" plant and is a broad-spectrum African folk medicine plant. This compound is known for its antiviral (HBV, HSV, Fowlpox virus), anti-inflammatory, anticonvulsant activities. Borkotoky and colleagues concluded that Beta-Amyrin showed a high binding affinity with the binding energy of -9.4 kcal/mol with transmembrane and C-terminal domains of SARS-CoV-2. These two domains are conserved and essential for virus assembly [21].

β-caryophyllene: β-caryophyllene is an oily liquid and a type of bicyclic sesquiterpenes. It is one of the common phytochemicals found in abundance in *Ocimum spp., Cinnamomum spp., Piper nigrum., Cannabis sativa, Syzygium aromaticum, Origanum vulgare, Rosmarinus officinalis,* and *Lavandula angustifolia* and in essential oils of many other plants. It is known for its antiviral (HSV, dengue virus), anticancer, antifungal, and anti-inflammatory activities. Narkhede and colleagues revealed that β-caryophyllene showed a good affinity for M^{Pro} with a binding energy of -7.2 kcal/mol. It also showed good drug-like properties [22].

CURCUMINOIDS

Curcuminoids are linear diarylheptanoids that constitute curcumin, demethoxycurcumin and bisdemethoxycurcumin with several known pharmacological properties. The curcumin is the principal constituent of the yellow pigment of *Curcuma longa* and is the main bioactive substance (Table **2**).

Curcumin: Curcumin is a diarylheptanoid and a natural phytopolylphenol pigment. It is found in *Curcuma longa,* a medicinal herb known for its pharmacological and biological properties across the world. It has been used for centuries in Indian and other Asian traditional medicine for treating various ailments. It is also the main constituent of Indonesian traditional medicine, the "Jamu" formulas. It is generally not related with any type of toxicity and is classified in "Generally Recognized as Safe" group by the FDA. It is known for its antiviral (SARS, influenza, coxsackievirus, hepatitis, HIV, HSV, Chikungunya, dengue, Zika viruses, *etc.*), antioxidant, anti-inflammatory, antibacterial, anti-cancer and several other properties.

Several studies have also been carried out to investigate the anti-SARS-CoV-2 activities of Curcumin [11 - 13, 16]. Utomo and colleagues concluded that Curcumin has a strong binding affinity with the residues of protease, spike and RBD-ACE-2 of SARS-CoV-2 with binding affinities of -11.82, -8.39 and -9.04 kcal/mol, respectively [12]. Another investigation also found that Curcumin interacted significantly with protease with a binding affinity of -8.15 kcal/mol and a high full fitness score. Maurya and colleagues also showed that Curcumin interacted with spike protein with good interactions and binding energy (MolDock score -141.36 kcal/mole) [23]. Another report also showed that Curcumin has a good affinity for protease with a binding energy of -7.4 kcal/mol [13]. These studies suggested that Curcumin may act as both viral entry and replication inhibitor and thus is one of the most potential anti-SARS-CoV-2 compound.

TANNIN

Tannins are natural polyphenols having an astringent taste which are divided into three groups, *i.e.* phlorotannins, hydrolysable tannins and condensed tannins. Furthermore, based on the structural properties, tannins are also categorized as condensed tannins, complex tannins, gallotannins, and ellagitannins. It is present mainly in the plant-based material, including food and beverages. The applications of tannins are vast and can be exploited in the food, pharmaceuticals, nutraceutical and cosmetology industries. Recently, various significant properties like potential medicinal agents (sore throat, fever, asthma, dysentery, intestinal disorders, inflammations, *etc.*), antiseptics, metal chelators, inhibitors of harmful pro-oxidative enzymes and of lipid peroxidation process, including many others, have been documented in the humans which makes them appropriate candidates for nutraceutical and pharmaceuticals industries [29].

Tannin or tannic acid is found in several plants such as *Nigella sativa, Camellia Sinensis, Syzygium cumini, Krameria triandra L, Quercus infectoria, Castanea sativa, Ocimum basilicum* and Algae, including several others. It is known for its antiviral (CoVs, RSV, Polio, HIV, HSV *etc.*), antioxidant, anti-inflammatory, anti-carcinogenic, analgesic and antimicrobial properties. Several studies have also been carried out to investigate the anti-SARS-CoV-2 activities of Tannin [30, 31]. A study by Tazeen and colleagues found that Tannin interacted with eleven different residues of helicase protein with a high binding affinity of -9.9 kcal/mol. These residues were from the DEAD-like helicase region of its core domain, which is involved in ATP-dependent RNA or DNA unwinding. Further, other interacting residues were predicted to be part of DNA binding sites of the helicase core domain. Tannin also showed remarkable interaction and high binding energy of -9.4 kcal/mol with several residues of receptor binding motif, which directly interacts with the ACE2 receptor in the host. Tannin also showed the highest affinity for RdRp with binding energy as -11.2 kcal/mol and interacted with several residues of catalytic and N-terminal domain. Tannin also showed very high inhibitory potential values against the helicase and RdRp [32]. Khalifa and colleagues studied 19 different hydrolysable tannins and concluded that castalin, pedunculagin and tercatain interacted strongly with catalytic dyad (Cys145 and His41) and receptor binding site of the protease of SARS-CoV-2. Thus, tannins might serve as potential leading inhibitor molecules for drug development and additional optimization process to combat COVID-19 [33].

Table 2. Potential antiviral phytochemicals against SARS-CoV-2 using *in-silico* approaches.

S. No.	Compound	Plant	Type	Reported Activities of Compound	Studied Protein	Reference
1	Tannin	*Nigella sativa, Camellia sinesis, Ocimum basilicum, Syzygium cumini, Quercus infectoria, Castanea sativa, Punica granatum*	Tannins	Antiviral (SARS-CoV, MERS-CoV), analgesic, anticancer antioxidant, anti-inflammatory	Spike, RdRp, Helicase	[32]
2	Castalin	*Punica granatum, Juglans, Phyllanthus emblica, Combretum glutinosum*	Tannins	Antiviral (SARS-CoV, MERS-CoV)	Protease	[33]

(Table 2) cont.....

S. No.	Compound	Plant	Type	Reported Activities of Compound	Studied Protein	Reference
3	Pedunculagin	*Punica granatum, Juglans, Phyllanthus emblica, Combretum glutinosum*	Tannins	Antiviral (SARS-CoV, MERS-CoV)	Protease	[33]
4	Tercatain	*Punica granatum, Juglans, Phyllanthus emblica, Combretum glutinosum*	Terpene	Antiviral (SARS-CoV, MERS-CoV)	Protease	[33]
5	Dithymoquinone	*Nigella sativa*	Terpene	Antiviral (SARS-CoV)	Spike, RdRp, Helicase	[32]
6	Theaflavin digallate	*Camellia sinensis*	Phenol	Antiviral (SARS-CoV), anticancer	Protease	[34]
7	Bonducellpin D	*Caesalpinia minax*	Terpenoids	Antiviral (SARS-CoV, MERS-CoV)	Protease	[20]
8	Caesalmin B	*Caesalpinia minax*	Terpenoids	Antiviral	Protease	[20]
9	Amaranthin	*Amaranthus tricolor, Amaranthus caudatus*	Lectin	Antiviral, anticancer anti-inflammatory antimicrobial	Protease	[24]
10	Methylrosmarinate	*Hyptis atrorubens Poit, Dracocephalum forrestii*	Phenolic compound	Antimicrobial, metalloproteinases Inhibitor	Protease	[24]
11	Calceolarioside B	*Fraxinus sieboldiana, Lepisorus contortus, Forsythia fructus*	Phenolic compound	Anticancer, antiviral	Protease	[24]
12	Hypericin	*Hypericum species*	Aromatic hydrocarbon	Antiviral, anti-neoplastic, immuno-stimulating activities	Protease	[24]
13	7-Deacetyl-7-benzoylgedunin	*Azadirachta indica*	Terpenoids	Anticancer	Envelope	[21]
14	24-Methylenecycloartanol	*Azadirachta indica*	Terpenoids	Antioxidant, anticancer	Envelope	[21]
15	Phytosterol	*Azadirachta indica*	Sterols	Anticancer, immune system modulators, anti-inflammatory	Membrane	[21]

(Table 2) cont.....

S. No.	Compound	Plant	Type	Reported Activities of Compound	Studied Protein	Reference
16	Beta-Amyrin	*Azadirachta indica, Aspergillus nidulans*	Terpenoids	Antiviral, anti-inflammatory, anticonvulsant	Membrane	[21]
17	24-Methylenecycloartan-3-one	*Azadirachta indica*	Terpenoids	Anticancer	Membrane	[21]
18	Eseential oil [(E, E)- α-farnesene, (E)-β-farnesene, (E, E)-farnesol	*Essential oil, Malus domestica, Matricaria recutita, Zingiber ocinale Roscoe*	Terpene	Antiviral, anti-inflammatory, antimicrobial	Nsp15	[19]
19	Cannabinoids	*Cannabis spp.*	Cannabinoids	Antiviral, anti-inflammatory	Spike	[11]
20	Epigallocatechin	*Camellia sinensis, Prunus domestica, Allium cepa, Corylus avellana*	Polyphenol	Antioxidant, anti-inflammatory	Spike, Protease	[13]
21	Epigallocatechin gallate	*Camellia sinensis, Malus domestica, Prunus domestica, Allium cepa, Corylus avellana*	Polyphenol	Antioxidant, anti-inflammatory, anti-proliferative	Spike, Protease	[11, 13]
22	Curcumin	*Curcuma longa*	Curcuminoid (Polyphenol)	Antioxidant, anti-inflammatory, antibacterial	Spike, Protease	[12, 13, 16, 23]
23	Demethoxycurcumin	*Curcuma longa*	Curcuminoid	Antioxidant, antiviral, anti-inflammatory		[13]
24	Brazilin	*Paubrasilia echinata, Caesalpinia sappan, Caesalpinia violacea, Haematoxylum brasiletto*	Catechols	Anti-Inflammatory, antioxidant, antibacterial	Protease	[12]

(Table 2) cont.....

S. No.	Compound	Plant	Type	Reported Activities of Compound	Studied Protein	Reference
25	Brazilin	*Paubrasilia echinata, Caesalpinia sappan, Caesalpinia violacea, Haematoxylum brasiletto*	Catechols	Anti-Inflammatory, antioxidant, antibacterial	Protease	[12]
26	Betulinic acid	*Compounds found in range of TCM, Crateva religiosa*	Terpenoid	Antiviral, Anticancer antiretroviral, antimalarial, anti-inflammatory	Protease	[14]
27	Homoharringtonine	*Cephalotoxus fortunei*	Alkaloid	Antiviral (MERS-CoV), Antitumor	SARS-CoV-2/ Vero cell line	[35, 36]
28	Emetine	*Ipecac root*	Emetin	Antiviral (hCoV), protein synthesis inhibitor	SARS-CoV-2/ Vero cell line	[35]
29	Neoandrographolide (AGP3)	*Andrographis paniculata*	Terpenoids	Antiviral, anticancer, antimicrobial	Spike, RdRp Protease,	[37]
30	Nimbin	*Azadirachta indica*	Terpenoids	Anti-Inflammatory, antimicrobial	Spike	[23]
31	Saikosaponin V	*Bupleurum spp., Heteromorpha spp. and Scrophularia scorodonia (TCM)*	Saikosaponins (Terpenoid)	Antiviral, anti tumor, anti-inflammatory, anticonvulsant, anti-nephritis, hepatoprotective	Spike, NS15	[17]
32	Saikosaponin U	*Bupleurum spp., Heteromorpha spp. and Scrophularia scorodonia (TCM)*	Saikosaponins (Terpenoid)	Antiviral, anti tumor, anti-inflammatory, anticonvulsant, anti-nephritis, hepatoprotective	Spike, NS15	[17]
33	EGCG	*Camellia sinensis*	Polyphenols	Antiviral	RdRp	[15]
34	10-Hydroxyusambarensine	*Strychnos usambarensis Loganiaceae*	Indole alkaloids	Antibacterial	Protease	[38]
35	Cryptoquindoline	*Cryptolepis sanguinolenta Periplocaceae*	Cryptolepines (Alkaloids)	Antibacterial, antifungal, antimalarial, antioxidant anti-inflammatory, antiamoebic	Protease	[37]

(Table 2) cont.....

S. No.	Compound	Plant	Type	Reported Activities of Compound	Studied Protein	Reference
36	6-Oxoisoiguesterin	*Bisnorterpenes species*	Terpenoids	Antibacterial	Protease	[38]
37	22-Hydroxyhopan-3- one	*Cassia siamea*	Terpenoids	Chemical markers	Protease	[38]
38	Oolonghomobisflavan-A	*Camellia sinensis*	Catechins	Antioxidant	Protease	[26]
39	Theaflavin-3-O-gallate	*Camellia sinensis*	Polyphenols	Antioxidant	Protease	[26]
40	Glycyrrhizin	*Glycyrrhiza uralensis, G. glabra, G.inflate*	Saponin	Antiviral, anticancer antitumor, anti-inflammatory	Protease	[22] [16]
41	Bicylogermecrene	*Eucalyptus, Lantana Camara, Aloysia gratissima*	Terpenoids	Antimicrobial, antibacterial, antifungal, antiviral	Protease	[22]
42	Tryptanthrine	*Strobilanthes cusia*	Alkaloid	Antiviral (hCoV), antibacterial	Protease	[22]
43	Indican	*Isatis indigotica, Indigofera*	Indole	Antiviral (SARS-CoV)	Protease	[22]
44	Indigo	*Isatis indigotica*	Organic compound	Antiviral (SARS-CoV), anti-cancer	Protease	[22]
45	Crysophanic acid	*Citri reticulatae Pericarpium, Aloe vera*	Anthraquinone (Flavanone)	Anti-Inflammatory, antiviral	Protease	[22]
46	Rhein	*Aloe barbadensis, Rheum palmatum*	Anthraquinone	Antiviral, anticancer antimicrobial, anti-inflammatory, antioxidant	Protease	[22]
47	Berberine	*Berberis vulgaris, Berberis aristata, Mahonia aquifolium*	Benzylisoquinoline alkaloids	Antioxidant, antiviral anti-inflammatory	Protease	[22]

(Table 2) cont.....

S. No.	Compound	Plant	Type	Reported Activities of Compound	Studied Protein	Reference
48	β-caryophyllene	*Sssential oil, Ocimum spp., Cinnamomum spp., Piper nigrum, Cannabis sativa, Syzygium aromaticum, Origanum vulgare, Rosmarinus officinalis, Lavandula angustifolia*	Bicyclic sesquiterpene	Antiviral, anticancer, antifungal, anti-inflammatory	Protease	[22]
49	Asiatic acid	*Centella asiatica*	Terpenoids	Antiviral, antioxidant, anti-inflammatory, antitumor, antimicrobial	Protease, Spike, NSP9	[27]
50	Withaferin	*Withania somnifera*	Withanolides (steroids)	Anticancer, antiviral, immunomodulator, anti-inflammatory	Protease, Spike, NSP9	[27]
51	Withanone	*Withania somnifera*	Withanolides (steroids)	Anti-Inflammatory, antioxidant, anticancer	Protease	[39]
52	Caffeic acid phenethyl ester	*Honeybee hive propolis*	Phenolic compound	Antiviral, antioxidant antibacterial, anti-inflammatory, anticarcinogenic	Protease	[39]
53	Hederagenin	*Nigella sativa, Momordica dioica, Luffa cylindrica*	Terpenoids	Anti-Inflammatory, anticancer, antiviral antimutagenic	Protease	[16]
54	Oleanolic acid	*Thymus vulgaris, Rosmarinus officinalis, Olea europaea, Syzygium samarangense*	Terpenoids	Antiviral, anticancer, antitumor, anti-inflammatory	Protease	[16]

(Table 2) cont.....

S. No.	Compound	Plant	Type	Reported Activities of Compound	Studied Protein	Reference
55	Rosmarinic acid	*Ocimum basilicum, Ocimum enuiflorum, Melissa officinalis, Rosmarinus officinalis, Salvia officinalis, Thymus vulgaris, Mentha piperita*	Polyphenol	Antiviral, anticancer antioxidant, anti-inflammatory	Protease	[16]
56	Ursolic acid	*Malus domestica, Ocimum basilicum, Vaccinium myrtillus, Vaccinium xycoccos, Rosmarinus officinalis, Thymus vulgaris, Mentha piperita, Prunus domestica*	Terpenoids	Antiviral, anticancer, antioxidative, anticarcinogenic, *anti*□inflammatory	Protease	[16]
57	Carnosol	*Rosmarinus officinalis*	Terpene	Anticancer, antiviral, antioxidative, anti-inflammatory, anti-microbial	Protease	[40]
58	Arjunglucoside-I	*Terminalia chebula*	Terpene	Anti-inflammatory, antiproliferative, antioxidant	Protease	[40]
59	Rosmanol	*Rosmarinus officinalis*	Terpene	Antioxidant, anticancer	Protease, Spike, NSP9, NS15	[40, 41]
60	Isothymol (Carvacol)(essential oil)	*Ammoides verticillata, Trachyspermum ammi, Nigella sativa, Origanum vulgare*	Terpene	Antiviral, antifungal, antibacterial	ACE2 receptor	[18]
61	Acetylglucopetunidin	-	Phenolic compound	Antiviral (SARS-CoV)	Protease	[28]

(Table 2) cont.....

S. No.	Compound	Plant	Type	Reported Activities of Compound	Studied Protein	Reference
62	Ellagic acid	*Punica granatum, Rubus idaeus, Fragaria ananassa, Vaccinium subg. Oxycoccus*	Catechols	Antiviral (SARS-CoV), antioxidant, antiproliferative, anti-inflammatory	Protease	[28]
63	Arzanol	*Helichrysum italicum*	Phenol	Anti-inflammatory, antiviral, antioxidant	Protease, Spike, NSP-9, NS15	[41]
64	d-viniferin	*Vitis vinifera, Rheum maximowiczii*	Stilbenoid	Anti-tussive	Protease, Spike, RdRp	[9]
65	Phyllaemblicin B	*Phyllanthus emblica*	Terpenoids	Antiviral	Protease, Spike, RdRp	[9]
66	Scalarane	*Hyrtios erectus*	Terpene	Anti-inflammatory, antibacterial, antiviral	Protease, Spike, RdRp	[9]
67	Mangiferin	*Mangifera indica*	Xanthone	Antiviral, analgesic anthelminthic, anti-inflammatory	Spike	[23]

PROMISING ANTIVIRAL POTENTIALS OF PLANTS

From reviewed literature on plants and compounds, we have discussed some significant plants with potential antiviral phytochemicals against COVID-19 (Tables **1** and **2**). These plants, including fruits, vegetables and seeds, are easily available and are used in human diet regularly. They include *Malus domestica* (Apple), *Azadirachta indica* (Neem), *Vitis vinifera* (Black grapes), *Glycyrrhiza glabra* (Licorice), *Curcuma longa* (Turmeric), *Camellia Sinensis* (Black, oolong, and green tea), *Ocimum basilicum* (Basil), *Nigella sativa* (Black seeds), *Origanum vulgare* (Oregano), *Caesalpinia minax, Matricaria Chamomile* (Chamomile), *and Trachyspermum ammi* (Caraway or Ajwain).

Camellia Sinensis (Black/Oolong/Green Tea)

Camellia Sinensis, commonly known as tea plant, is used to make most traditional caffeinated teas, such as oolong black green and white tea. It was originated in China and other tropical and subtropical regions of the world. It contains several phytoconstituents such as antioxidants, steroids, flavonoids, tannins, terpenes, lipid, and polyphenols, including many others. It is known for its medicinal properties including antiviral (anti-SARS), anti-inflammatory, antioxidant, antibacterial, anticancer, anti-helminthic, antimicrobial, as stimulant, and for detoxification. Peele and colleagues studied the compound Theaflavin digallate (TFDG), a natural antioxidant phenol of Camellia Sinensis against the SARS-CoV-2. They concluded that it interacted with very high affinity with active site residues of M^{Pro} and thus can be tested as a potent antiviral in *in vivo* experiments against COVID-19 [34]. Epigallocatechin gallate, another important polyphenol found in high quantity in Camellia Sinensis showed significant interactions with spike glycoproteins and M^{Pro} [11, 13]. Importantly, in a previous study, Epigallocatechin gallate was reported to inhibit the proteolytic activity of SARS-CoV [11]. *Theaflavin*, a flavonoid present in Camellia Sinensis, which is known to exhibit anti-SARS activity previously, also showed inhibitory potential against the RdRp of SARS-CoV-2 [14]. Additionally, three important phytochemicals of oolong tea, *Oolonghomobisflavan-A* (catechins), *Theasinensin-D* (flavonoids) and *Theaflavin-3-O-gallate* (polyphenol) with known antioxidant and antiviral activities also showed significant interactions with M^{Pro} of SARS-CoV-2 [26]. Interestingly, Oolonghomobisflavan-A showed better inhibitory potential against the M^{Pro} as compared to some repurposed drugs currently under trials (*Lopinavir Atazanavir, and Darunavir*) [26]. Further, Apigenin also showed a potential affinity for the RdRp and M^{Pro} and Quercetin for M^{Pro}, as reported by different studies [15, 16].

Vitis vinifera (Grapevine or Black grapes)

Vitis vinifera is commonly known as grapevine with fruits that are known as "black grapes". Grape is the second largest fruit grown in the world, especially in the Mediterranean region. *Vitis vinifera*, its seed and extract are already known for its several pharmacological properties, including antiviral (MERS-CoV, hepatitis and influenza viruses), anti-inflammatory, anti-oxidative, antimicrobial, cardioprotective, hepatoprotective, and neuroprotective activities. It contains numerous bioactive phytochemicals such as polyphenols, flavonoids, terpenes, anthocyanins, procyanidins, proanthocyanidins and resveratrol [42, 43]. Joshi and colleagues studied several compounds, including many anti-tussive molecules. Interestingly, the top anti-tussive compounds like d-viniferin, Chrysanthemin, Myritilin and Myricitrin are present in *Vitis vinifera* extract. This is a key ingredient of Ayurvedic antitussive remedies, immunity and energy boosters like Chyawanprash [9]. Qamar and colleagues also found that Myricitrin has a significant affinity for protease of SARS-CoV-2, thus being a potential antiviral candidate [24]. Another study identified that this plant had good binding affinities and exhibited good interactions with residues of spike and M^{Pro} of SARS-CoV-2 as compared to control antiviral, Nelfinavir.

Malus domestica (Apple)

Malus domestica is one of the healthiest and a popular fruit of human diet with evidence that indicates that it has been cultivated since ancient times. Currently, China is the largest producer of this plant. It is loaded with powerful bioactive phytochemicals such as antioxidants (including quercetin, catechins, phlorizin, and chlorogenic acids), pectin, flavonoids, terpenoids, polyphenols, alkaloids, isoprenoid glycosides and many others. This plant is also known for its substantial antioxidant activities due to the presence of phytochemicals. These phytoconstituents are also known to exhibit antiviral, anti-inflammatory, antimicrobial and anticancer activities [44]. Ramaiah and colleagues concluded that the compounds Apigenin, Quercetin and Ursolic acid interacted significantly with the residues of M^{Pro} of SARS-CoV-2 [16]. Another report also concluded that Apigenin interacted with the RdRp of SARS-CoV-2 [15]. In another study by Tallei and colleagues, it was revealed that Epigallocatechin gallate, a polyphenol showed an affinity for the spike glycoprotein of SARS-CoV-2. Furthermore, another report suggested that some components of essential oil such as (E, E)-α-farnesene, (E)-β-farnesene, and (E, E)-farnesol, also found in *Malus domestica,* exhibit significant affinity for the SARS-CoV-2 endoribonucleoase (Nsp15) [11].

Azadirachta indica (Neem)

Azadirachta indica is commonly known as neem or 'Divine Tree', or 'Nature's Drugstore', a well-known medicinal plant, especially found in the Indian subcontinent. *Azadirachta indica* has been comprehensively used in the Unani, Ayurveda, and Homeopathic medicine system since ancient times. The United Nations declared this plant as the tree of the 21st century. It consists of several important phytochemicals such as alkaloids, flavonoids, saponins, terpenoids, polyphenol, sterols, carotenoids, steroids and ketones. Due to the presence of several essential phytochemicals, it has tremendous pharmacological properties such as antiviral (Influenza virus, HSV, HIV), antioxidant, anti-inflammatory, immuno-modulator, anti-allergenic, anti-fungal, anti-cancer, anti-malarial, anti-bacterial, anti-carcinogenic and others [45]. Borkotoky and colleagues extensively studied several compounds of this plant to identify potential inhibitors against Membrane (M) and Envelope (E) proteins of SARS-CoV-2 [21]. The author identified a few common compounds which interacted with biologically critical residues of M and E protein with strong and stable binding affinities required for assembly. The compounds were also predicted to have good pharmacokinetic properties, thus indicating their potential to inhibit the function of the studied proteins. The identified compounds were several terpenoids (Nimbolin A, Nimocin, 7-Deacetyl-7-benzoylgedunin, 24-Methylenecycloartanol, Cycloeu-calenone, Beta-Amyrin, 24-Methylenecycloartan-3-one) and sterols (phytosterol).

In another study, the Nimbin, a triterpenoid found in the *Azadirachta indica* showed a significant binding affinity for the spike glycoprotein and the ACE2 receptor of SARS-CoV-2 with good pharmacokinetic properties [23].

Glycyrrhiza glabra (Licorice)

Glycyrrhiza glabra is a legume plant which occurs naturally in the Europe, Middle Eastern region and parts of Asia. It is used as a flavoring agent, natural sweetener and in medicinal remedies since thousands of years. *Glycyrrhiza glabra* has been extensively used to treat cough (anti-tussive), colds, asthma around the world since ancient times. It contains active compounds, including flavonoids, glycyrrhizin, glycyrrhetinic acid, isoflavonoids, triterpenoids and chalcones, among others. It exhibits immuno-modulatory, antiviral (SARS-CoV, HIV, HSV, hepatitis, influenza, Varicella zoster viruses), antioxidant, anti-inflammatory, antimicrobial, anti-hepatotoxic, and anti-mutagenic properties [46]. Ramaiah and colleagues studied some essential phytoconstituents of this plant, including flavonoids (Liquiritigenin, Glycoumarin and Glabridin) and saponin (Glycyrrhizin). All these compounds showed significant interaction and stable affinity with M^{Pro} of SARS-CoV-2 [16]. Further, the study by Islam and colleagues also found that Glabridin and Glycyrrhizin have a good binding affinity and strong interactions with catalytic residues of M^{Pro} of SARS-CoV-2. The ADMET and pharmacokinetics study also indicated their efficacy to act as a potential drug molecule [10].

Nigella sativa (Black Seed)

Nigella sativa is a widely used medicinal plant found in Southwest Asia, Southern Europe, and North Africa and is cultivated in many countries like Saudi Arabia, Middle Eastern Mediterranean region, Pakistan, Turkey, India, Syria and South Europe. The *Nigella* seeds and oil have a long history of folklore usage in Arabian and Indian civilization as both medicine and food and are very popular in traditional medicine systems such as Ayurveda, Unani and Tibb, and Siddha. It has been shown to possess a wide spectrum of biological and therapeutic potential, including antiviral (CoVs, Influenza, HIV, HCV *etc.*), antioxidant, anti-inflammatory, immunomodulatory, analgesics, antimicrobial, anti-cancer, fever, bronchodilator, gastroprotective, hepatoprotective, and several other properties [47, 48].

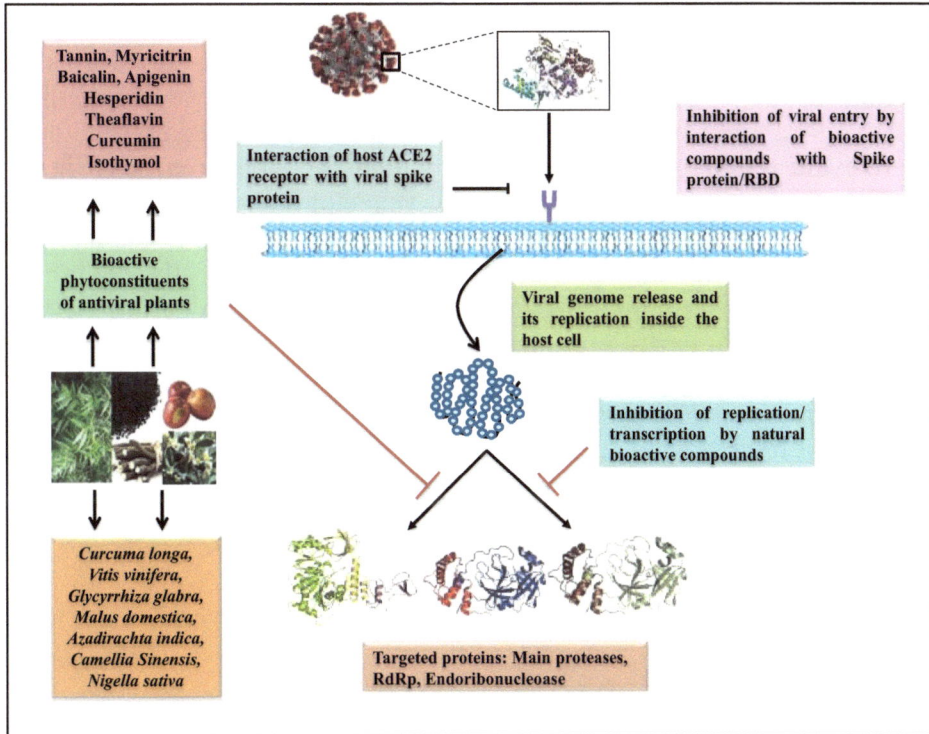

Fig. (2). Potential antiviral compounds targeting proteins of SARS-CoV-2 at different stages of the viral life cycle.

Tazeen and co-workers studied some significant compounds of *Nigella,* including Dithymoquinone (major bioactive component), Tannin and Rutin. All these compounds showed significant interactions and inhibitory potential and a strong affinity with several residues of receptor-binding domain (spike), RdRp and helicase of SARS-CoV-2 [32]. Das and coworkers also showed strong and stable binding affinities of *Nigella sativa* component (Rutin) against the protease and spike protein [13]. Some other studies also showed significant inhibitory potentials of *Nigella sativa* compounds such as isothymol (essential oil), hederagenin and some tannins (castalin, pedunculagin, tercatain) against the receptor-binding domain (spike) and protease of SARS-CoV-2 [16, 18, 34]. Due to its evidence-based healing power, it is considered as one of the top ranked herbal medicines and thus can be further explored to combat the COVID-19, to enhance immune system and also for general well-being.

CONCLUDING REMARKS

The ongoing COVID-19 pandemic has compelled the research scientist towards the identification of therapeutics against SARS-CoV-2 on an urgent basis. In this context, the perusal of the scientific literature on anti-SARS-CoV-2 activity of medicinal plants and their phytochemicals has generated valuable information on their future usage as possible therapeutic agents. We have reviewed different pharmacological and therapeutic properties of these plants and their compounds that were evaluated in recent studies using computational approaches (Fig. **2**). As these compounds are present in many fruits, vegetables and herbs which are used commonly in human diets, it may help to provide the first line of defense against the disease. Even if they may or may not inhibit the virus directly, they might be able to potentiate other antiviral compounds or provide relief from COVID-19 symptoms due to their essential healing properties. Further, they can also be taken as immune system rejuvenator in the daily diet as they have low systemic toxicity. However, further comprehensive *in-vitro* and *in-vivo* experiments are needed to validate their efficacy against COVID-19 infection. In addition, the synergistic effects of standard antivirals and natural compounds in prophylaxis against this respiratory infection is another aspect that can be studied in future investigations.

CONSENT FOR PUBLICATION

Not Applicable.

CONFLICT OF INTEREST

The author declares no conflict of interest, financial or otherwise.

ACKNOWLEDGEMENT

Ayesha Tazeen and Zoya Shafat are supported by Research Fellowship by the University Grants Commission (UGC), Government of India. Farah Deeba and Md Imam Faizan are supported by Research Fellowship by the Indian Council of Medical Research (ICMR), Government of India. The research in our laboratory is funded by the Council of Scientific and Industrial Research (CSIR), India (37(1697)17/EMR-II) and Central Council for Research in Unani Medicine (CCRUM), Ministry of Ayurveda, Yoga and Naturopathy, Unani, Siddha and Homeopathy (AYUSH) (F.No.3-63/2019-CCRUM/Tech).

REFERENCES

[1]   Hussain W, Haleem KS, Khan I, *et al.* Medicinal plants: a repository of antiviral metabolites. Future Virol 2017; 12(6): 299-308.
[http://dx.doi.org/10.2217/fvl-2016-0110]

[2]   Sumner J. The natural history of medicinal plants. USA: Timber press 2000.

[3]   Collins M. Medieval herbals: the illustrative traditions. University of Toronto Press 2000.

[4]   Saad B, Said O. Greco-Arab and Islamic herbal medicine: traditional system, ethics, safety, efficacy, and regulatory issues. John Wiley & Sons 2011.
[http://dx.doi.org/10.1002/9780470944363]

[5]   Kamboj VP. Herbal medicine. Curr Sci 2000; 78(1): 35-9.

[6]   Mohanraj K, Karthikeyan BS, Vivek-Ananth RP, *et al.* IMPPAT: A curated database of Indian Medicinal Plants, Phytochemistry And Therapeutics. Sci Rep 2018; 8(1): 4329.
[http://dx.doi.org/10.1038/s41598-018-22631-z] [PMID: 29531263]

[7]   Jassim SA, Naji MA. Novel antiviral agents: a medicinal plant perspective. J Appl Microbiol 2003; 95(3): 412-27.
[http://dx.doi.org/10.1046/j.1365-2672.2003.02026.x] [PMID: 12911688]

[8]   Vaijwade DN, Kulkarni SR, Sanghai NN. Screening of antiviral compounds from plants—a review. J Pharm Res 2014; 8(8): 1050-8.

[9]   Joshi RS, Jagdale SS, Bansode SB, *et al.* Discovery of potential multi-target-directed ligands by targeting host-specific SARS-CoV-2 structurally conserved main protease. J Biomol Struct Dyn 2020; 1-16.
[http://dx.doi.org/10.1080/07391102.2020.1760137] [PMID: 32329408]

[10]   Islam R, Parves MR, Paul AS, *et al.* A molecular modeling approach to identify effective antiviral phytochemicals against the main protease of SARS-CoV-2. J Biomol Struct Dyn 2020; 1-12.
[http://dx.doi.org/10.1080/07391102.2020.1761883] [PMID: 32340562]

[11]   Tallei TE, Tumilaar SG, Niode NJ, *et al.* Potential of Plant Bioactive Compounds as SARS-CoV-2 Protease (Mpro) and Spike (S) Glycoprotein Inhibitors: A Molecular Docking Study. Preprint. 2020.
[http://dx.doi.org/10.1155/2020/6307457]

[12]   Utomo RY, Meiyanto E. Revealing the potency of citrus and galangal constituents to halt SARS-CoV-2 infection. Preprints 2020; 2020030214.

[13]   Das S, Sarmah S, Lyndem S, Singha Roy A. An investigation into the identification of potential inhibitors of SARS-CoV-2 main protease using molecular docking study. J Biomol Struct Dyn 2020; 1-11.
[http://dx.doi.org/10.1080/07391102.2020.1763201] [PMID: 32362245]

[14]   Mani JS, Johnson JB, Steel JC, *et al.* Natural product-derived phytochemicals as potential agents against coronaviruses: A review. Virus Res 2020; 284: 197989.
[http://dx.doi.org/10.1016/j.virusres.2020.197989] [PMID: 32360300]

[15]   Singh S, Sonawane A, Sadhukhan S. Plant-derived natural polyphenols as potential antiviral drugs against SARS-CoV-2 *via* RNA-dependent RNA polymerase (RdRp) inhibition: An in-silico analysis. J Biomol Struct Dyn. 2020 Jul 28:1-16.
[http://dx.doi.org/10.1080/07391102.2020.1796810] [PMID: 32720577]

[16]   Sampangi-Ramaiah MH, Vishwakarma R, Shaanker RU. Molecular docking analysis of selected natural products from plants for inhibition of SARS-CoV-2 Protease. Curr Sci 2020; 118(7): 1087-92.

[17]   Sinha SK, Shakya A, Prasad SK, *et al.* An *in-silico* evaluation of different Saikosaponins for their potency against SARS-CoV-2 using NSP15 and fusion spike glycoprotein as targets. J Biomol Struct Dyn 2020; 1-12.
[http://dx.doi.org/10.1080/07391102.2020.1762741] [PMID: 32345124]

[18]   Abdelli I, Hassani F, Bekkel Brikci S, Ghalem S. *In silico* study the inhibition of angiotensin converting enzyme 2 receptor of COVID-19 by *Ammoides verticillata* components harvested from Western Algeria. J Biomol Struct Dyn 2020; 1-14.
[http://dx.doi.org/10.1080/07391102.2020.1763199] [PMID: 32362217]

[19]   Silva JKRD, Figueiredo PLB, Byler KG, Setzer WN. Essential Oils as Antiviral Agents. Potential of Essential Oils to Treat SARS-CoV-2 Infection: An *In-Silico* Investigation. Int J Mol Sci 2020; 21(10): 3426.
[http://dx.doi.org/10.3390/ijms21103426] [PMID: 32408699]

[20]   Gurung AB, Ali MA, Lee J, Farah MA, Al-Anazi KM. Unravelling lead antiviral phytochemicals for

the inhibition of SARS-CoV-2 M^{pro} enzyme through *in silico* approach. Life Sci 2020; 255: 117831.
[http://dx.doi.org/10.1016/j.lfs.2020.117831] [PMID: 32450166]

[21]   Borkotoky S, Banerjee M. A computational prediction of SARS-CoV-2 structural protein inhibitors from *Azadirachta indica* (Neem). J Biomol Struct Dyn 2020; 1-17.
[http://dx.doi.org/10.1080/07391102.2020.1774419] [PMID: 32462988]

[22]   Narkhede RR, Pise AV, Cheke RS, Shinde SD. Recognition of natural products as potential inhibitors of COVID-19 main protease (Mpro): *in-silico* evidences. Nat Prod Bioprospect 2020; 10(5): 297-306.
[http://dx.doi.org/10.1007/s13659-020-00253-1] [PMID: 32557405]

[23]   Maurya VK, Kumar S, Prasad AK, Bhatt MLB, Saxena SK. Structure-based drug designing for potential antiviral activity of selected natural products from Ayurveda against SARS-CoV-2 spike glycoprotein and its cellular receptor. Virus Disease 2020; 31(2): 179-93.
[http://dx.doi.org/10.1007/s13337-020-00598-8] [PMID: 32656311]

[24]   Structural basis of SARS-CoV-2 3CLpro and anti-COVID-19 drug discovery from medicinal plants. J Pharm Anal. 2020 Aug; 10(4): 313-9.
[http://dx.doi.org/10.1016/j.jpha.2020.03.009] [PMID: 32296570]

[25]   Aanouz I, Belhassan A, El-Khatabi K, Lakhlifi T, El-Ldrissi M, Bouachrine M. Moroccan Medicinal plants as inhibitors against SARS-CoV-2 main protease: Computational investigations. J Biomol Struct Dyn 2020; 1-9.
[http://dx.doi.org/10.1080/07391102.2020.1758790] [PMID: 32306860]

[26]   Bhardwaj VK, Singh R, Sharma J, Rajendran V, Purohit R, Kumar S. Identification of bioactive molecules from tea plant as SARS-CoV-2 main protease inhibitors. J Biomol Struct Dyn 2020; 8: 1-10.
[http://dx.doi.org/10.1080/07391102.2020.1766572] [PMID: 32397940]

[27]   Azim KF, Ahmed SR, Banik A, Khan MM, Deb A, Somana SR. Screening and druggability analysis of some plant metabolites against SARS-CoV-2: An integrative computational approach. Inform Med Unlocked 2020; p. 100367.
[http://dx.doi.org/10.1016/j.imu.2020.100367] [PMID: 32537482]

[28]   Sayed AM, Khattab AR. Nature as a treasure trove of potential anti-SARS-CoV drug leads: a structural/mechanistic rationale. RSC Adv 2020;10(34):19790-802.
[http://dx.doi.org/10.1039/D0RA04199H]

[29]   Singh AP, Kumar S. Applications of tannins in industry. Tannins-Structural Properties. Biological Properties and Current Knowledge. IntechOpen 2019.
[http://dx.doi.org/10.5772/intechopen.85984]

[30]   Vilhelmova-Ilieva N, Galabov AS, Mileva M. Tannins as antiviral agents. IntechOpen 2019.
[http://dx.doi.org/10.5772/intechopen.86490]

[31]   Mohammed N, Al-Ani RT, Mohammed S. Antibacterial Activity of Tannins Extracted from Some Medicinal Plants *in vitro*. Al-Anbar Medical Journal 2008; 6(1): 1-7.

[32]   Tazeen A, Deeba F, Alam A, *et al.* Virtual screening of potential therapeutic inhibitors against spike, helicase and polymerase of SARS-CoV-2 (COVID-19). Coronaviruses 2020; 1: 1.
[http://dx.doi.org/10.2174/2666796701999200826114306]

[33]   Khalifa I, Zhu W, Mohammed HHH, Dutta K, Li C. Tannins inhibit SARS-CoV-2 through binding with catalytic dyad residues of 3CL^{pro} : An *in silico* approach with 19 structural different hydrolysable tannins. J Food Biochem 2020; e13432.
[http://dx.doi.org/10.1111/jfbc.13432] [PMID: 32783247]

[34]   Peele KA, Potla Durthi C, Srihansa T, *et al.* Molecular docking and dynamic simulations for antiviral compounds against SARS-CoV-2: A computational study. Inform Med Unlocked 2020; 19: 100345.
[http://dx.doi.org/10.1016/j.imu.2020.100345] [PMID: 32395606]

[35]   Choy KT, Wong AY, Kaewpreedee P, *et al.* Remdesivir, lopinavir, emetine, and homoharringtonine

inhibit SARS-CoV-2 replication in vitro. Antivir Res 2020; p. 104786.
[http://dx.doi.org/10.1016/j.antiviral.2020.104786] [PMID: 32251767]

[36]   Ianevski A, Yao R, Fenstad MH, *et al.* Potential antiviral options against SARS-CoV-2 infection. Viruses 2020; 12(6): 642.
[http://dx.doi.org/10.3390/v12060642] [PMID: 32545799]

[37]   Murugan NA, Pandian CJ, Jeyakanthan J. Computational investigation on *Andrographis paniculata* phytochemicals to evaluate their potency against SARS-CoV-2 in comparison to known antiviral compounds in drug trials. J Biomol Struct Dyn 2020; 15: 1-12.
[http://dx.doi.org/10.1080/07391102.2020.1777901] [PMID: 32543978]

[38]   Gyebi GA, Ogunro OB, Adegunloye AP, Ogunyemi OM, Afolabi SO. Potential inhibitors of coronavirus 3-chymotrypsin-like protease (3CL^pro): an *in silico* screening of alkaloids and terpenoids from African medicinal plants. J Biomol Struct Dyn 2020; 1-13.
[http://dx.doi.org/10.1080/07391102.2020.1764868] [PMID: 32367767]

[39]   Kumar V, Dhanjal JK, Kaul SC, Wadhwa R, Sundar D. Withanone and caffeic acid phenethyl ester are predicted to interact with main protease (M^pro) of SARS-CoV-2 and inhibit its activity. J Biomol Struct Dyn 2020; 1-13.
[http://dx.doi.org/10.1080/07391102.2020.1772108] [PMID: 32431217]

[40]   Umesh KD, Kundu D, Selvaraj C, Singh SK, Dubey VK. Identification of new anti-nCoV drug chemical compounds from Indian spices exploiting SARS-CoV-2 main protease as target. J Biomol Struct Dyn 2020; 1-9.
[http://dx.doi.org/10.1080/07391102.2020.1763202] [PMID: 32362243]

[41]   Salman S, Shah FH, Idrees J, *et al.* Virtual screening of immunomodulatory medicinal compounds as promising anti-SARS-COV-2 inhibitors. Future Virol 2020; 10.2217/fvl-2020-0079.
[http://dx.doi.org/10.2217/fvl-2020-0079]

[42]   Pasqua G, Simonetti G. Antimicrobial and antiviral activities of grape seed extracts. In: Lorenzo Rodriguez JM, Ruiz DF, Eds. Grape seeds. New York: Nova Science Publishers 2016; pp. 211-3.

[43]   Odimegwu DC, Ukachukwu UG. Antiviral natural products against hepatitis-a virus. In: Streba CT, Vere CC, Rogoveanu I, Tripodi V, Lucangioli S, Eds. Hepatitis A and other Associated Hepatobiliary Diseases. London: IntechOpen 2020.
[http://dx.doi.org/10.5772/intechopen.91869]

[44]   Liaudanskas M, Viškelis P, Raudonis R, Kviklys D, Uselis N, Janulis V. Phenolic composition and antioxidant activity of Malus domestica leaves. Sci World J 2014; 2014.
[http://dx.doi.org/10.1155/2014/306217]

[45]   Ramadass N, Subramanian N. Study of phytochemical screening of neem (Azadirachta indica). Int J Zool Stud 2018; 3: 209-12.

[46]   Bhat H, Sampath P, Pai R, Bollor R, Baliga M, Fayad R. Indian medicinal plants as immunomodulators: scientific validation of the ethnomedicinal beliefs. Bioactive Food as Dietary Interventions for Arthritis and Related Inflammatory Diseases: Bioactive Food in Chronic Disease States 2012; 22: 215.

[47]   Ahmad A, Husain A, Mujeeb M, *et al.* A review on therapeutic potential of Nigella sativa: A miracle herb. Asian Pac J Trop Biomed 2013; 3(5): 337-52.
[http://dx.doi.org/10.1016/S2221-1691(13)60075-1] [PMID: 23646296]

[48]   Molla S, Azad AK, Al Hasib AA, Hossain MM, Ahammed S, Rana S. A review on antiviral effects of Nigella sativa L. PharmacologyOnline. Newsletter 2019; 2: 47-53.

CHAPTER 10

Drug Repurposing Candidates and Therapeutic Approaches towards the Treatment of COVID-19

Arshi Islam[1], Nazish Parveen[1], Abu Hamza[1], Nazim Khan[1], Syed Naqui Kazim[1], Anwar Ahmed[2,3] and Shama Parveen[1,*]

[1] *Centre for Interdisciplinary Research in Basic Sciences, Jamia Millia Islamia, New Delhi, India*

[2] *Centre of Excellence in Biotechnology Research, College of Science, King Saud University, Riyadh, Saudi Arabia*

[3] *Department of Biochemistry, College of Science, King Saud University, Riyadh, Saudi Arabia*

Abstract: The current outbreak of the novel coronavirus disease known as COVID-19 caused by the newly identified coronavirus strain SARS-CoV-2 has become a prominent health problem worldwide. Therefore, there is an urgent requirement to uncover the specified preventive measures to control the spread of the disease. Different therapeutic approaches such as administration of corticosteroids, vitamins, trace elements, immune enhancers and convalescent plasma recovery can be good alternatives, but the current emergent situation demands specified treatment. The development of vaccines will require longer durations; therefore, deployment of existing drugs as a repurposing approach remains a great option to combat this pathogenic virus. WHO includes different categories of drug treatment options such as antivirals, antimalarial, antiparasitic, antifungal anti-inflammatory, immunosuppressants, inhibitors of kinase and protease monoclonal antibodies immunomodulators, ACE inhibitors and others. Antiviral drugs such as remdesivir, lopinavir/ritonavir, favipiravir, umifenovir and antimalarial drugs such as chloroquine/hydroxy-chloroquine, and several combinations of these drugs are being utilized in different clinical trials and have shown efficacy in the treatment of COVID-19. We have reviewed a general outline about these drugs in the present chapter along with the strategies that may be deployed in the identification of further antiviral agents. However, the side effects associated with their administration and their minimal and maximum dosage norms require special attention. Therefore, the safety and efficacy criteria for the available drugs need confirmation *via* further clinical trials.

Keywords: Arbidol, Chloroquine, COVID-19, Favipiravir, Hydroxy-chloroquine, Lopinavir, Remdesivir, Ritonavir, Therapeutics.

---

* **Corresponding author Shama Parveen:** Centre for Interdisciplinary Research in Basic Sciences, Jamia Millia Islamia, New Delhi, India; E-mails: sparveen2@jmi.ac.in and shamp25@yahoo.com

INTRODUCTION

In late December 2019, an illness of respiratory infections of unknown cause emerged in Wuhan, Hubei province of China. The genome sequence analysis revealed a novel severe acute respiratory syndrome-related coronavirus SARS-CoV-2, formerly known as 2019-nCoV, as the cause of this emerging respiratory illness [1]. The respiratory infection caused by SARS-CoV-2 is named coronavirus disease 2019 or COVID-19. The earlier identified strains of human coronavirus *i.e*, SARS-CoV and MERS-CoV were found zoonotic in origin and reported as the causative agent of severe respiratory infections outbreak from China in 2003 and Saudi Arabia in 2012, respectively [2]. At present, COVID-19 has spread its tentacles worldwide and was later declared as pandemic [3]. Therefore, the present situation of the COVID-19 emergency demands the critical need of potential control strategies for the protection of the people who are at high risk of infection.

The Available Therapeutic Options

Currently, the emerging viral disease, COVID-19 embarks global health with no specific treatments available. However, general treatments, which include maintenance of nutritional elements and administration of immune enhancers, become an efficient way of providing supportive care to the affected individuals [4]. Prior to administration, the nutritional status of the affected individuals should be monitored against nutrition or trace elements to determine its appropriate dosage and minimal risk of side effects associated with it [4]. Many medicinal plants that are part of the Unani and Ayurvedic medicine system under the AYUSH Ministry, Government of India have reported antiviral, anti-inflammatory, antioxidant and immune-modulatory properties. These are plant-derived natural compounds or their combination that can thus be used as nutritional supplements to enhance the sagging immune system in the context of the ongoing COVID-19 pandemic. Alternatively, Traditional Chinese Medicines (TCM) is also based on the plant system. These can also be an effective treatment for COVID-19 since they also possess efficient antiviral activity and provide symptomatic relief as well [5]. In addition, convalescent plasma or passive immune therapy can be given for the treatment of severe and critical cases [4]. Convalescent plasma usually becomes a great option when no specific vaccine or drug is available for the emerging infection [6]. These kinds of general treatment may be extremely helpful in the maintenance and recovery of the patients. However, the current pandemic scenario of COVID-19 warrants an urgent need for vaccines and specified antiviral drugs.

One cannot rule out the existence of generic antiviral treatments that include corticosteroids. Corticosteroids were efficiently used for the treatment of SARS in China and Hong Kong. The reason for their use in SARS illness is that in acute respiratory viral infections, the early response cytokines such as IFN-γ, TNF, IL-1, and IL-6 contribute to tissue damage [7, 8] and corticosteroid treatment may repress this cytokine storm [9]. One such corticosteroid named dexamethasone is widely used and has anti-inflammatory and immunosuppressant effects. It was tested in patients with COVID-19 in the United Kingdom's national clinical trial RECOVERY and was found to have benefits for seriously ill patients [10].

The formulation of vaccines against COVID-19 will take some time; therefore rapid deployment of anti-COVID-19 drugs can be proved as a great therapy to combat the severity of the disease. However, the ongoing pandemic and global emergency of COVID-19 makes the drug therapy development pathway unacceptable as it owes higher costs and longer durations [11]. Therefore, the repurposing of the existing drugs such as those for influenza, hepatitis B (HBV), hepatitis C (HCV), malaria, HIV and other pathogens with an expedition in antiviral treatments can result as an efficient therapeutic option against COVID-19 emergency [12].

Strategies for the Development of an Antiviral Drug

There are three strategies that can be envisaged to discover a potential antiviral drug against this emerging viral pathogen [13]. The first method involves the testing of broad-spectrum antivirals using standard assays [14]. The productive advantage of using these drugs lies in their known pharmacokinetics and pharmacodynamics properties such as, metabolic characteristics, dosages used, potential efficacy, side effects and drug regimens. However, being broad-spectrum and hence non-specific, they may possess adverse side reactions, which should not be underestimated. The second approach utilizes existing compounds for antiviral therapy. The identification of these antiviral compounds is done *via* high throughput screening of chemical libraries or molecular databases [15]. The selected compounds are further evaluated by antiviral assays. The third strategy is based on the development of new specific or targeted drugs [16]. However, this approach will require comprehensive information on genome, biophysical properties and pathology of SARS-CoV-2, which further poses a challenge for the scientific community. A general outline in Fig. (**1**) briefly describes the types of antiviral treatments and drugs available at present against COVID-19 and the strategies that can be envisaged for the development of antiviral drugs.

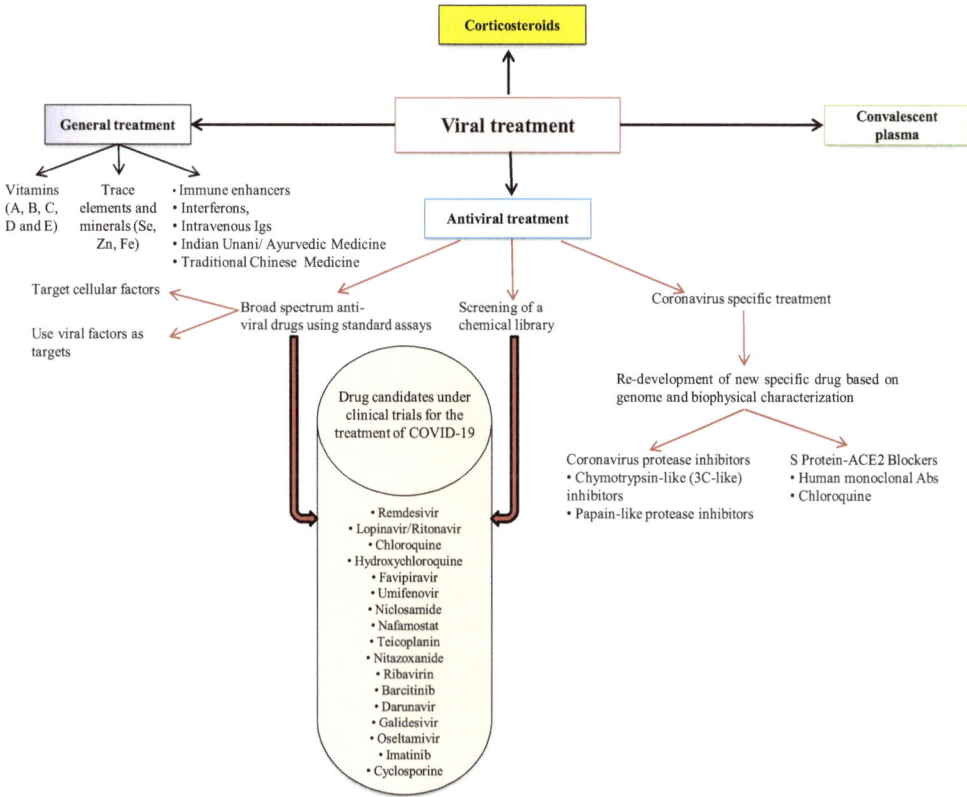

Fig. (1). The available therapeutic options and the antiviral development strategies for the treatment of COVID-19.

Several clinical studies are registered for the discovery of an effective treatment against COVID-19 [12]. The drug repurposing is definitely a potential therapeutic approach for the treatment of the current pandemic of COVID-19. This strategy has provided pharmaceuticals with several candidate drugs. Here, we are reviewing some of the antiviral and well known antimalarial drugs having promising antiviral treatment capacity and are currently under clinical trials for the treatment of COVID-19. These include remdesivir, lopinavir/ritonavir, chloroquine/ hydroxychloroquine, favipiravir (T-705, Avigan), and umifenovir (arbidol).

REMDESIVIR

Remdesivir is a broad spectrum monophosphoramidate prodrug of a nucleoside analog GS-5734, initially developed to combat the infections caused by Ebola and Marburg viruses [17, 18]. However, the *in vivo* and *in vitro* models of the drug had also been reported with efficacy against human coronaviruses that cause serious respiratory illness *i.e.*, SARS-CoV and MERS-CoV [17, 19]. The active form of remdesivir (GS-441524) incorporates itself into nascent viral RNA by the enzyme RNA-dependent RNA polymerases (RdRps), causing its premature termination. It has been speculated in a study that the active form of remdesivir cannot be excised by nsp14-ExoN, which is possibly the cause of this viral replication arrest [20].

In a recent *in vitro* study by Wang and colleagues, remdesivir effectivity was found at low micromolar concentration *i.e.* 0.77 µM, which was potential enough for the blockage of SARS-CoV-2 infection. The half-cytotoxic concentration (CC50) and selectivity index (SI) was found as > 100 µM and > 129.87 respectively [17]. The clinical condition of the first case of COVID-19 in the USA was improved following the intravenous administration of remdesivir [21]. Since then, there has been much interest developed in this antiviral drug and many clinical trials have been registered against it. To assess the efficacy and safety of remdesivir in patients affected with COVID-19, a randomized/double-blinded, placebo-controlled, and multicentered, phase 3 clinical trial study was initiated on 5th of February, 2020 in China (clinical trial no. NCT04252664 and NCT04257656). On 2nd of May, FDA gave emergency use authorization to employ investigational drug remdesivir in the treatment of patients infected with COVID-19 [22]. However, this is a remedy in such an emergency to build a complete picture of how this drug works, many clinical trials are underway.

LOPINAVIR/RITONAVIR *(LPV/RTV)*

The protease inhibitor lopinavir, is usually given in the therapy and prevention of HIV-1. The oral bioavailability of lopinavir is known to be less efficient for an effective response due to the catabolic phenomena by the enzyme system cytochrome P450 (particularly 3A4 isoenzyme) [23]. Thus, ritonavir, another protease inhibitor, is given in combination with lopinavir, as a booster which significantly increases its half-life by inhibiting cytochrome P450 [13, 23]. The *in vitro* analyses have revealed that *LPV/RTV* exerts antiviral effects by inhibiting the replication process of SARS and MERS-CoV [24].The main target of these inhibitors in coronaviruses, is 3C-like protease or 3CLpro, which helps in the processing of the translation product (polypeptide) from the genomic RNA into its protein components [25]. In a study contrasting the treatment of SARS, it was shown that the use of LPV/RTV with ribavirin was associated with a better outcome [26]. A study from South Korea has reported a triple combination therapy of LPV/RTV, ribavirin and IFN-α2 as a successful treatment against MERS-CoV infection [27]. According to the present Chinese guidelines for the COVID-19 treatment, a PO 50 mg-200 mg dose twice in a day for not more than

10 days should be administered [28]. The *LPV/RTV* is used as a single agent regimen when combined with either interferon-α or ribavirin. However, no efficacy was found in a randomized open-label study which includes two arms: one was *LPV/RTV* and the other was the standard care. The study includes 199 patients of COVID-19 (Clinical Trial Number: ChiCTR2000029308). Moreover, no significant benefit in regard to overall mortality or in the reduction in viral load was observed [29].

CHLOROQUINE/HYDROXYCHLOROQUINE

Chloroquine and hydroxychloroquine (CQ/HCQ) both are traditional antimalarial drugs derived from quinoline molecule. The mechanism of action of these antimalarial drugs is not well understood. However, some direct and indirect mechanisms have been proposed that illustrates their immunomodulatory effects [30]. Both HCQ and CQ interfere with lysosomal and transcriptional activity at the molecular level. They have also been shown to disrupt the stability of the membrane, autophagy and in the alteration of signaling pathways [30]. Both the drugs have a large volume distribution, long half-life, slow commencement of the action and prolonged effects after drug discontinuation.

Some previous studies have reported the direct antiviral effect of chloroquines in flavivirus, retrovirus and coronaviruses [31 - 33]. It has been said that in the human body, chloroquine phosphate gets converted into chloroquine to play its therapeutic effect. A recent *in vitro* study has shown that chloroquine, with EC50 as 1.13 μmol/L and SI > 88 can effectively inhibit SARS-CoV-2 at the cellular level [17]. The *in vivo* clinical trial studies have also shown the promising results of the two drugs. Following the results of these initial clinical trial studies the National Health Commission of the People's Republic of China published recommendations regarding treatment with chloroquine. They have suggested 500 mg chloroquine phosphate and 300 mg chloroquine, two times in a day for not more than 10 days [28]. Though the results seem promising but there are certain side effects associated with the use of CQ/HCQ which limits the long-term use of these drugs, such as renal toxicity [34]. Therefore, an accurate prescription is required in people with renal or liver failure.

FAVIPIRAVIR

A pyrazine carboxamide derivative (6-fluoro-3-hydroxy-2-pyrazinecarboxamide), favipiravir is known as a broad spectrum oral antiviral drug. The drug was initially approved as a therapeutic option in the treatment of influenza virus in Japan [35]. This prodrug gets converted into its active form which is ibofuranosyl-5'-triphosphate (T-705-RTP) following ribosylation and phosphorylation intracellularly [35]. This active form of favipiravir competes with the purine nucleosides for the incorporation into viral RNA and that's how it inhibits the enzyme RNA dependent RNA polymerase (RdRp) of the RNA viruses [36].

Based on its mechanism of action of inhibiting the RdRp enzyme of RNA viruses and safety data in some clinical studies, it is considered as one of the efficient candidates in the treatment of COVID-19. No preclinical and *in vitro* studies are available yet. However, clinical trials are underway against this drug to check its safety and efficacy in SARS-CoV-2 infection. A clinical study carried out in Shenzhen (ChiCTR2000029600), with the recruitment of 80 patients have shown a shorter period of viral clearance in favipiravir arm than the control one [37]. Another clinical study which is multicentered (ChiCTR200030254) also reported effective control against COVID-19 following favipiravir administration [38]. Recently, In India, the Pharmaceutical Company Glenmark, has remarked the results obtained from the Phase 3 clinical trial study of favipiravir against the COVID-19 treatment. The study included mild to moderate patients who received favipiravir tablets 3,600 mg (1,800 mg BID) (Day 1) + 1,600 mg (800 mg BID) (Day 2 or later) up to of 14 days, along with standard supportive care. The study is evident to consider using the drug favipiravir in milder infections of symptomatic patients of COVID-19 [39].

UMIFENOVIR (ARBIDOL)

Umifenovir (arbidol) is one of the potential candidates for an antiviral treatment in respiratory viral infections. The drug was initially licensed in Russia and China for prophylaxis, and treatment for influenza virus. Currently, the drug is approved by Drug Controller General of India (DCGI) for clinical trials in COVID-19 treatment at the Council of Scientific and Industrial Research (CSIR) [40]. Previous studies on arbidol had shown blocking of viral fusion against influenza A and B and hepatitis C virus [41]. The *in vitro* studies have shown that arbidol most likely inhibits the entry and replication of the hepatitis C virus [42]. In addition, the derivative arbidol mesylate have shown the antiviral activity against the SARS-CoV in the cultured cells where it was found more effective than the arbidol itself [43]. Another derivative, arbidol hydrochloride, blocks the virus replication by inhibiting the fusion mechanism of viral membrane with the host cells [24]. Arbidol is being used in a clinical trial for COVID-19 treatment (ChiCTR2000029573). The drug has been added into the NHC Guidelines for the Diagnosis and Treatment of COVID-19 (6th and 7th editions) in China, where it is recommended as an oral administration for adults at a dose of 200 mg, 3 times per day for no more than 10 days [44]. The current dosage of arbidol may not possibly attain an ideal therapeutic efficacy against SARS-CoV-2, and therefore, needs to be elevated however, such a regimen will require verifications *via* further clinical trial studies [45].

A summary of potential antiviral/anti-malarial agents is given in Table **1**, providing a brief description of their action mechanism and the pathogen they are associated with.

Table 1. Details about the potential drug candidates for COVID-19 treatment.

Antiviral/ Anti-malarial Agent	Key Feature	Mechanism of Action	Viral Pathogen	References
Remdesivir (RDV)	Nucleoside analogue	Inhibits RNA dependent RNA polymerase enzyme	SARS-CoV-2 MERS-CoV SARS-CoV	[46, 47]
Lopinavir/ Ritonavir	Protease inhibitor	Inhibits 3CLpro	SARS-CoV-2 MERS-CoV SARS-CoV	[29]
Chloroquine/ Hydroxy-chloroquine	Antimalarial drug	Increase pH of endosomes, interfere with membrane stability, alter signaling pathways and transcriptional activity, interfere with the glycosylation of cellular receptors, ACE-2 of SARS-CoV	SARS-CoV-2 MERS-CoV SARS-CoV	[30, 48, 49]
Favipiravir	Nucleoside analogue	Inhibits RdRp enzyme, prevents replication	SARS-CoV-2 Influenza	[50]
Arbidol	Broad spectrum antiviral	Impede the trimerization of SARS-CoV-2 spike glycoprotein	SARS-CoV-2 Influenza	[51]

World Health Organization has classified the type of drug treatment available for the COVID-19. The classification includes specific and broad spectrum antivirals (Interferons, Interleukin-2, Favipiravir, Umifenovir, Remdesivir, LPV/RTV), antimalarial (CQ/HCQ), antiparasitic (Niclosamide, Nitazoxanide), antibiotic (Carrimycin, Teicoplanin, Azithromycin), antifungal (Itraconazole), anti-inflammatory (Dexamethasone), immunosuppressants (Thalidomide), inhibitors of kinase and protease (Imatinib mesylate, CamostatMesilate), monoclonal antibodies (Eculizumab), immunomodulators (CD24), ACE inhibitors (Losartan), antiarrhythmic (Amiodarone), vasodilator (Angiotensin 1-7), anticoagulant (Rivaroxaban), NSAID (Ibuprofen), mucolytic, antidepressant and others [52]. The classification also includes many non-drug candidates. The drug safety and efficacy criteria in different stages of the infection requires further clinical trial studies with accuracy in their dosage so as to minimize the side effects associated with their long-term usage.

CONCLUDING REMARKS

In this article, we have briefly described the therapeutic options that are available at present to combat the severity of the emerging infectious disease COVID-19. These options include general treatment, convalescent plasma and antiviral treatment using drug repurposing and generation of specific COVID-19 drugs. Out of all these options, it is supposed that drugs that can directly interact with SARS-CoV-2 or targets host ACE2 receptor molecule will be proved as the most effective approach against COVID-19. Nonetheless, redevelopment of such specified drugs with antiviral and anti-inflammatory properties would show better antiviral effects but on the cost of longer duration and high performance for the evaluation of clinical trials. Drug repurposing remains an alternative approach in such an emergency of COVID-19. However, the development of vaccines is always a finite aid against disease, and there are various efforts in progress to develop these vaccines against SARS-CoV-2.

CONSENT FOR PUBLICATION

Not Applicable.

CONFLICT OF INTEREST

The author declares no conflict of interest, financial or otherwise.

ACKNOWLEDGEMENTS

Arshi Islam and Abu Hamza are supported by the Senior Research Fellowship of Indian Council of Medical Research (ICMR), Government of India. The research in our laboratory is funded by the Council of Scientific and Industrial Research (CSIR), India (37(1697)17/EMRII) and Central Council for Research in Unani Medicine (CCRUM), Ministry of Ayurveda, Yoga and Naturopathy, Unani, Siddha and Homeopathy (AYUSH) (F.No. 3-63/2019-CCRUM/Tech). The authors also extend their appreciation to the Centre of Excellence in Biotechnology Research, Deanship of Scientific Research, King Saud University, Riyadh, Saudi Arabia, for support.

REFERENCES

[1]   Zhu N, Zhang D, Wang W, *et al.* A novel coronavirus from patients with pneumonia in China, 2019. N Engl J Med 2020; 382(8): 727-33.
[http://dx.doi.org/10.1056/NEJMoa2001017] [PMID: 31978945]

[2]   Cui J, Li F, Shi ZL. Origin and evolution of pathogenic coronaviruses. Nat Rev Microbiol 2019; 17(3): 181-92.
[http://dx.doi.org/10.1038/s41579-018-0118-9] [PMID: 30531947]

[3]   Islam A, Ahmed A, Naqvi IH, *et al.* Emergence of deadly severe acute respiratory syndrome

coronavirus-2 during 2019–2020. VirusDis 2020; 31: 128-36.
[http://dx.doi.org/10.1007/s13337-020-00575-1] [PMID: 32292802]

[4]   Zhang L, Liu Y. Potential interventions for novel coronavirus in China: A systematic review. J Med Virol 2020; 92(5): 479-90.
[http://dx.doi.org/10.1002/jmv.25707] [PMID: 32052466]

[5]   Ren JL, Zhang AH, Wang XJ. Traditional Chinese medicine for COVID-19 treatment. Pharmacol Res 2020; 155: 104743.
[http://dx.doi.org/10.1016/j.phrs.2020.104743] [PMID: 32145402]

[6]   Marano G, Vaglio S, Pupella S, *et al.* Convalescent plasma: new evidence for an old therapeutic tool? Blood Transfus 2016; 14(2): 152-7.
[PMID: 26674811]

[7]   Van Reeth K, Van Gucht S, Pensaert M. Correlations between lung proinflammatory cytokine levels, virus replication, and disease after swine influenza virus challenge of vaccination-immune pigs. Viral Immunol 2002; 15(4): 583-94.
[http://dx.doi.org/10.1089/088282402320914520] [PMID: 12513929]

[8]   Cheung CY, Poon LL, Lau AS, *et al.* Induction of proinflammatory cytokines in human macrophages by influenza A (H5N1) viruses: a mechanism for the unusual severity of human disease? Lancet 2002; 360(9348): 1831-7.
[http://dx.doi.org/10.1016/S0140-6736(02)11772-7] [PMID: 12480361]

[9]   Oba Y, Lee N, Sung J. The use of corticosteroids in SARS. N Engl J Med 2003; 348(20): 2034-5.
[http://dx.doi.org/10.1056/NEJM200305153482017] [PMID: 12748321]

[10]   The Economic Times. Health Ministry adds steroid dexamethasone in COVID-19 treatment protocol.
https://economictimes.indiatimes.com/industry/healthcare/biotech/pharmaceuticals/health-ministr-
-adds-steroid-dexamethasone-in-co-
id-19-treatment%20protocol/articleshow/76660072.cms?from=mdr

[11]   Lythgoe MP, Rhodes CJ, Ghataorhe P, Attard M, Wharton J, Wilkins MR. Why drugs fail in clinical trials in pulmonary arterial hypertension, and strategies to succeed in the future. Pharmacol Ther 2016; 164: 195-203.
[http://dx.doi.org/10.1016/j.pharmthera.2016.04.012] [PMID: 27133570]

[12]   Lythgoe MP, Middleton P. Ongoing clinical trials for the management of the covid-19 pandemic. Trends Pharmacol Sci 2020; 41(6): 363-82.
[http://dx.doi.org/10.1016/j.tips.2020.03.006] [PMID: 32291112]

[13]   Lu H. Drug treatment options for the 2019-new coronavirus (2019-nCoV). Biosci Trends 2020; 14(1): 69-71.
[http://dx.doi.org/10.5582/bst.2020.01020] [PMID: 31996494]

[14]   Chan JF, Chan KH, Kao RY, *et al.* Broad-spectrum antivirals for the emerging Middle East respiratory syndrome coronavirus. J Infect 2013; 67(6): 606-16.
[http://dx.doi.org/10.1016/j.jinf.2013.09.029] [PMID: 24096239]

[15]   Dyall J, Coleman CM, Hart BJ, *et al.* Repurposing of clinically developed drugs for treatment of Middle East respiratory syndrome coronavirus infection. Antimicrob Agents Chemother 2014; 58(8): 4885-93.
[http://dx.doi.org/10.1128/AAC.03036-14] [PMID: 24841273]

[16]   Wang C, Xu P, Zhang L, Huang J, Zhu K, Luo C. Current strategies and applications for precision drug design. Front Pharmacol 2018; 9: 787.
[http://dx.doi.org/10.3389/fphar.2018.00787] [PMID: 30072901]

[17]   Wang M, Cao R, Zhang L, *et al.* Remdesivir and chloroquine effectively inhibit the recently emerged novel coronavirus (2019-nCoV) *in vitro*. Cell Res 2020; 30(3): 269-71.
[http://dx.doi.org/10.1038/s41422-020-0282-0] [PMID: 32020029]

[18]   Warren TK, Jordan R, Lo MK, *et al.* Therapeutic efficacy of the small molecule GS-5734 against Ebola virus in rhesus monkeys. Nature 2016; 531(7594): 381-5.
[http://dx.doi.org/10.1038/nature17180] [PMID: 26934220]

[19]   Sheahan TP, Sims AC, Graham RL, *et al.* Broad-spectrum antiviral GS-5734 inhibits both epidemic and zoonotic coronaviruses. Sci Transl Med 2017; 9(396): eaal3653.
[http://dx.doi.org/10.1126/scitranslmed.aal3653] [PMID: 28659436]

[20]   Gordon CJ, Tchesnokov EP, Feng JY, Porter DP, Götte M. The antiviral compound remdesivir potently inhibits RNA-dependent RNA polymerase from Middle East respiratory syndrome coronavirus. J Biol Chem 2020; 295(15): 4773-9.
[http://dx.doi.org/10.1074/jbc.AC120.013056] [PMID: 32094225]

[21]   Holshue ML, DeBolt C, Lindquist S, *et al.* Washington State 2019-nCoV Case Investigation Team. First case of 2019 novel coronavirus in the United States. N Engl J Med 2020; 382(10): 929-36.
[http://dx.doi.org/10.1056/NEJMoa2001191] [PMID: 32004427]

[22]   The Economic Times. FDA allows emergency use of anti-viral vaccine Remdesivir to treat COVID-19 patients. https://economictimes.indiatimes.com/news/international/world-news/fda allows-emergenc--use-of-anti-viral-vaccine-remdesivir-to-treat-covid-19-patients/articleshow/75501209.cms

[23]   Sham HL, Kempf DJ, Molla A, *et al.* ABT-378, a highly potent inhibitor of the human immunodeficiency virus protease. Antimicrob Agents Chemother 1998; 42(12): 3218-24.
[http://dx.doi.org/10.1128/AAC.42.12.3218] [PMID: 9835517]

[24]   Wu C, Liu Y, Yang Y, *et al.* Analysis of therapeutic targets for SARS-CoV-2 and discovery of potential drugs by computational methods. Acta Pharm Sin B 2020; 10(5): 766-88.
[http://dx.doi.org/10.1016/j.apsb.2020.02.008] [PMID: 32292689]

[25]   Morse JS, Lalonde T, Xu S, Liu WR. Learning from the past: possible urgent prevention and treatment options for severe acute respiratory infections caused by 2019-nCoV. ChemBioChem 2020; 21(5): 730-8.
[http://dx.doi.org/10.1002/cbic.202000047] [PMID: 32022370]

[26]   Chu CM, Cheng VC, Hung IF, *et al.* Role of lopinavir/ritonavir in the treatment of SARS: initial virological and clinical findings. Thorax 2004; 59(3): 252-6.
[http://dx.doi.org/10.1136/thorax.2003.012658] [PMID: 14985565]

[27]   Kim UJ, Won EJ, Kee SJ, Jung SI, Jang HC. Combination therapy with lopinavir/ritonavir, ribavirin and interferon-α for Middle East respiratory syndrome. Antivir Ther 2016; 21(5): 455-9.
[http://dx.doi.org/10.3851/IMP3002] [PMID: 26492219]

[28]   Dong L, Hu S, Gao J. Discovering drugs to treat coronavirus disease 2019 (COVID-19). Drug Discov Ther 2020; 14(1): 58-60.
[http://dx.doi.org/10.5582/ddt.2020.01012] [PMID: 32147628]

[29]   Cao B, Wang Y, Wen D, *et al.* A trial of lopinavir–ritonavir in adults hospitalized with severe Covid-19. N Engl J Med 2020; 382(19): 1787-99.
[http://dx.doi.org/10.1056/NEJMoa2001282] [PMID: 32187464]

[30]   Schrezenmeier E, Dörner T. Mechanisms of action of hydroxychloroquine and chloroquine: implications for rheumatology. Nat Rev Rheumatol 2020; 16(3): 155-66.
[http://dx.doi.org/10.1038/s41584-020-0372-x] [PMID: 32034323]

[31]   Randolph VB, Winkler G, Stollar V. Acidotropic amines inhibit proteolytic processing of flavivirus prM protein. Virology 1990; 174(2): 450-8.
[http://dx.doi.org/10.1016/0042-6822(90)90099-D] [PMID: 2154882]

[32]   Neely M, Kalyesubula I, Bagenda D, Myers C, Olness K. Effect of chloroquine on human immunodeficiency virus (HIV) vertical transmission. Afr Health Sci 2003; 3(2): 61-7.
[PMID: 12913796]

[33]   Vincent MJ, Bergeron E, Benjannet S, *et al.* Chloroquine is a potent inhibitor of SARS coronavirus infection and spread. Virol J 2005; 2(1): 69.
[http://dx.doi.org/10.1186/1743-422X-2-69] [PMID: 16115318]

[34]   Mavrikakis M, Papazoglou S, Sfikakis PP, Vaiopoulos G, Rougas K. Retinal toxicity in long term hydroxychloroquine treatment. Ann Rheum Dis 1996; 55(3): 187-9.
[http://dx.doi.org/10.1136/ard.55.3.187] [PMID: 8712882]

[35]   Furuta Y, Komeno T, Nakamura T. Favipiravir (T-705), a broad spectrum inhibitor of viral RNA polymerase. Proc Jpn Acad, Ser B, Phys Biol Sci 2017; 93(7): 449-63.
[http://dx.doi.org/10.2183/pjab.93.027] [PMID: 28769016]

[36]   Furuta Y, Takahashi K, Kuno-Maekawa M, *et al.* Mechanism of action of T-705 against influenza virus. Antimicrob Agents Chemother 2005; 49(3): 981-6.
[http://dx.doi.org/10.1128/AAC.49.3.981-986.2005] [PMID: 15728892]

[37]   Cai Q. Experimental treatment with Favipiravir for COVID-19: an open-label control study. Engineering (Beijing). 2020 Oct; 6(10): 1192-98.
[http://dx.doi.org/10.1016/j.eng.2020.03.007] [PMID: 32346491]

[38]   Chen C, Zhang Y, Huang J. Favipiravir *versus* arbidol for COVID-19: a randomized clinical trial. medRxiv 2020.
[http://dx.doi.org/10.1101/2020.03.17.20037432]

[39]   Express Pharma. Glenmark announces top-line results from Phase 3 clinical trial of favipiravir for COVID-19 treatment. https://www.expresspharma.in/covid19-updates/glenmark-announces-top- line-results-from-phase-3-clinical-trial-of-favipiravir-for-covid-19-treatment/.Accessed2020.

[40]   The Indian Express. https://indianexpress.com/article/india/favipiravir-umifenovir-drugs-now- in-clinical-trials-to-treat-covid-19-6466919/

[41]   Boriskin YS, Leneva IA, Pécheur EI, Polyak SJ. Arbidol: a broad-spectrum antiviral compound that blocks viral fusion. Curr Med Chem 2008; 15(10): 997-1005.
[http://dx.doi.org/10.2174/092986708784049658] [PMID: 18393857]

[42]   Pécheur EI, Borisevich V, Halfmann P, *et al.* The synthetic antiviral drug arbidol inhibits globally prevalent pathogenic viruses. J Virol 2016; 90(6): 3086-92.
[http://dx.doi.org/10.1128/JVI.02077-15] [PMID: 26739045]

[43]   Khamitov RA, Loginova SIa, Shchukina VN, Borisevich SV, Maksimov VA, Shuster AM. Antiviral activity of arbidol and its derivatives against the pathogen of severe acute respiratory syndrome in the cell cultures. Vopr Virusol 2008; 53(4): 9-13.
[PMID: 18756809]

[44]   National Health Commission of the People's Republic of China. http://www.nhc.gov.cn/yzygj/ s7653p/202001/f492c9153ea9437bb587ce2ffcbee1fa. shtml

[45]   Wang X, Cao R, Zhang H, *et al.* The anti-influenza virus drug, arbidol is an efficient inhibitor of SARS-CoV-2 *in vitro*. Cell Discov 2020; 6(1): 28.
[http://dx.doi.org/10.1038/s41421-020-0169-8] [PMID: 32373347]

[46]   Wang Y, Zhang D, Du G, *et al.* Remdesivir in adults with severe COVID-19: a randomised, double-blind, placebo-controlled, multicentre trial. Lancet 2020; 395(10236): 1569-78.
[http://dx.doi.org/10.1016/S0140-6736(20)31022-9] [PMID: 32423584]

[47]   Eastman RT, Roth JS, Brimacombe KR, *et al.* Remdesivir: A review of its discovery and development leading to emergency use authorization for treatment of COVID-19. ACS Cent Sci 2020; 6(5): 672-83.
[http://dx.doi.org/10.1021/acscentsci.0c00489] [PMID: 32483554]

[48]   Singh R, Vijayan V. Chloroquine: A potential drug in the COVID-19 scenario. Transactions of the Indian National Academy of Engineering 2020; 1-2.

[49]   Hashem AM, Alghamdi BS, Algaissi AA, *et al.* Therapeutic use of chloroquine and

hydroxychloroquine in COVID-19 and other viral infections: A narrative review. Travel Med Infect Dis 2020; 35: 101735.
[http://dx.doi.org/10.1016/j.tmaid.2020.101735] [PMID: 32387694]

[50] Du YX, Chen XP. Favipiravir: pharmacokinetics and concerns about clinical trials for 2019-nCoV infection. Clin Pharmacol Ther 2020; 108(2): 242-7.
[http://dx.doi.org/10.1002/cpt.1844] [PMID: 32246834]

[51] Vankadari N. Arbidol: A potential antiviral drug for the treatment of SARS-CoV-2 by blocking trimerization of the spike glycoprotein. Int J Antimicrob Agents 2020; 56(2): : 105998..
[http://dx.doi.org/10.1016/j.ijantimicag.2020.105998] [PMID: 32360231]

[52] World Health Organization. COVID 19 candidate treatments. https://www.who.int/publications/m/item/covid-19-candidate-treatments

CHAPTER 11

COVID-19 Vaccine Development: Challenges and Current Scenarios

Nazish Parveen[1]**, Arshi Islam**[1]**, Nazim Khan**[1]**, Anwar Ahmed**[2,3]**, Irshad H. Naqvi**[4] **and Shama Parveen**[1,*]

[1] *Centre for Interdisciplinary Research in Basic Sciences, Jamia Millia Islamia, New Delhi, India*

[2] *Centre of Excellence in Biotechnology Research, College of Science, King Saud University, Riyadh, Saudi Arabia*

[3] *Department of Biochemistry, College of Science, King Saud University, Riyadh, Saudi Arabia*

[4] *Dr. M.A. Ansari Health Centre, Jamia Millia Islamia, New Delhi, India*

Abstract: The ongoing situation of COVID-19 pandemic entails us towards the development of a prophylactic vaccine as a public health priority. The emergence of SARS-CoV-2 in Wuhan, China during December 2019 marked the third introduction of a highly pathogenic Coronavirus into human population in the twenty-first century. Knowledge from the former vaccine candidates of SARS-CoV and MERS-CoV has unlocked the door for the developers to accelerate the global vaccine development pathway for ongoing COVID-19 pandemic, soon after the online publication of SARS-CoV-2 genomic sequence. The vaccine development pipeline for COVID-19 shows a promising result by utilizing various platforms (nucleic acid, viral vector, recombinant protein, live attenuated viruses, inactivated viruses and virus like particles) with different strategies. Surprisingly till now, we have about 190 vaccine candidates in the clinical and pre-clinical pipeline till 31st August 2020. Approximately, 39 of these vaccine candidates are impending into the human clinical trials after showing significant safety data in preclinical studies of which, 8 vaccine candidates are running in final phase3 stage. Three of them have got an emergency approval for limited or early use. At least 8 candidate vaccines have been developed from India, from which 2 of them have entered phase2 trials. Already existing tuberculosis vaccines are also being tested in clinical trials bridging the gap before a potential COVID-19 vaccine is developed. This chapter highlights the obstacles for implementation of vaccine development for SARS-CoV-2. One of the impediments is identification of high-risk population including frontline health care workers, elderly individuals and persons with pre-existing chronic diseases. We have also provided a comprehensive overview about

* **Corresponding author Shama Parveen:** Centre for Interdisciplinary Research in Basic Sciences, Jamia Millia Islamia, New Delhi, India; E-mails: sparveen2@jmi.ac.in and shamp25@yahoo.com

the COVID-19 vaccine candidates that are in preclinical and clinical stages of development. Thus, fast track clinical trials of many candidates are implemented in different geographical regions promising a prophylactic vaccine against SARS-CoV-2.

Keywords: COVID-19, Clinical trial, Clinical pipeline, Challenges, SARS CoV-2, Pre-clinical trial, Vaccine development.

INTRODUCTION

Coronaviruses are one of the critical pathogens, affecting humans (mainly respiratory system) and vertebrates. The world witnessed a rapid outbreak of Coronavirus infection that became pandemic, putting global public health in peril from the very beginning of twenty-first century. This century had already experienced the emergence of two formerly identified Coronaviruses. The commencement of Coronavirus emergence as a severe acute respiratory syndrome (SARS-CoV) occurred in China during 2002-2003 [1, 2]. After 10 years, in 2012 an outbreak of Middle East Respiratory Syndrome (MERS-CoV) took place in Saudi Arabia. At the end of 2019, another mysterious ongoing outbreak of Coronavirus was reported in the city of Wuhan, China, (epicentre of COVID-19) that manifests respiratory like ailments [3]. WHO on 11th February 2020 named the disease as "the Corona Virus Disease-2019; **COVID-19**" and the pathogen was designated as a 2019 novel Coronavirus (**2019-nCoV**) that was later named as **SARS CoV-2**. On 11th March 2020, WHO declared COVID-19 as a pandemic [2].

Most of the affected individuals manifest mild respiratory illness (fever, cough, difficulty in breathing) but some of the individuals show severe manifestations like respiratory bilateral interstitial pneumonia which advance to respiratory failure [4]. Moreover, some patients have also been reported with hypo/dysgeusia (loss of sense of smell), hypo/anosmia (loss of sense of taste) and gastrointestinal problems as early symptoms of the infection. However, more severe illness has been demonstrated with health care workers and in the individuals of older age, immunocompromised and those with chronic health conditions. This pathogen is extremely contagious, transmitted from either infected asymptomatic or symptomatic individuals through the droplets of saliva or discharge from the nose [5].

Coronavirus belongs to the family Coronaviridae and the genus beta-Coronavirus (β-CoVs). β-CoVs are enveloped viruses with positive sense single stranded RNA genome (+mRNA). They show eminently higher mutation rate due to the constant transcription errors as well as RNA Dependent RNA Polymerase (RdRP) jump.

The genome consists of functional and structural proteins (surface glycoprotein or spike (S), envelope (E), matrix (M), and nucleocapsid (N)) [6]. Of these structural proteins, the S protein imparts a vital role in the host cell attachment [7, 8]. Receptor binding domain (RBD), a key part of S protein helps in initial attachment of virus to the host cell surface. SARS-CoV-2 uses the same ACE2 (angiotensin converting enzyme 2) human receptor, which is abundantly present on the mucosal epithelial cells of respiratory tract and lung parenchyma [9 - 12]. A recent analysis suggested that SARS-CoV-2 has lower pathogenicity rate (about 3%) than SARS-CoV (10%) and MERS-CoV (40%) [13]. Furthermore, it has higher transmissibility rate (R0:1.4–5.5) than both SARS-CoV (R0:2–5) and MERS-CoV (R0: <1) [13].

Till 31st August 2020, WHO reported over 29,107,970 confirmed cases of COVID-19 with 926,910 deaths in 216 countries and territories across the world [14]. By the mid of April 2020, several short approaches like good hygiene practices, social distancing and quarantine methods have been implemented to lessen the transmission of SARS-CoV-2. Other approaches include the implementation of therapeutic drugs (remdesivir, favipiravir, hydroxychloroquine, combination of lopinavir and ritonavir and many more) to reduce the effect of viral attack. The most promising approach being followed to minimize the impact of SARS-CoV-2 is the development of a prophylactic vaccine. Due to the current pandemic situation, COVID-19 vaccine is concurrently needed all over the world. In this review, we describe some of the major vaccine candidates in the clinical pipeline and the obstacles behind the implementation of vaccine.

VACCINES

There was a rapid acceleration in the expansion of SARS-CoV-2 globally and the announcement of outbreak as a public health emergency of international concern by the WHO. This prompted the research scientists to accelerate the development process for safe and efficacious vaccine. Development of a vaccine is a complex, cost-effective and a time-consuming process. Traditionally it takes about a period of 12-15 years to produce a licensed vaccine [15]. Due to the risk of failure and high expenses, developers should pursue a paradigm (sequential steps) for vaccine development with various halts to check its safety and efficiency. The safety of the vaccine is first evaluated in the laboratories with animal models (rats or monkeys). If the vaccine shows no disease in animal models, then the testing is progressed towards humans in different phases with gradually rise in number of subjects (Fig. **1**). But during this Covid-19 pandemic, a fast-tracked paradigm with 12-18 months of timeline was suggested with a quick start and many shortened steps. Moreover, few steps will be carried out in parallel before safety data will be obtained from a previous step, thus leading to a high financial risk to the developers and manufacturers. For example, human phase1 clinical trial will be executed in parallel with the animal studies.

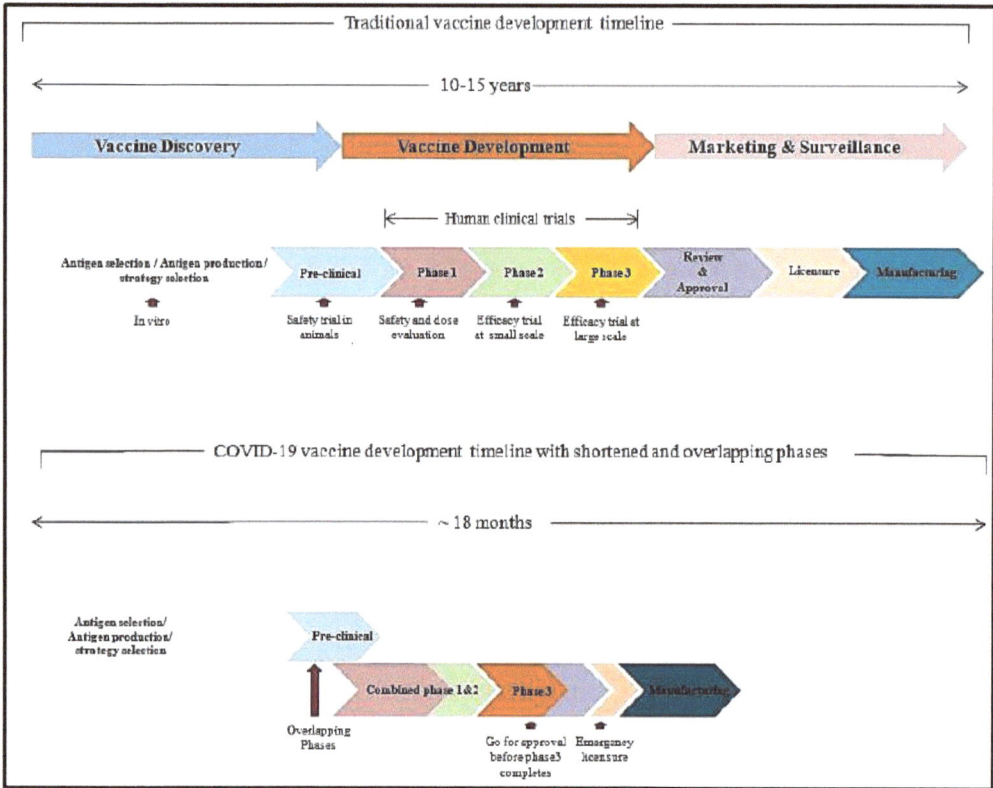

Fig. (1). Differences between the traditional vaccine Vs COVID-19 vaccine development pathway (The COVID-19 vaccine development time will be accelerated by conducting multiple steps simultaneously at financial risk without knowing the results from previous step. Reduction in the timeline will leads to shortened clinical trial phases to evaluate safety and efficacy of the vaccine).

Currently, no vaccine against COVID-19 is available. Even though numerous vaccine candidates have been discovered for SARS-CoV and MERS-CoV, still none of them have been approved yet. However, more than 190 potential vaccine candidates against SARS-CoV-2 using different platform and strategies are in the clinical pipeline globally.

Most of the candidates are in preclinical trials and it might take a year to start phase1 clinical trials except for those funded by Coalition for Epidemic Preparedness Innovations (CEPI). Most of the vaccine candidates in human clinical trials are from China as compared with other countries. Some of the vaccine candidates are running in human clinical trial, while some others will begin these imminently. Even though, if safety results of human trials will be satisfactory, there may be various obstacles in the implementation of the vaccine.

OBSTACLES IN THE IMPLEMENTATION OF COVID-19 VACCINE

Due to the current pandemic situation, COVID-19 vaccine is concurrently needed all over the world. Therefore, clinical and serological assays will be required to judge which population or areas are at higher risk after the vaccine is approved to be used for the public. A globally fair allocation system will be formed during vaccine development.

Infelicitously, the main obstacles accompanying the implementation of COVID-19 vaccine are numerous. One of the major obstacles is the observation of immunopotentiation (increased infectivity) after immunization with whole virus or even complete spike protein with previous SARS and MERS vaccine candidates [16]. The rationale behind this discovery remains unexplained. Hence, it will be critical to meticulously monitor a safety profile of COVID-19 vaccine prior to the commencement of human trials. Another obstacle is the selection of the target population; health care workers, immunocompromised individuals or those suffering from health problems like diabetes, hypertension or asthma and the individuals above 60 years are at a higher risk of infection [17]. Consequently, this type of vulnerable population can be preferred for clinical trials.

Still another obstacle will be the accessibility of vaccine on time for this ongoing pandemic of COVID-19. However, it should be stock-pilled (accumulated and maintained for future use). Due to these peculiar obstacles, COVID-19 vaccine candidates in the clinical pipeline must incorporate these key features that are summarized in Fig. (2). The global vaccine community will provide financial and technical support needed for the vaccine development, large scale manufacturing, deployment and fair allocation system which are critical to addressing the COVID-19 pandemic as well as future pandemic preparedness. The challenge remains with the possibility of the occurrence of a new major outbreak of Coronavirus in future. Moreover, the most improbable if the pandemic ends prior to the COVID-19 vaccine developed. In addition, the vaccine should be economical enough to be afforded by the developing countries.

ANTIGEN SELECTION FOR VACCINE DEVELOPMENT

A prophylactic vaccine acts by displaying unique antigens from virus to the immune system, seeking out to train the immune system for the expeditious generation of a significant number of antibodies at the time of actual infection [15]. The future candidate vaccines against COVID-19 might have the same strategies and the target antigen as in the SARS and MERS vaccine studies that are outlined in Table **1**. Selection or design of antigen is essential for optimum immune response apart from the mode of strategy or the adjuvant to enhance the immune response [18]. Different vaccines have distinct characteristics with respect to the type of antigen, immune response (humoral or cell mediated) generated and the location of eliciting the immune response.

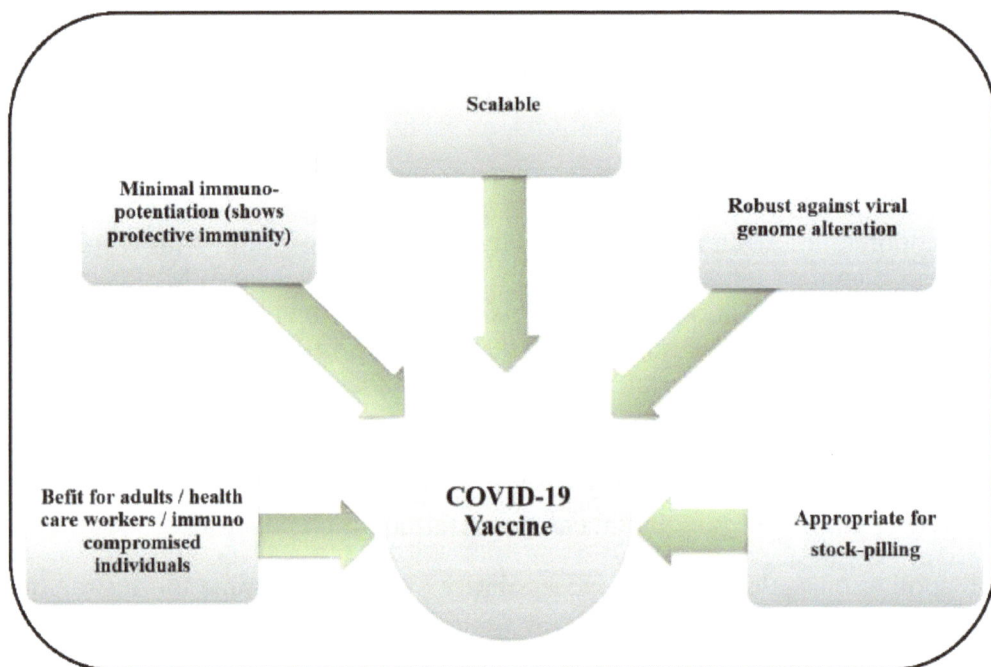

Fig. (2). Key features of COVID-19 vaccine.

Table 1. Target antigens and vaccine platforms employed in SARS and MERS vaccine development.

Antigen	Vaccine Platform	Pros	Cons	Stage	References
Full length spike or S1 protein	DNA vaccine	Easy to construct, Safe, Induces both cell mediated and humoral immune response, Inexpensive	Relatively produces lesser immune response, Potent delivery system is required, May be toxic due to repeated doses	Phase 2	[26]
Full length spike or S1 protein	Viral vector vaccine	Induces active and specific immune response	Pre-existing immunity in humans may cause inflammation or harmful immune response	Phase 1	[26, 27]

(Table 1) cont.....

Antigen	Vaccine Platform	Pros	Cons	Stage	References
Whole virus	Inactivated vaccine	Rapid production, Virus structure intact, Potent immune response, formulated with various adjuvant to boost immune response	Comparatively unsafe, May cause hypersensitivity	Phase 1	[28]
Whole virus	Live attenuated vaccine	Rapid production, Virus structure intact, Potent immune response, formulated with various adjuvant to boost immune response	Comparatively unsafe, Risk of reverting virulence, Not suitable for infants and immunocompromised individuals	Phase 1	[26]
Full length spike, RBD, Nucleo-capsid	Subunit vaccine	Safe, Minimizing undesirable side effects at infection site, Induces potent and safe immune response, Consistent production	Required suitable adjuvant, not always cost effective	Phase 1	[26, 29, 30]
RBD, co-expression of S1, M, E	VLPs	Variety of expression system required, Induces neutralizing Antibodies and protection, Preserved virus structure	Required optimal components for VLP formation	Phase 1	[31, 32]

In the view of recent findings, it has been demonstrated that SARS-CoV-2 binds to the same ACE2 receptor found on mucosal epithelial cells of human lungs in a similar manner as former SARS-CoV [9, 19] and shows 89% nucleotide similarity [20] with SARS like Coronavirus. Previous efforts made in the development of a vaccine against SARS and MERS, will open the door for the companies or universities to expedite COVID-19 vaccine development. The technologies and the antigens employed in the vaccination studies for SARS-CoV and MERS-CoV have their own pros and cons that are summarized in Table **1**.

Full-length spike (S) protein perhaps is the most potent antigen for vaccine development as it could generate neutralizing antibodies, resulting in inhibition of host cell attachment, hence infection [21 - 23]. However, immunopotentiation was also observed with SARS-CoV and MERS-CoV vaccine candidates using inactivated vaccine or subunit vaccine strategies. Among the various technology platforms in the clinical pipeline is the nucleic acid-based vaccines proved to be the most progressed one. Moreover, it was the first candidate vaccine entering the phase1 clinical trial. Development in the technologies has been created to enhance the stability and the efficacy of protein expression in mRNA or other nucleic acid-based vaccines, which leads to robust and protective immune response [24, 25].

ONGOING VACCINE DEVELOPMENT FOR COVID-19

With expeditious emergence of infection and with its ability to become pandemic within a few weeks, battle of developing a therapeutic vaccine against SARS-CoV-2 has been flared up in many countries. The platform technologies that have been applied for SARS and MERS for which clinical safety data already exist may unlock a faster route for the progression of COVID-19 vaccine into clinical trials. As of now, we are not having any approved therapeutic vaccine against COVID-19. However, more than 190 prophylactic vaccine candidates are in the pre-clinical and clinical pipeline globally using wide array of technology platforms till 31st August 2020. Fig. (**3**) shows the distribution of COVID-19 vaccine candidates according to different vaccine platform. About 151 vaccine candidates are in preclinical stage and would probably take about a year to start phase 1 clinical trial excluding those funded by CEPI (Coalition for Epidemic Preparedness Innovations). In fact, 39 vaccine candidates have commenced their human clinical trial (Table **2**). Some other candidates were reported to impending into the milestone of human trials by the end of 2020. Some of the investigators are also testing efficacy of tuberculosis vaccine over COVID-19 infection. But information about the vaccine candidates of COVID-19 in the developmental pipeline is very preliminary. So we have highlighted the major COVID-19 vaccine strategies that are publicly available on the websites or other documents including biocentury.com, clinicaltrialsarena.com, covid-19 vaccine tracker, and WHO [33 - 36].

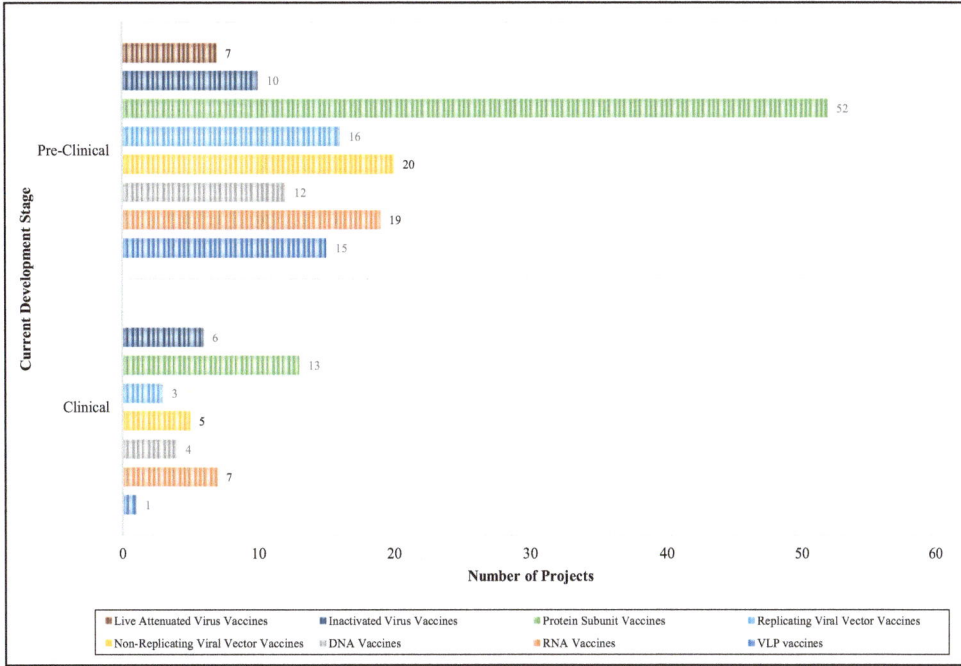

Fig. (3). Graphical representation of COVID-19 vaccine candidates by different vaccine platforms in clinical pipeline (other efforts include pre-existing tuberculosis vaccine to fight against COVID-19). As of 31 August 2020, 190 candidates are undergoing development, of which 39 vaccine candidates will enter human clinical trial.

Till date, at least 39 candidate vaccines against COVID-19 infection are being evaluated for safety profile data in clinical trials (Table **2**). The researchers are trying various inventive technology platform for vaccine development. The most feasible for speeding up in the clinical trials are the vector-based, inactivated virus followed by nucleic acid-based vaccine platforms. China is leading with maximum number of candidates that are being evaluated in human trials.

Currently, 8 vaccine candidates (Sputnik-V, Ad5-nCoV, AZD1222, BBIBP-CorV, CoronaVac, mRNA-1273, BNT162 and Wuhan's inactivated vaccine) have moved into the phase 3 clinical trial. Recently the 3 most advanced Sputnik-V, Ad5-nCoV and CoronaVac vaccine candidates have got an emergency approval for early or limited use before obtaining results from phase 3 trial. CVnCoV, NVX-CoV2373, COVAXIN and a recombinant subunit vaccine by China are in phase2 clinical trial. At least 15 teams are conducting combined phase 1/2 clinical trial including LV-SMENP-DC, GX-19, INO-4800, AG0301-COVID-19, Jassen's vaccine, QazCovid, Epivac Corona *etc* while 14 other vaccine candidates are in phase1 clinical study to evaluate an optimal dose that can be administered safely to the individuals (Fig. **4**).

Table 2. Description of COVID-19 vaccine candidates in clinical pipeline.

Vaccine Candidate	Vaccine Platform	Researcher / Developer	Vaccine Characteristics	Status
BCG vaccine	Tuberculosis vaccine	Mercks	Tuberculosis Vaccine to evaluate its efficacy against COVID-19	Phase 4
VMP1002	Tuberculosis vaccine	Max Planck Institute	Genetically modified BCG vaccine, Tuberculosis Vaccine to evaluate its efficacy against COVID-19	Phase 3
Sputnik-V	Non-replicating Viral vector	Gameleya Research Institute	Genetically modified adenoviral vector expressing S protein, Combination of Ad5 and Ad26	Phase 3 (approved for early use)
Ad5-nCoV	Non-replicating Viral vector	Can Sino Biological lnc. / Beijing Institute of Biotechnology	Replication defective Adenovirus type 5 vector expressing S protein	Phase 3 (approved for limited use)
AZD1222	Non-replicating Viral vector	University of Oxford /AstraZeneca	Genetically modified Adenoviral vector expressing S protein	Phase 3
CoronaVac	Inactivated vaccine	Sinovac / Dynavax	Formalin inactivated, Adjuvanted with CpG 1018™	Phase 3 (approved for limited use)
Wuhan's inactivated vaccine	Inactivated vaccine	Wuhan's Institute of Biological Products / Sinopharm	Heat killed SARS-CoV2	Phase 3
BBIBP-CorV	Inactivated vaccine	Beijing Institute of Biological Products / Sinopharm	Unknown	Phase 3
mRNA-1273	RNA	Moderna Therapeutics / NIAID	LNP encapsulated mRNA encoding S protein of SARS-CoV-2	Phase 3
BNT162	RNA	BioNTech / Fosun Pharma / Pfizer	mRNA encoding S protein	Phase3
Recombinant Subunit vaccine	Protein subunit	Anhui ZhifeiLongcom Biopharmaceutical / Institute of Microbiology, Chinese Academy of Sciences	Recombinant viral S protein (RBD Dimer), Adjuvanted	Phase 2
NVX-CoV2373	Protein subunit	Novavax	Full length recombinant S protein based nanoparticle, Adjuvanted with Matrix-M	Phase 2

(Table 2) cont.....

Vaccine Candidate	Vaccine Platform	Researcher / Developer	Vaccine Characteristics	Status
COVAXIN	Inactivated vaccine	Bharat Biotech / ICMR / NIV	Heat killed Sars-CoV2	Phase 2
CVnCoV	RNA	CureVac	LNP encapsulated mRNA encoding S protein of SARS-CoV2	Phase 2
Inactivated vaccine	Inactivated	Institute of Medical Biology / Chinese Academy of Medical Science	Unknown	Phase 1/2
QazCovid	Inactivated	Research Institute for Biological Safety Problems, Kazakhstan	Inactivated SARS-CoV-2	Phase 1/2
LV-SMENP-DC	Replicating viral vector	Shehzhen Geno-immune Medical Institute	Based on minigene (conserved domain of S protein), DCs altered with lentiviral vector expressing minigene, Delivered with antigen specific CTLs	Phase 1/2
Jassens vaccine	Non-replicating viral vector	Jhonsons and Jhonsons	S protein expressed in recombinant Adenoviral vector	Phase 1/2
GX-19	DNA	Genexine	DNA encoding S protein of SARS-CoV2, Based on Genexineplatform(GX-19)	Phase 1/2
AG0301-COVID-19	DNA	Anges Inc. / Osaka university / Takara Bio	Plasmid DNA, Adjuvanted	Phase 1/2
INO-4800	DNA	Inovio Pharmaceuticals	Plasmid DNA encoding S protein, Delivered through electroporation	Phase 1/2
DNA Vaccine	DNA	Zydus Cadila	Plasmid DNA encoding S protein of SARS-CoV2	Phase1/2
RNA vaccine	RNA	Arcturus therapeutics / Duke-NUS	Based on STARR™ technology platform, Self-amplifying RNA delivered with LUNAR system	Phase 1/2
RNA vaccine	RNA	Imperial college of London	Self-amplifying RNA, LNP incapsulated	Phase 1/2
Subunit vaccine	Protein subunit	Sanofi / GSK	S protein inserted in Baculovirus vector Adjuvanted with CpG 1018	Phase 1/2
Subunit vaccine	Protein subunit	Kentucky Bio Processing (KBP)	Antigens produced in tobacco plants	Phase 1/2

(Table 2) cont.....

Vaccine Candidate	Vaccine Platform	Researcher / Developer	Vaccine Characteristics	Status
Subunit vaccine	Protein Subunit	West China Hospital, Sichuan University	RBD (Baculovirus production expressed in Sf9 cells)	Phase 1/2
EpiVacCorona	Protein Subunit	Russian biological research centre, Vector Institute	Small peptides of S protein	Phase 1/2
Subunit vaccine	Protein subunit	FBRI SRC VB VECTOR / Rospotrebnadzor / Koltsovo	Based on S protein of SARS-CoV2	Phase 1/2
Subunit vaccine	Protein subunit	Queensland university / GSK / Dynavax	Molecular Clamp stabilized S protein	Phase 1
COVAX-19	Protein subunit	Vaxine / Flinders University	Based on S protein of SARS-CoV2	Phase 1
SCB-2019	Protein subunit	Clover Biopharmaceuticals / GSK / Dynavax	Trimeric S protein similar to native SARS-CoV2, Adjuvanted with CpG 1018™ & ASO3	Phase 1
Subunit vaccine	Protein Subunit	Adimmune	RBD of S protein of SARS-CoV-2	Phase 1
Soberana1	Protein subunit	Instituto Finlay de Vacunas, Cuba	RBD + Adjuvant	Phase 1
Subunit vaccine	Protein Subunit	Medigen Vaccine Biologics Corporation/NIAID/Dynavax	S-2P protein + CpG 1018	Phase 1
RNA vaccine	RNA	Academy of Military Medical Sciences / Suzhou Abogen Biosciences / Walvax Biotechnology	Based on mRNA	Phase 1
RNA vaccine	RNA	People's Liberation Army (PLA) Academy of Military Sciences/Walvax Biotech	Based on mRNA	Phase 1
Vector vaccine	Replicating viral vector	Pasteur Institute / Themis / Pittsburg university	Measles vector expressing S protein	Phase 1
Pathogen specific-aAPC vaccine	Replicating viral vector	Shehzhen Geno-immune Medical Institute	Artificial APC modified with LV minigene	Phase 1
GRAd-COV2	Non-Replicating Viral Vector	ReiThera/LEUKOCARE/Univercells	Replication defective Simian Adenovirus (GRAd) encoding S	Phase 1
VLP Vaccine	Virus like particle	Medicago	Plant based VLP	Phase 1

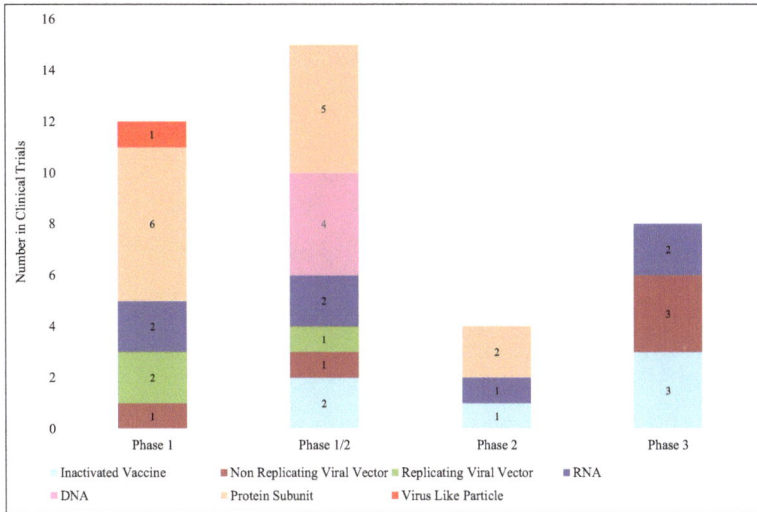

Fig. (4). Graphical representation of COVID-19 vaccine candidates in different phases of clinical trials. As of 31st August 2020, 39 vaccine candidates will enter human clinical trial.

A remarkable feature of COVID-19 vaccine development pipeline is the wide array of technology platform being assessed, comprising of viral vector (replicating and non-replicating), nucleic acid (DNA and RNA), protein subunit, live attenuated virus, inactivated virus and virus like particle approaches. Some of these platforms are not even used before in already existing licensed vaccines. In the view of vaccine candidates listed in Table **2**, the novel DNA or RNA based platform exhibits higher resilience to manipulate antigen and potential for speed. Some of the platforms may be more appropriate for distinct population (like immunocompromised individuals, elderly people, children's and pregnant women's). Some platforms could implement the adjuvant with vaccine candidates to boost the immune response.

Viral Vector Vaccine

Viral vector based vaccines use live virus as a vector to deliver DNA (antigen) of the target virus into the human cell. A virus such as measles or adenovirus is genetically engineered so that it can produce Coronavirus proteins in the body. These viruses are weakened therefore they cannot cause disease. There are two types: Replicating viral vector vaccines (those that can still replicate within host cells) and Non-replicating viral vector vaccines (those that cannot replicate within the host cells because replicating genes have been disabled). These vaccines can enhance the immunogenicity in human cell without the use of an adjuvant [37]. About 8 viral vector based vaccines are at different stages of clinical trials. A brief description of these vaccine candidates is given below.

Sputnik-V (Approved for Early Use)

The Gameleya Research Institute in Russia has developed a non-replicating viral vector based vaccine candidate for COVID-19 named Gam-COVID-Vac, later renamed as Sputnik-V. It is a combination of two genetically engineered adenoviruses (Ad5 and Ad26) with SARS-CoV-2 gene encoding S protein [35]. On 4th September 2020, a combined phase 1/2 trial results were published showing immune response with mild side effects [38]. Russian health care regulator had approved the Sputnik-V for early use prior to the commencement of phase3 trial. Medical experts declared that this as a risky move. Recently phase 3 clinical trials were also launched for this candidate [39].

Ad5-nCoV (Approved for Limited Use)

Ad5-nCoV is a recombinant novel Coronavirus (SARS-CoV-2) vaccine co-developed by Can Sino Biological and Beijing Institute of Biotechnology. The vaccine is based on Can Sino Bio's replication defective type 5 adenoviral vector, which is used for the expression of spike (S) protein of the SARS-CoV-2. Previously this adenoviral technology platform was successfully used in developing the first approved Ebola vaccine in China during 2017. Preclinical study of Ad5-nCoV vaccine candidate showed a robust and safe immune response in animal models.

Preliminary safety data of phase1 trial including 108 healthy individuals aged between 18-60 years at Tongi hospital in Wuhan, China (the epicenter of COVID-19) has been published in May [40, 41]. Unprecedently on 25th June, 2020 the Chinese military has approved the Ad5-nCoV to use for year as a "specially needed drug". Currently its phase 3 trial is ongoing in Saudi Arabia [42].

AZD1222

It is an Adenovirus vector-based vaccine developed at the University of Oxford in a partnership with AstraZeneca. The vaccine candidate consists of a genetic code for an immunogenic S protein within a modified chimpanzee adenoviral vector AZD1222 (previously known as ChAdOx1). This results in the expression of S protein after vaccination. Phase 1 clinical trial with 110 individuals aged 18-55 years has been conducted in multiple areas across Oxford, London and Southampton [43]. The volunteers will be randomly administered with either AZD1222 or a control licensed vaccine MenACWY (vaccine for meningitis). The study showed positive results with no adverse side effects. The vaccine will be delivered intramuscularly. A Phase 2b/3 clinical trial was started in England by recruiting approximately 10,000 healthy individuals [44] as well as phase 3 trial involving 30,000 volunteers in Brazil, South Africa and the United States [45].

Janssen Vaccine

Johnson & Johnson, a multinational company, has flared up the vaccine development program for COVID-19 as soon as genomic sequence of SARS-CoV-2 was published under its division, Janssen's Pharmaceuticals [46]. The company uses adenoviral vector (Janssen's AdVac®) analogous to the platform used in their Ebola vaccine as well as their HIV and ZIKA vaccine candidates [47]. Janssen's vaccine is based on recombinant adenovirus 26 (Ad26), whose replicating mechanism has been disabled so that it could not lead to common cold. The S protein of SARS-CoV-2 was inserted into the vector. The company expects to begin the phase1 clinical trial by September 2020 and the prophylactic vaccine might be available for use in early 2021. The company has launched a phase 1/2 trials in July and a Phase 3 trial will be launched in September with 60,000 participants in Latin America [36].

GRAd-COV2

ReiThera, a biotechnological company, has developed a vaccine for COVID-19 based on adenoviral vector that infects gorillas and named it GRAd-COV2. In July 2020, the company has launched a phase1 clinical trial in collaboration with Lazzaro Spallanzani National Institute for Infectious Disease in Rome [48].

LV-SMENP-DC

Shehzhen Geno-immune produces a vaccine based on a minigene, which was engineered by the insertion of conserved structural and protease domain of S protein of the SARS-CoV-2 into a lentiviral vector system (NHP/TYF) to express the viral antigens (SMENP minigene). Dendritic cells were then modified by LV-SMENP minigene and immune modulatory genes to formulate this candidate against COVID-19 infection. The candidate (expressing COVID-19 antigens) vaccine will be administered with cytotoxic T lymphocytes (CTLs). A combined phase1/2 study of the vaccine was started on 24 March, 2020 [49]. It is an open label study including 100 healthy individuals of 6 months to 80 years of age to evaluate the efficacy of COVID-19 LV-DC and T cell vaccine. Each subject will be administered subcutaneously with 5×10^8 cells of LV-DC vaccine and 1×10^8 CTLs *via* intravenous infusion method (controlled administration).

aAPC

An artificial APC (antigen presenting cell) vaccine candidate was also produced by Shehzhen Geno-immune against COVID-19. The vaccine is based on the LV minigenes and the immune modulatory genes to modify the artificial APC. Phase1 clinical trial of the vaccine was started on 15th February 2020 [50]. Like LV-DC vaccine, it is also an open label study involving 100 volunteers of 6 months to 80 years of age to evaluate its safety and efficiency. Each subject will receive subcutaneously 5×10^8 cells of the vaccine.

University of Pittsburg collaborated with **Pasteur Institute** and **Themis** for developing a vaccine based on a recombinant Measles vector (rMV). Measles vaccine is modified to express S protein of SARS-CoV-2 on its surface [36].

Whole Virus Vaccines

Whole virus vaccine includes live-attenuated or inactivated vaccine using whole virus particles which are fully damaged by heat, chemical or radiations. These types of vaccines needed an extended safety profile. At least 6 vaccines are developed by using SARS-CoV-2 in a weakened or inactivated form. These vaccines are being evaluated for safety profile and efficacy in different stages of clinical trials. A brief description of these vaccine candidates is given below.

CoronaVac (Approved for Limited Use)

It is a formalin inactivated vaccine candidate developed by Sinovac. Dynavax supported the candidate by deploying its patented adjuvant system (CpG 1018™). Phase 2 clinical trials were initiated in parallel with phase1. A total of 743 individuals were enrolled at a single centre with 143 healthy individuals at phase 1 and 600 at phase 2 of 18-59 years of age, with two dose vaccination of distinct concentration [51, 52]. It is a randomized, placebo controlled and double-blinded study. Results of the study showed positive immune response. Sinovac has launched phase 3 clinical trial in Brazil and Indonesia. The study involves 8870 healthy individuals of 18-59 years who were scheduled to be injected with the vaccine or placebo [53]. In July the vaccine has got an emergency approval for limited use [36]. Sinovac has agreed with Indonesia to supply 40 million vaccine doses by March 2021.

Inactivated Novel Coronavirus Pneumonia Vaccine

Wuhan Institute of Biological Products has developed an inactivated novel Coronavius pneumonia vaccine under Sinopharm (China National Pharmaceuticals) using heat killed SARS-CoV-2. Combined Phase1/2 clinical trials were initiated on 12th April 2020 by enrolling 96 individuals in three different age groups [54]. The result from the phase1 study showed an effective neutralizing antibody response. Recently the companies have launched the phase3 clinical trial in the United Arab Emirates by recruiting 15,000 healthy adults [55]. In August, Sinopharm announced that the vaccine will be available for public use by the end of this year.

BBIBP-CorV

Beijing Institute of Biological Products has developed a second inactivated vaccine under Sinopharm (China National Pharmaceuticals). A phase 3 trial, including 5,000 healthy individuals, has been started in United Arab Emirates [56].

Inactivated SARS-CoV-2 Vaccine

Institute of Medical Biology, together with Chinese Academy of Medical Sciences, developed an inactivated vaccine. A combined phase1/2 trial was executed on 15th May 2020 to evaluate the safety and immunogenicity of the inactivated SARS-CoV-2 vaccine of distinct doses [57]. The study involves 942 healthy individuals of 18-59 years. Phase 2 trial was also initiated in June.

COVAXIN

The vaccine has been developed by an Indian company Bharat Biotech situated in Hyderabad in association with National Institute of Virology (NIV) and Indian Council of Medical Research (ICMR). It is an indigenous inactivated SARS-CoV-2 vaccine. The candidate is based on genetically modified and inactivated rabies virus vaccine which carries genes for the S protein of SARS-CoV-2. COVAXIN will be India's first vaccine to enter human clinical trial. The vaccine candidate has been approved for a combined phase1/2 clinical trial by Drug Controller General of India (DGCI) of India. The clinical trials of this vaccine have been started in India [58]. Traditionally these trials take months which goes along with phase 3 trial. Moreover, these clinical trials must be followed by analysis and verification of the vaccine candidate before it is approved for public use.

QazCovid

Kazakhastan, a central nation of Asia has developed an inactivated SARS-CoV-2 vaccine and named it QasCovid. Their Research Institute of Biological Safety Problems has launched a combined phase 1/2 clinical trial in August [59].

Nucleic acid vaccines

Nucleic acid-based vaccines consist of a genetic sequence (DNA or mRNA) encoding the antigen in a recombinant plasmid. These recombinant plasmids are inserted directly into the patient's cell, which leads to the induction of a strong cell mediated as well as humoral immune response without the help of adjuvant unlike traditional vaccines [60]. Many biotechnological companies are leading with nucleic acid vaccine platforms for SARS CoV-2. Most of these SARS-CoV-2 vaccines encode Spike protein. These nucleic-acid based vaccines are easy to develop in very less time, but no licensed vaccine has used this approach. About 11 nucleic-acid based vaccines are in different stages of clinical trials. A brief description of these vaccine candidates is given below.

mRNA-1273

The vaccine was manufactured by Moderna Therapeutics (USA National Institute of Allergy and Infectious Diseases) funded by CEPI. It is the first American vaccine to enter in the human trial. It is based on mRNA which is encapsulated in a lipid like nanoparticle (LNP). The mRNA-1273 vaccine candidate showed promising results in phase 1 study which was published online on 14th July 2020 [61, 62]. Thus, it was permitted to enter the phase 2 trials, enrolling 600 participants of 18 years and older. It is a randomized, placebo controlled and dose confirmation study for the evaluation of safety and immunogenicity of the candidate. The company has launched phase 3 clinical trials by enrolling 30,000 participants on 27th July 2020 [63], after obtaining promising results from the phase2 clinical trial.

BNT162

It is an mRNA-based vaccine developed by Biopharmaceuticals New Technologies (BioNTech). The company also announced its tactical partnership with two large pharmaceutical companies (Fosun Pharma and Pfizer) to accelerate the global development and accessibility of its vaccine candidate. BioNTech and Fosun Pharma collaborated to produce BNT162 vaccine candidates in China. Moreover, BioNTech also made an alliance with Pfizer for the co-development and distribution of this vaccine candidate in other parts of the world. The company has initiated the combined phase1/2 clinical trials for the candidate by enrolling 200 healthy individuals of aged between 18-55 years in Germany [49, 50]. BNT162 exhibiting promising results with some side effects (like sleeping disturbance and sore arms) during phase1/2 clinical trial. A phase 2/3 trial with 30,000 volunteers in the United States and other countries including Argentina, Brazil, and Germany has been started on 27th July [64].

Chinese researchers at the Academy of Military Medical Sciences in collaboration with **Suzhou Abogen Biosciences and Walvax Biotechnology** have developed a vaccine candidate based on mRNA which encodes for S protein of SARS-CoV-2. The vaccine showed a protective immune response in monkeys during preclinical studies. Phase1 clinical trial was also started in July to evaluate the safety and immunogenicity of the vaccine candidate in humans [65].

Self-amplifying RNA Vaccine for COVID-19

Researchers at Imperial College of London produced a self-amplifying RNA vaccine to fight against COVID-19 infection. The vaccine is based on chemically derived mRNA molecule which codes for spike protein of SARS-CoV-2. Phase 1/2 clinical trial of the candidate vaccine was recruited on 15th June 2020 to evaluate the safety of the vaccine and its effect on the immune system [66].

Arcturus therapeutics *and* ***Duke-NUS*** Medical School is collaborating for the development of the COVID-19 vaccine based on the Arcturus proprietary STARR™ technology platform. The technology combines a self-amplifying RNA molecule with LUNAR® delivery system (a nanoparticle based delivery system) in a lipid solution, so that proteins will be expressed inside the human cell leading to the induction of protective immune response [67]. Phase 1/2 trial at Singapore General Hospital was launched in August 2020 [68].

CVnCoV

CureVac developed an mRNA-based vaccine candidate named CVnCoV against COVID-19 by using its proprietary mRNA-based platform. They used non-modified nucleotides for the formation of mRNA which encodes for full length S protein and is made up of lipid nanoparticle (LNP) [35]. The company has initiated the phase 1 clinical trial for the optimization of the dosage and safety profile of the vaccine candidate by recruiting 168 healthy adults [69]. Phase 2 trial was also launched in August 2020 [70].

GX-19

Genexine Inc, a biotechnological company in South Korea, has developed a DNA based vaccine candidate against COVID-19 called GX-19. The company received an approval to initiate a combined Phase 1/2 clinical trial of GX-19 vaccine candidate [71]. A total of 190 healthy individuals aged 18-50 years with 40 people in phase 1 and 150 in phase 2 clinical trial have been enrolled. The study is designed as a placebo-controlled, randomized and double blinded [72].

INO-4800 DNA Vaccine

INOVIO Pharmaceuticals, funded by Coalition for Epidemic Preparedness Innovations (CEPI), is one of the foremost companies in developing the Coronavirus vaccine. They constructed a DNA (INO-4800) through their modern DNA medicine platform just after the publication of genomic sequence. DNA medicine platform consists of optimized DNA plasmids which is a small circular double stranded DNA designed by the computer sequencing technology to induce a specific immune response. The vaccine is delivered through company's proprietary CELLECTRA® 3PSP (small, handly and a portable device for the intra-dermal delivery of vaccine) followed by electroporation. Phase 1 clinical trial was initiated on 6th April 2020 [58]. It is an open-label study involving 40 healthy individuals in 2 different areas of the USA. The vaccine will be administered intradermally in 2 doses that will be given 4 weeks apart. Further, human trials will be conducted in China and South Korea. It is expected that the results of the phase 1 trial will be presented by fall of 2020 [73, 74]. The company plans to progress into combined phase2/3 clinical trials following the safety profile and immunogenicity data from phase 1 study [36].

AG0301-COVID19

Anges, a Japanese biotechnological company in collaboration with Osaka University and Takara Bio has developed a vaccine based on DNA which encodes S protein of SARS-CoV-2. A phase1/2 study has begun with 20 subjects aged 20-65 years [75].

bacTRL-Spike

Symvivo developed a monovalent bacTRL-Spike vaccine candidate based on genetically altered probiotic bacteria (*Bifidobacterium longum*), which colonizes into the human gut. The bacteria attach itself to the epithelial cells of the intestine where it will replicate constitutively and secrete plasmid DNA encoding spike protein of SARS-CoV-2. The vaccine is currently being evaluated in the phase1 clinical trial by recruiting 84 subjects at different doses against the placebo. The vaccine will be administered orally [76].

Zydus Cadila DNA Vaccine

Indian Biopharmaceutical company Zydus Cadila situated in Ahmedabad has also developed a vaccine against COVID-19 by two distinct approaches. One includes the development of DNA vaccine against the S protein of the SARS-CoV2. The second is the modification of a live attenuated recombinant measles vector (rMV) based vaccine against COVID-19 infection [33, 34]. After showing satisfactory results from preclinical studies, Zydus Cadila's DNA vaccine against COVID-19 has been approved for combined phase1/2 clinical trial by Drug Controller General of India (DGCI) of India. It is India's second vaccine to start human trials [77].

Subunit Vaccines

Subunit vaccine contains only the specific part of virus (protein, sugar, or a capsid), eliciting a strong immune response by targeting the specific part of the virus. However, there is a limitation with these types of vaccines, as they required one or more booster doses to provide immune protection against the disease and an adjuvant to boost the immune response [78]. About 13 research teams are working on SARS-CoV-2 protein subunit (whole Spike protein or RBD) vaccines. A brief description of these vaccine candidates is given below.

Recombinant subunit vaccine for COVID-19

Anhui Zhifei Longcom Biopharmaceuticals has collaborated with Institute of Microbiology of the Chinese Academy of Sciences to develop a vaccine candidate based on recombinant viral proteins (RBD domain of S protein) and adjuvants to enhance the immune response. The candidate vaccine is running in the phase1 trial with 50 healthy individuals [79]. The candidate also received an approval to progress into the phase 2 clinical trial on 10th July 2020 [80].

NVX-CoV2373

Novavax funded by CEPI has developed a protein-based vaccine candidate by using its proprietary nanoparticle technology. Novavax patented adjuvant Matrix-M™ was also integrated in this vaccine candidate. Preclinical studies of the vaccine candidate have shown neutralizing antibody response against SARS-CoV-2 to a higher extent as well as potent immune response. Novavax has initiated the combined phase1/2 clinical trials of the candidate on 25th May 2020 [81]. It is a placebo-controlled phase 1 study including approximately 131 healthy individuals. A phase 2 clinical trial was launched on 17th August in South Africa [82].

Sanofi and GSK have collaborated to produce an adjuvanted vaccine by deploying the GSK's proprietary adjuvant technology. Sanofi will provide its S-protein antigen of SARS-CoV-2. The DNA sequence against S protein is inserted into the Baculovirus vector. It is based on Sanofi's former licensed recombinant product of influenza virus [83]. Sanofi has also collaborated with Biomedical Advanced Research and Development **(BARDA)** to initiate the development of its recombinant protein-based vaccine candidate for COVID-19. They have launched a combined phase1/2 clinical trial in September [84].

Kentucky BioProcessing (KBP) division of BAT (British American Tobacco) is developing a vaccine candidate by cloning a portion of genetic sequence to create a potential antigen. The gene encoding the antigen was inserted into the tobacco plants for reproduction, the plant was harvested, the protein was then extracted and purified for clinical testing [83]. The company had launched a combined phase1/2 clinical trial in July after obtaining promising results in preclinical studies [85].

University of Queensland funded by Coalition for Epidemic Preparedness innovations (CEPI) is constructing viral surface proteins (spike protein) by using 'Molecular clamp' technology which blocks the spike protein to display it more easily to our immune system and neutralizes the virus [86]. A Phase 1 clinical trial is ongoing with 120 healthy individuals aged 18-55 years old [87].

COVAX-19

Vaxine, a biopharmaceutical company and Flinders University in Australia has developed a monovalent recombinant subunit vaccine named as COVAX-19. It becomes Australia's first vaccine candidate to enter human trial [35]. The phase1 clinical trial has started by recruiting 40 healthy individuals aged 18-65 years. The vaccine candidate or placebo will be administered as two doses three weeks apart [88].

SCB-2019

Clover Biopharmaceuticals has designed a recombinant subunit vaccine candidate based on the S protein by its proprietary Trimer-Tag© technology platform [35]. The vaccine candidate is based on the trimeric S protein, which is similar to the virus indigenous S protein. The candidate was developed *via* a mammalian cell culture system. The company has cGMP biomanufacturing facilities for large scale production of the vaccine. Clover is also collaborating with Dynavax and GSK for the appraisal of its COVID-19-S-Trimer vaccine candidate. Dynavax and GSK offered its CpG 1018 and ASO3 adjuvants, respectively, to enhance the immune response. The adjuvant CpG 1018 is also used in Dynavaxformer USA approved HEPLISAV-B ® vaccine (adult hepatitis B vaccine). Phase1 clinical trial of SCB-2019 was started on 19th June 2020 by enrolling 150 subjects. Each subject will receive the vaccine along with either CpG 1018 adjuvant or ASO3 adjuvant [89].

Medigen, a Taiwan based company is developing a subunit vaccine in collaboration with **Dynavax**. The vaccine consists of S protein of SARS-CoV-2 and an adjuvant from Dynavax. A phase1 clinical trial has been registered to start in September 2020 [90]. Another Taiwan based company **Adimmune** has also developed a subunit vaccine based on RBD domain of S protein of SARS-CoV-2. They have launched phase 1 clinical trial in August 2020 [36].

Soberana1

Finlay Vaccine Institute situated in Havana developed a subunit vaccine candidate known as Soberana1 based on RBD of S protein of SARS-CoV-2. The vaccine also contains an adjuvant to boost immune response. The company has launched phase 1 clinical trial in August 2020 [36].

EpiVacCorona

Russia has developed its second COVID-19 vaccine named EpiVacCorona at Russian biological research Centre known as Vector Institute. The vaccine is based on small peptides of SARS-CoV-2 Spike protein. A combined phase1/2 clinical trial has been launched in August 2020 [36].

Virus Like Particle (VLP) Based Vaccine

Empty virus shell mimics the virus structure but are not infectious due to the absence of genetic material. VLP based vaccines are safe and efficacious as compare to traditional virus-based vaccines. These vaccines have several benefits such as these particles resemble like native viruses, hence manifests repetitive antigens on its surface. They are replication incompetent which makes it safer to be employed in immunocompromised individuals [91].

Medicago has developed a VLP vaccine candidate by deploying its proprietary plant based technology platform. The company is also producing an antibody candidate to combat COVID-19 infection [92]. The vaccine candidate is also tested with adjuvants from GSK and Dynavax. Phase1 clinical trial has been initiated with 180 healthy subjects after showing protective immune response in mice during preclinical studies [93]. The company is also planning to initiate phase 2 trial by October 2020.

Tuberculosis Vaccine in Clinical Trial

In the race of producing COVID-19 vaccine, some of the researchers are also investigating the previously existing tuberculosis vaccine as a possible quick fix. Human clinical trials of tuberculosis vaccines are ongoing to evaluate its effectiveness against COVID-19 infection.

BCG vaccine

BCG is a live attenuated vaccine that consists of Bacillus of Calmette and Guerin strain of *Mycobacterium bovis* to prevent tuberculosis infection. Moreover, it is postulated that BCG vaccines can also assist in the prevention of viral respiratory infection. Countries with regular BCG vaccination appears to have less severe pandemic. According to the researchers of BCG, this may be since the vaccine is an immune system enhancer.

Phase 3 clinical studies in Australia and Netherlands are ongoing to investigate the efficacy of BCG vaccination in lowering the prevalence and severity of COVID-19 infection. An open-label, randomized controlled phase 3 study in Australia is running by recruiting 4,170 healthcare workers (directly involved with COVID-19 patients) into two groups [94]. On the other hand, Netherland recruited 1500 healthcare workers in placebo-controlled, multi-centered phase3 clinical trial [95].

VPM1002 Vaccine

The VPM1002 is based on a BCG vaccine, which is genetically modified for better immune response. The vaccine is developed at the Max Planck Institute for Infection Biology. A phase 3 study of this candidate is ongoing to evaluate whether it is also effective for COVID-19 infection or not [96]. The study is being conducted in several hospitals of Germany involving healthcare workers and older individuals. It is a double-blinded, randomized, placebo controlled, multi-centred study involving 2 groups of individuals being administered a single dose of the vaccine or placebo. The study is expected to be concluded by the mid of 2020.

Vaccine Candidates in Preclinical Trial

Till 31st August 2020, at least 151 vaccine candidates of COVID-19 are in preclinical trial, of which some of them will enter phase1 clinical trials imminently by the end of 2020. Different technology platforms are being evaluated for the development of vaccine for COVID-19 ranging from nucleic acid (DNA and RNA), virus-like particle, peptide, viral vector (replicating and non-replicating), recombinant protein, live attenuated virus and inactivated virus approaches. Table **3** summarizes all the major COVID-19 vaccine candidates in preclinical trials. However, few of them are described briefly here [33 - 36].

Table 3. Description of COVID-19 vaccine candidates in preclinical trial.

Developer/Researcher	Vaccine Platform	Vaccine Description	Status
Applied DNA / Takis Biotech	DNA	PCR based linear DNA vaccine	Pre-clinical (human trial began by end of April 2020)
Korolinska Institute / Cobra Biologics ("OPEN CORONA" project)	DNA	DNA vaccine administered through electroporation	Pre-clinical (human trial beginning in 2021)

(Table 3) cont.....

Developer/Researcher	Vaccine Platform	Vaccine Description	Status
Entos Pharmaceuticals	DNA	Fusogenix delivery system (lipid based)	Pre-clinical
Ege University	DNA	DNA vaccine	Pre-clinical
Immuno Therapeutics / Epivax / Pharma Jet	DNA	Plasmid DNA Needle free delivery system	Pre-clinical
University of Waterloo	DNA	Bacteriophage based Administered Intranasally	Pre-clinical
BioNet Asia	DNA	DNA vaccine	Pre-clinical
Chula Vaccine Research Center	DNA	DNA vaccine administered through electroporation	Pre-clinical
National Research Centre, Egypt	DNA	Plasmid DNA Encoding RBD domain of S protein &N protein	Pre-clinical
MediphageBioceuticals/University of Waterloo	DNA	msDNA (multicopy single-stranded DNA)	Pre-clinical
Scancell/University of Nottingham/Nottingham Trent University	DNA	Plasmid DNA Encoding S1, S2 and RBD domain of S protein &N protein	Pre-clinical
DIOSynVax Ltd / University of Cambridge	DNA	DNA vaccine administered through multiple delivery system	Pre-clinical
CanSino Biologics/Precision NanoSystems	RNA	LNP encapsulated mRNA	Pre-clinical
Gennova	RNA	Self-amplifying RNA	Pre-clinical
Selcuk University	RNA	mRNA based	Pre-clinical
Greenlight Biosciences	RNA	mRNA based	Pre-clinical
IDIBAPS-Hospital Clinic, Spain	RNA	mRNA based	Pre-clinical
Sanofi Pasteur / Translate Bio	RNA	LNP encapsulated mRNA Multiple RNA construct	Pre-clinical
Fudan university / Shanghai Jiao Tong University / RNA Cure Bio Pharma	RNA	LNP encapsulated mRNA encoding VLP	Pre-clinical
Fudan university / Shanghai Jiao Tong University / RNA Cure Bio Pharma	RNA	LNP encapsulated mRNA encoding RBD	Pre-clinical
BIOCAD	RNA	Liposome encapsulated mRNA	Pre-clinical
Centro Nacional Biotecnologia (CNB-CSIC),Spain	RNA	mRNA derived from replication defective SARS-CoV2	Pre-clinical
University of Tokyo / Daiichi-Sankyo	RNA	LNP encapsulated RNA	Pre-clinical

(Table 3) cont.....

Developer/Researcher	Vaccine Platform	Vaccine Description	Status
Tongji university / Stermina Therapeutics / Curevac	RNA	mRNA based	Pre-clinical
FBRI SRC VB VECTOR, Rospotrebnadzor, Koltsovo	RNA	mRNA encoding S protein	Pre-clinical
eThe RNA immunotherapies	RNA	mRNA based Adjuvanted Administered intranasally	Pre-clinical
RNA immune Inc.	RNA	Multiple mRNA candidates	Pre-clinical
China CDC / Tongji University / Stermina	RNA	mRNA based	Pre-clinical
Chula Vaccine Research Center / University of Pennsylvania	RNA	Liposome encapsulated mRNA	Pre-clinical
Green light Biosciences	RNA	mRNA	Pre-clinical
IDIBAPS-Hospital Clinic, Spain	RNA	mRNA	Pre-clinical
Pittsburgh school of Medicine	Protein Subunit (PittCoVac)	S1 Subunit Based on Micro-needle array (MNA) Foremost study published in EBIO Medicine	Pre-clinical
University of Virginia	Protein Subunit	S subunit Intranasal liposomal formulation Adjuvanted with GLA/3M052	Pre-clinical
Mynvax	Protein Subunit	RBD domain of S protein	Pre-clinical
Izmir Biomedicine and Genome Center	Protein Subunit	Recombinant S protein	Pre-clinical
Bogazici University	Protein Subunit	Peptide based Novel adjuvant system	Pre-clinical
Oncosec Medical Inc.	Protein Subunit (CoRVax 12)	Based on oncosec's former TAVO™ candidate and DNA encoding S protein of SARS-CoV-2 Delivered through electroporation	Pre-clinical
Soligenix /Hawai university	Protein Subunit	Antigenic portion of S protein Adjuvanted Thermostable	Pre-clinical (Phase1 trial begun in middle of 2020)
IMV Inc.	Protein Subunit	LNP formulated peptide antigen DPX delivery system (Dry lipid based)	Pre-clinical (Phase1 trial begins)

(Table 3) cont.....

Developer/Researcher	Vaccine Platform	Vaccine Description	Status
Helix Biogen Consult, Ogbomoso / Trinity Immonoefficient Laboratory, Ogbomoso, Oyo State, Nigeria.	Protein Subunit	S Subunit	Pre-clinical
National Research Centre, Egypt	Protein Subunit	Based on subunit of S, N, M & S1 protein	Pre-clinical
Boston children's hospital	Protein Subunit	S protein Adjuvanted Specific for older population	Pre-clinical
Generex / Epivax	Protein Subunit	Epitopic region of S protein, predicted through li-Key peptide technology	Pre-clinical
VIDO-InterVac / University of Saskatchewan	Protein Subunit	Microsphere peptides based Adjuvanted	Pre-clinical
Baylor college of Medicine	Protein Subunit	RBD domain of S protein	Pre-clinical
Vaxil Bio	Protein Subunit	Based on signal peptide of Vaxil Bio's tuberculosis vaccine VaxHit Bioinformatics tool	Pre-clinical
Flow pharma	Protein Subunit	FlowVax vaccine based on killer T-cell	Pre-clinical (non-human primates)
Innovax Biotech / Xiamen university	Protein Subunit (COVID-19 XWG-3)	Recombinant truncated S protein Pandemic adjuvant system	Pre-clinical
Sanofi / GSK	Protein Subunit	S protein inserted in Baculovirus vector Adjuvanted with CpG 1018	Pre-clinical (human trial begun in 2020)
Sanofi / BARDA	Protein Subunit	Recombinant S protein	Pre-clinical
Lake Pharma Inc.	Protein Subunit	S protein nanoparticle	Pre-clinical
Oncogen	Protein subunit	Synthetic full-length S and M protein Based on cancer neo-antigen vaccination therapy	Pre-clinical
Heat Biologics Inc / Miami university	Protein subunit	Antigen bounds to gp96 backbone	Preclinical
University of Alberta	Protein subunit	S protein based	Pre-clinical
MIGAL Research Institute	Protein subunit	Recombinant IBV vaccine expresses chimeric proteins consists of structural domain of S and N protein Oral vaccine	Pre-clinical

Developer/Researcher	Vaccine Platform	Vaccine Description	Status
Sorrento Therapeutics	Protein subunit (ST1-6991)	Cellular vaccine S1 subunit Based on replication defective human erythroleukemia K562	Pre-clinical
AdaptVac (PREVENT-nCoV consortium)	Protein subunit	Capsid virus like particles (cVLP)	Pre-clinical
Ligandal Inc.	Protein subunit	Peptide scaffolds mimic the ligand binding with ACE2 receptor of host cell	Pre-clinical
National Institute of Infectious Disease, Japan	Protein subunit	S protein Adjuvanted	Pre-clinical
WRAIR/USAMRIID	Protein subunit	S protein	Pre-clinical
AnyGo Technology	Protein subunit	Recombinant S1 protein	Pre-clinical
ExpreS·ion Biotechnologies /Adapt Vac	Protein subunit	Capsid virus like particles (cVLP) expressed *via* Drosophilla S2 insect cell	Pre-clinical
Osaka University / BIKEN / National Institute of Biomedical Innovation, Japan	Protein subunit	Recombinant protein-based virus like particles Adjuvanted	Pre-clinical
Biological E ltd	Protein subunit	RBD of S protein Adjuvanted	Pre-clinical
AJ Vaccines	Protein subunit	S protein	Pre-clinical
Epivax / university of Georgia	Protein subunit	S protein	Pre-clinical
Saint-Petersburg scientific research institute of vaccine and serum	Protein subunit	Recombinant protein nanoparticle based on S protein and other epitopes	Pre-clinical
Lomonosov Moscow State University	Protein subunit	Multivalent vaccine Based on structurally modified spherical like particles of Tobacco mosaic virus (TMV)	Pre-clinical
Yisheng Biopharma	Protein subunit	Recombinant S protein	Pre-clinical
BaiyaPhytopharm/ Chula Vaccine Research Center	Protein subunit	RBD of S protein fused with Fc portion of IgG Adjuvanted	Pre-clinical
University of San Martin and CONICET, Argentina	Protein subunit	S protein	Pre-clinical
Chulalongkorn University / GPO, Thailand	Protein subunit	RBD of S protein fused with Fc portion of IgG Adjuvanted vaccine	Pre-clinical

(Table 3) cont.....

Developer/Researcher	Vaccine Platform	Vaccine Description	Status
Quadram Institute Biosciences	Protein subunit	Outer membrane vesicle (OMV) nanoparticles produced by genetically modified probiotic gut bacteria	Pre-clinical
Axon Neuroscience SE	Protein subunit	Peptides derived from S protein	Pre-clinical
EpiVax	Protein subunit (EPV-CoV-19)	Protein Subunit	Pre-clinical
MOGAM Institute for Biomedical Research / GC Pharma	Protein subunit	S protein	Pre-clinical
Neovii/ Tel Aviv University	Protein subunit	Based on RBD of S protein	Pre-clinical
Intravacc / Epivax	Protein subunit	Outer membrane vesicles (OMV) peptide	Pre-clinical
Intravacc / Epivax	Protein subunit	Outer membrane vesicles (OMV) subunit	Pre-clinical
BiOMViSSrl / University of Trento	Protein subunit	Outer membrane vesicles (OMV) subunit	Pre-clinical
ImmunoPrecise	Protein subunit	S protein based Epitope screening	Pre-clinical
FarmacológicosVeterinarios SAC (FARVET SAC) / Universidad Peruana Cayetano Heredia (UPCH)	Protein subunit	RBD protein expressed in Baculovirus + FAR Squalene adjuvant	Pre-clinical
Applied Biotechnology Institute, Inc	Protein subunit	Heat stable subunit Oral formulation	Pre-clinical
ID Pharma	Non-replicating viral vector	S protein expressed *via* Sendai virus vector	Pre-clinical
Vaxart	Non-replicating viral vector	Oral vaccine	Pre-clinical
Vabiotech	Non-replicating viral vector	Recombinant S protein expressed *via* IC-BEVS	Pre-clinical
Ankara University	Non-replicating viral vector	S protein expressed in recombinant Adenoviral vector	Pre-clinical
National Research Centre, Egypt	Non-replicating viral vector	S protein expressed in Influenza, H1N1 vector	Pre-clinical
Massachusetts Eye and Ear / Massachusetts General Hospital / AveXis	Non-replicating viral vector (AAVCOVID)	Adenovirus based	Pre-clinical

Developer/Researcher	Vaccine Platform	Vaccine Description	Status
Geovax/ Bravovax	Non-replicating viral vector	MVA encoded VLPs	Pre-clinical (human trial to begin by end of 2020)
Altimmune / Alabama University	Non-replicating viral vector (AdCOVID)	Adenovirus based NasoVax vaccine manifesting S protein of SARS-CoV2	Pre-clinical
Greffex	Non-replicating viral vector	Adenoviral vector Grevac™ plug-And-Play technology.	Pre-clinical
DZIF-German Centre for Infection Research	Non-replicating viral vector	MVA (Modified Vaccinia Ankara) encoded S protein	Pre-clinical
Centro Nacional Biotecnologia (CNB-CSIC), Spain	Non-replicating viral vector	MVA (Modified Vaccinia Ankara) manifesting S protein	Pre-clinical
Erciyes University	Non-replicating viral vector	Adeno5-based vaccine manifesting S protein of SARS-CoV2	Pre-clinical
Stabilitech Biopharma Ltd	Non-Replicating Viral Vector	S protein expressed in Adenoviral vector Oral vaccine	Pre-clinical
Valo Therapeutics Ltd	Non-replicating viral vector	Adenovirus based peptides like HLA	Pre-clinical
University of Manitoba	Non-replicating viral vector	Based on Dendritic cell	Pre-clinical
National Center for Genetic Engineering and Biotechnology (BIOTEC) /GPO, Thailand	Non-replicating viral vector	S protein expressed in inactivated Flu-based vaccine Adjuvanted	Pre-clinical
University of Georgia / University of Iowa	Non-replicating viral vector	S protein expressed in Parainfluenza virus 5 (PIV5)	Pre-clinical
IDIBAPS-Hospital Clinic, Spain	Non-replicating viral vector	MVA (Modified Vaccinia Ankara) manifesting S protein Adjuvanted	Pre-clinical
Stabilitech Biopharma Ltd	Non-replicating viral vector	S protein expressed in inactivated flu vaccine	Pre-clinical
ImmunityBio, Inc. & NantKwest, Inc.	Non-replicating viral vector	2nd Gen E2b- Ad5 expressing Spike, RBD, Nucleocapsid proteins Administered subcutaneously & Orally	Pre-clinical

(Table 3) cont.....

Developer/Researcher	Vaccine Platform	Vaccine Description	Status
Fundação Oswaldo Cruz and Instituto Buntantan	Replicating viral vector	Antigenic part of S protein expressed through attenuated influenza virus	Pre-clinical
FarmacológicosVeterinarios SAC (FARVET SAC) / Universidad Peruana Cayetano Heredia (UPCH)	Replicating viral vector	RBD expressed in Oral Salmonella enteritidis (3934Vac)	Pre-clinical
KU Leuven	Replicating viral vector	Yellow Fever 17D (YF17D) Vector	Pre-clinical
Cadila Healthcare Limited	Replicating viral vector	Measles Vector	Pre-clinical
FBRI SRC VB VECTOR / Rospotrebnadzor / Koltsovo	Replicating viral vector	Based on rMV (Measles Vector)	Pre-clinical
Tonix Pharmaceuticals	Replicating viral vector (TNX-1800)	Horse pox virus vaccine manifests S protein of SARS-CoV2	Pre-clinical
AVI/Merck	Replicating viral vector	S protein of SARS-CoV- 2 expressed by Replication-competent VSV chimeric virus technology (VSVΔG)	Pre-clinical
Hong Kong University	Replicating viral vector	Weakened Influenza vector expressing RBD of S protein	Pre-clinical
Israel Institute for Biological Research/Weizmann Institute of Science	Replicating viral vector	VSV (Vesicular stomatitis virus) vector expressing S protein	Pre-clinical
UW–Madison/FluGen/Bharat Biotech	Replicating viral vector	Based on M2-deficient single replication (M2SR) influenza vector	Pre-clinical
FBRI SRC VB VECTOR / Rospotrebnadzor / Koltsovo	Replicating viral vector	Based on recombinant Influenza A virus, Intranasal vaccine	Pre-clinical
Biocad / IEM	Replicating viral vector	Live viral vector vaccine based on attenuated influenza virus backbone Administered intranasally	Pre-clinical
Intravacc/ Wageningen Bioveterinary Research/Utrecht Univ	Replicating viral vector	Newcastle disease virus vector (NDV) expressing S protein	Pre-clinical
The Lancaster University, UK	Replicating viral vector	Avian paramyxovirus vector (APMV) expressing S protein	Pre-clinical
University of Western Ontario	Replicating viral vector	VSV (Vesicular stomatitis virus) vector expressing S protein	Pre-clinical

(Table 3) cont.....

Developer/Researcher	Vaccine Platform	Vaccine Description	Status
Aurobindo	Replicating viral vector	VSV (Vesicular stomatitis virus) vector expressing S protein	Pre-clinical
DZIF-German Centre for Infection Research	Live attenuated Virus	Measles vector expressing S and N protein	Pre-clinical
IAVI / Batavia	Live attenuated Virus	VSV (Vesicular stomatitis virus) vector expressing S protein	Pre-clinical
Codagenix	Live attenuated Virus	Codon deoptimization to attenuate virus	Pre-clinical
Indian Immunologicals Ltd / Griffith University	Live attenuated Virus	Codon deoptimization to attenuate virus	Pre-clinical
University of Western Ontario	Live attenuated Virus	VSV (Vesicular stomatitis virus) vector expressing S protein	Pre-clinical
Mehmet Ali Aydinlar University / AcıbademLabmed Health Services A.S.	Live attenuated Virus	Codon deoptimization to attenuate virus	Pre-clinical
UW–Madison / FluGen / Bharat Biotech	Live attenuated Virus	M2-deficient single replication (M2SR) influenza vector	Pre-clinical
Osaka university / BIKEN / NIBIOHN	Inactivated virus	TBD	Pre-clinical
Chinese centre for Disease control and prevention (CDC)	Inactivated virus	Unknown	Pre-clinical
Institute of Medical Biology / Chinese Academy of Medical Sciences	Inactivated virus	Unknown	Pre-clinical
Valneva /Dynavax	Inactivated virus	Formaldehyde inactivated Adjuvanted with CpG 1018	Pre-clinical
Beijing Minhai Biotechnology Co., Ltd.	Inactivated virus	Unknown	Pre-clinical
Research Institute for Biological Safety Problems, Rep of Kazakhstan	Inactivated virus	Unknown	Pre-clinical
KM Biologics	Inactivated virus	Inactivated Adjuvanted with alum	Pre-clinical
Selcuk University	Inactivated virus	Unknown	Pre-clinical
Erciyes University	Inactivated virus	Inactivated	Pre-clinical
National Research Centre, Egypt	Inactivated virus	Inactivated whole virus	Pre-clinical
Middle East Technical University	Virus like particle	Unknown	Pre-clinical
Ufovax	Virus like particle	Sprotein based nanoparticle (1C-SApNP)	Pre-clinical

(Table 3) cont.....

Developer/Researcher	Vaccine Platform	Vaccine Description	Status
Imophoron Ltd and Bristol University's Max Planck Centre	Virus like particle	ADDomer platform Artificial single VLP Multiepitope display Thermostable vaccine	Pre-clinical
iBio / cc pharming	Virus like particle	Plant derived VLP	Pre-clinical
IrsiCaixa AIDS Research / IRTACReSA / Barcelona Supercomputing Centre / Grifols	Virus like particle	S protein integrated in HIV VLPs	Pre-clinical
Saiba GmbH	Virus like particle	VLP's expressing RBD of S protein	Pre-clinical
Mahidol University / The Government Pharmaceutical Organization (GPO)	Virus like particle	VLP Adjuvant	Pre-clinical
University of Sao Paulo	Virus like particle	VLPs peptides	Pre-clinical
Navarrabiomed / Oncoimmunology group	Virus like particle	Virus-like particles Delivered through Lentivirus and Baculovirus vehicles	Pre-clinical
VBI Vaccines Inc.	Virus like particle	Enveloped VLPs	Pre-clinical
Tulane University	Virus like particle	Unknown	Pre-clinical
BezmialemVakiUniversity	Virus like particle	Unknown	Pre-clinical
ARTES Biotechnology	Virus like particle	Unknown	Pre-clinical
OSIVAX	Virus like particle	Unknown	Pre-clinical
Doherty Institute	Virus like particle	Unknown	Pre-clinical

CONCLUDING REMARKS

No specific drug is available against the causative agent of COVID-19 pandemic. Therefore, existing antiviral drugs are used for the management of the patients. In addition, immune-enhancing supplements are also utilized to boost the sagging immune system of the human host. Further, **"social distancing"** is followed to minimize the human to human transmission of the infection. Therefore, development of a prophylactic vaccine is urgently needed since this currently ongoing pandemic is exaggerating all over the world. According to the recent analysis, there is also a prospect of COVID-19 disease becoming endemic in future. Thus, joint efforts of the scientific research community including virologists, immunologists, and clinicians are needed at this hour to formulate the vaccine against this respiratory pathogen at a pandemic speed.

CONSENT FOR PUBLICATION

Not Applicable.

CONFLICT OF INTEREST

The author declares no conflict of interest, financial or otherwise.

ACKNOWLEDGEMENTS

The research in our laboratory is funded by Council of Scientific and Industrial Research (CSIR), India (37(1697)17/EMR-II) and Central Council for Research in Unani Medicine (CCRUM), Ministry of Ayurveda, Yoga and Naturopathy, Unani, Siddha and Homeopathy (AYUSH) (F.No.3-63/2019-CCRUM/Tech). The authors also extend their appreciation to the Centre of Excellence in Biotechnology Research, King Saud University, Riyadh, Saudi Arabia for support.

REFERENCES

[1] Li Q, Guan X, Wu P, *et al.* Early transmission dynamics in Wuhan, China, of novel coronavirus-infected pneumonia. N Engl J Med 2020; 382(13): 1199-207.
[http://dx.doi.org/10.1056/NEJMoa2001316] [PMID: 31995857]

[2] WHO Director-General's remarks at the media briefing on 2019-nCoV on 11 February 2020. World Health Organization. 2020. Available from: https://www.who.int/dg/speeches/detail/who-directo--general-sremarks-at-the-media-briefing-on-2019-ncov-on-11-february2020

[3] Lau SK, Woo PC, Li KS, *et al.* Severe acute respiratory syndrome coronavirus-like virus in Chinese horseshoe bats. Proc Natl Acad Sci USA 2005; 102(39): 14040-5.
[http://dx.doi.org/10.1073/pnas.0506735102] [PMID: 16169905]

[4] Chen Y, Liu Q, Guo D. Emerging coronaviruses: Genome structure, replication, and pathogenesis. J Med Virol 2020; 92(4): 418-23.
[http://dx.doi.org/10.1002/jmv.25681] [PMID: 31967327]

[5] Rothe C, Schunk M, Sothmann P, *et al.* Transmission of 2019-nCoV infection from an asymptomatic contact in Germany. N Engl J Med 2020; 382(10): 970-1.
[http://dx.doi.org/10.1056/NEJMc2001468] [PMID: 32003551]

[6] Cui J, Li F, Shi ZL. Origin and evolution of pathogenic coronaviruses. Nat Rev Microbiol 2019; 17(3): 181-92.
[http://dx.doi.org/10.1038/s41579-018-0118-9] [PMID: 30531947]

[7] Tortorici MA, Veesler D. Structural insights into coronavirus entry. Adv Virus Res 2019; 105: 93-116.
[http://dx.doi.org/10.1016/bs.aivir.2019.08.002] [PMID: 31522710]

[8] Yang P, Wang X. COVID-19: a new challenge for human beings. Cell Mol Immunol 2020; 17(5): 555-7.
[http://dx.doi.org/10.1038/s41423-020-0407-x] [PMID: 32235915]

[9] Hoffmann M, Kleine-Weber H, Schroeder S, *et al.* SARS-CoV-2 cell entry depends on ACE2 and TMPRSS2 and is blocked by a clinically proven protease inhibitor. Cell 2020; 181(2): 271-80.
[http://dx.doi.org/10.1016/j.cell.2020.02.052] [PMID: 32142651]

[10] Wang Q, Zhang Y, Wu L, *et al.* Structural and functional basis of SARS-CoV-2 entry by using human ACE2. Cell 2020; 181(4): 894-904.
[http://dx.doi.org/10.1016/j.cell.2020.03.045] [PMID: 32275855]

[11] Li Y, Zhou W, Yang L, You R. Physiological and pathological regulation of ACE2, the SARS-CoV-2 receptor. Pharmacol Res 2020; 157: 104833.

[http://dx.doi.org/10.1016/j.phrs.2020.104833] [PMID: 32302706]

[12]   Lukassen S, Chua RL, Trefzer T, *et al.* SARS-CoV-2 receptor ACE2 and TMPRSS2 are primarily expressed in bronchial transient secretory cells. EMBO J 2020; 39(10): e105114.
       [http://dx.doi.org/10.15252/embj.2020105114] [PMID: 32246845]

[13]   Chen J. Pathogenicity and transmissibility of 2019-nCoV-A quick overview and comparison with other emerging viruses. Microbes Infect 2020; 22(2): 69-71.
       [http://dx.doi.org/10.1016/j.micinf.2020.01.004] [PMID: 32032682]

[14]   Coronavirus disease (COVID-2019) situation reports. WHO. 2020. Available from: https://www.who.int/emergencies/diseases/novel-coronavirus-2019/situation-reports

[15]   Han S. Clinical vaccine development. Clin Exp Vaccine Res 2015; 4(1): 46-53.
       [http://dx.doi.org/10.7774/cevr.2015.4.1.46] [PMID: 25648742]

[16]   Jiang S, Bottazzi ME, Du L, *et al.* Roadmap to developing a recombinant coronavirus S protein receptor-binding domain vaccine for severe acute respiratory syndrome. Expert Rev Vaccines 2012; 11(12): 1405-13.
       [http://dx.doi.org/10.1586/erv.12.126] [PMID: 23252385]

[17]   Huang C, Wang Y, Li X, *et al.* Clinical features of patients infected with 2019 novel coronavirus in Wuhan, China. Lancet 2020; 395(10223): 497-506.
       [http://dx.doi.org/10.1016/S0140-6736(20)30183-5] [PMID: 31986264]

[18]   Kamal AM, Mitrut P, Docea AO, *et al.* Double therapy with pegylated Interferon and Ribavirin for chronic hepatitis C. A pharmacogenenetic guide for predicting adverse events. Farmacia 2017; 65: 877-84.

[19]   Zhou P, Yang X-L, Wang X-G, *et al.* Discovery of a novel coronavirus associated with the recent pneumonia outbreak in humans and its potential bat origin. bioRxiv 2020.
       [http://dx.doi.org/10.1101/2020.01.22.914952]

[20]   Wu F, Zhao S, Yu B, *et al.* Complete genome characterisation of a novel coronavirus associated with severe human respiratory disease in Wuhan, China. bioRxiv 2020.
       [http://dx.doi.org/10.1101/2020.01.24.919183]

[21]   Al-Amri SS, Abbas AT, Siddiq LA, *et al.* Immunogenicity of Candidate MERS-CoV DNA Vaccines Based on the Spike Protein. Sci Rep 2017; 7: 44875.
       [http://dx.doi.org/10.1038/srep44875] [PMID: 28332568]

[22]   Du L, He Y, Zhou Y, Liu S, Zheng BJ, Jiang S. The spike protein of SARS-CoV--a target for vaccine and therapeutic development. Nat Rev Microbiol 2009; 7(3): 226-36.
       [http://dx.doi.org/10.1038/nrmicro2090] [PMID: 19198616]

[23]   Du L, Zhao G, He Y, *et al.* Receptor-binding domain of SARS-CoV spike protein induces long-term protective immunity in an animal model. Vaccine 2007; 25(15): 2832-8.
       [http://dx.doi.org/10.1016/j.vaccine.2006.10.031] [PMID: 17092615]

[24]   Pardi N, Hogan MJ, Porter FW, Weissman D. mRNA vaccines - a new era in vaccinology. Nat Rev Drug Discov 2018; 17(4): 261-79.
       [http://dx.doi.org/10.1038/nrd.2017.243] [PMID: 29326426]

[25]   Maruggi G, Zhang C, Li J, Ulmer JB, Yu D. mRNA as a Transformative Technology for Vaccine Development to Control Infectious Diseases. Mol Ther 2019; 27(4): 757-72.
       [http://dx.doi.org/10.1016/j.ymthe.2019.01.020] [PMID: 30803823]

[26]   Schindewolf C, Menachery VD. Middle East Respiratory Syndrome Vaccine Candidates: Cautious Optimism. Viruses 2019; 11(1): 1-17.
       [http://dx.doi.org/10.3390/v11010074] [PMID: 30658390]

[27]   Song F, Fux R, Provacia LB, *et al.* Middle East respiratory syndrome coronavirus spike protein delivered by modified vaccinia virus Ankara efficiently induces virus-neutralizing antibodies. J Virol

2013; 87(21): 11950-4.
[http://dx.doi.org/10.1128/JVI.01672-13] [PMID: 23986586]

[28]   Zhang N, Jiang S, Du L. Current advancements and potential strategies in the development of MERS-CoV vaccines. Expert Rev Vaccines 2014; 13(6): 761-74.
[http://dx.doi.org/10.1586/14760584.2014.912134] [PMID: 24766432]

[29]   Song Z, Xu Y, Bao L, *et al.* From SARS to MERS, Thrusting Coronaviruses into the Spotlight. Viruses 2019; 11(1): E59.
[http://dx.doi.org/10.3390/v11010059] [PMID: 30646565]

[30]   Yong CY, Ong HK, Yeap SK, Ho KL, Tan WS. Recent advances in the vaccine development against middle east respiratory syndrome-coronavirus. Front Microbiol 2019; 10: 1781.
[http://dx.doi.org/10.3389/fmicb.2019.01781] [PMID: 31428074]

[31]   Liu YV, Massare MJ, Barnard DL, *et al.* Chimeric severe acute respiratory syndrome coronavirus (SARS-CoV) S glycoprotein and influenza matrix 1 efficiently form virus-like particles (VLPs) that protect mice against challenge with SARS-CoV. Vaccine 2011; 29(38): 6606-13.
[http://dx.doi.org/10.1016/j.vaccine.2011.06.111] [PMID: 21762752]

[32]   Lokugamage KG, Yoshikawa-Iwata N, Ito N, *et al.* Chimeric coronavirus-like particles carrying severe acute respiratory syndrome coronavirus (SCoV) S protein protect mice against challenge with SCoV. Vaccine 2008; 26(6): 797-808.
[http://dx.doi.org/10.1016/j.vaccine.2007.11.092] [PMID: 18191004]

[33]   Pong W. A dozen vaccine programs under way as WHO declares coronavirus public health emergency. Biocentury 2020. Available from: https://www.biocentury.com/article/304328/industry-and-academiccenters-are-rushing-to-create

[34]   Draft landscape of COVID-19 candidate vaccines. WHO 2020. Available from: https://www.who.int/publications/m/item/draft-landscape-of-covid-19-candidate-vaccines

[35]   Duddu P. Coronavirus treatment: Vaccines/drugs in the pipeline for COVID-19. Clinical trials arena 2020. Available from: https://www.clinicaltrialsarena.com/analysis/coronavirus-mers-cov-drugs/

[36]   Corum J, Grady D, Wee S-L, Zimmer C. Coronavirus vaccine tracker. The New York Times , 2020 [Accessed 10 Sep 2020]; Available from: https://www.nytimes.com/interactive/2020/science/coronavirus-vaccine-tracker.html

[37]   Choi Y, Chang J. Viral vectors for vaccine applications. Clin Exp Vaccine Res 2013; 2(2): 97-105.
[http://dx.doi.org/10.7774/cevr.2013.2.2.97] [PMID: 23858400]

[38]   https://clinicaltrials.gov/ct2/show/NCT04436471?term=vaccine&cond=covid-19&draw=4

[39]   https://clinicaltrials.gov/ct2/show/NCT04530396?term=vaccine&cond=covid-19&draw=3

[40]   http://www.chictr.org.cn/showprojen.aspx?proj=51154

[41]   hictr.org.cn/showprojen.aspx?proj=52006

[42]   https://clinicaltrials.gov/ct2/show/NCT04526990?term=vaccine&cond=covid-19&draw=6

[43]   https://www.clinicaltrialsregister.eu/ctr-search/trial/2020-001072-15/GB

[44]   https://www.clinicaltrialsregister.eu/ctr-search/trial/2020-001228-32/GB

[45]   http://www.isrctn.com/ISRCTN89951424

[46]   https:// www.thepharmaletter.com/article/j-j-working-on-coronavirusvaccine

[47]   https:// clinicaltrials.gov/ct2/show/NCT02543567

[48]   https://clinicaltrials.gov/ct2/show/NCT04528641?term=vaccine&cond=covid-19&draw=8

[49]   https://clinicaltrials.gov/ct2/show/NCT04276896

[50]   https://clinicaltrials.gov/ct2/show/NCT04299724

[51]   https://clinicaltrials.gov/ct2/show/NCT04352608?term=Sinovac&cntry=CN&draw=2

[52]   https://clinicaltrials.gov/ct2/show/NCT04383574?term=covid-19&cond=vaccine&cntry=CN&draw=2

[53]   https://clinicaltrials.gov/ct2/show/NCT04456595?term=vaccine&cond=covid-19&draw=2

[54]   http://www.chictr.org.cn/showprojen.aspx?proj=52227

[55]   https://www.nytimes.com/interactive/2020/science/coronavirus-vaccine-tracker.html

[56]   http://www.chictr.org.cn/showprojen.aspx?proj=56651

[57]   https://clinicaltrials.gov/ct2/show/NCT04412538?term=vaccine&cond=covid-19&draw=2

[58]   https://www.bharatbiotech.com/covaxin.html

[59]   https://clinicaltrials.gov/ct2/show/NCT04530357?term=vaccine&cond=covid-19&draw=4

[60]   Li L, Petrovsky N. Molecular mechanisms for enhanced DNA vaccine immunogenicity. Expert Rev Vaccines 2016; 15(3): 313-29.
[http://dx.doi.org/10.1586/14760584.2016.1124762] [PMID: 26707950]

[61]   Phase   I.   2019.https://clinicaltrials.gov/ct2/show/NCT04283461?term=vaccine&cond=covid-19&draw=2

[62]   Jackson LA, Anderson EJ, Rouphael NG, *et al.* An mRNA Vaccine against SARS-CoV-2 — preliminary report. N Eng J Med 2020; 383(20): 1920-31.
[http://dx.doi.org/10.1056/NEJMoa2022483] [PMID: 32663912]

[63]   https://clinicaltrials.gov/ct2/show/NCT04405076?term=moderna&cond=covid-19&draw=2&rank=1

[64]   https://clinicaltrials.gov/ct2/show/NCT04368728?term=vaccine&cond=covid-19&draw=3

[65]   http://www.chictr.org.cn/showprojen.aspx?proj=55524

[66]   http://www.isrctn.com/ISRCTN17072692

[67]   https://ir.arcturusrx.com/news-releases/news-release-details/

[68]   https://clinicaltrials.gov/ct2/show/NCT04480957?term=vaccine&cond=covid-19&draw=10

[69]   https://clinicaltrials.gov/ct2/show/NCT04449276?term=vaccine&cond=covid-19&draw=6

[70]   https://clinicaltrials.gov/ct2/show/NCT04515147?term=vaccine&cond=covid-19&draw=11

[71]   https://www.biospectrumasia.com/news/37/16171/genexine-enters-human-trial-of-co-id-19-vaccine.html

[72]   https://clinicaltrials.gov/ct2/show/NCT04445389?term=vaccine&cond=covid-19&draw=3

[73]   McKay BLP. Drugmakers rush to develop vaccines against china virus. Wall St J 2020.
https://www.wsj.com/articles/drugmakers-rush-to-develop-vaccines-against-china-virus11579813026

[74]   Inovio selected by cepi to develop vaccine against new coronavirus inovio. Inovio Pharmaceuticals Inc , 2020 [Accessed on 28 January 2020]; Available from: http://ir.inovio.com/news-and-media/news/press-release-details/2020/Inovio-Selected-byCEPI-to-Develop-Vaccine-Against-New-Coronavirus/default.aspx

[75]   https://clinicaltrials.gov/ct2/show/NCT04463472?term=NCT04463472&draw=2&rank=1

[76]   https://clinicaltrials.gov/ct2/show/NCT04334980

[77]   https://pipelinereview.com/index.php/2020021773810/Vaccines/

[78]   Zhang N, Tang J, Lu L, Jiang S, Du L. Receptor-binding domain-based subunit vaccines against MERS-CoV. Virus Res 2015; 202: 151-9.
[http://dx.doi.org/10.1016/j.virusres.2014.11.013] [PMID: 25445336]

[79]   https://clinicaltrials.gov/ct2/show/NCT04445194?term=longcom&draw=2

[80]   https://clinicaltrials.gov/ct2/show/NCT04466085?term=NCT04466085&draw=2&rank1

[81]   https://clinicaltrials.gov/ct2/show/NCT04368988?term=vaccine&recrs=a&cond=covid-19&draw=2

[82]   https://clinicaltrials.gov/ct2/show/NCT04533399?term=vaccine&cond=covid-19&draw=7

[83]   https://www.coronavirustoday.com/coronavirus-vaccines-0

[84]   https://clinicaltrials.gov/ct2/show/NCT04537208?term=sanofi&cond=sars-cov-2&draw=2&rank=1

[85]   https://clinicaltrials.gov/ct2/show/study/NCT04473690?term=vaccine&cond=covid-19&draw=3

[86]   https: //www.uq.edu.au/news/article/2020/01/race-develop-coronavirus-vaccine

[87]   https://www.anzctr.org.au/Trial/Registration/TrialReview.aspx?id=379861&isReview=true

[88]   Recombinant M. Monovalent recombinant covid19 vaccine (COVAX19). Clinicaltrialsgov , 2020 [Accessed on 1 Jul 2020]; Available from: https://clinicaltrials.gov/ct2/show/NCT04453852

[89]   https://clinicaltrials.gov/ct2/show/NCT04405908?term=clover&cond=covid-19&draw=2&rank=1

[90]   https://clinicaltrials.gov/ct2/show/study/NCT04487210?term=vaccine&cond=covid-19&draw=7

[91]   Mohsen MO, Zha L, Cabral-Miranda G, Bachmann MF. Major findings and recent advances in virus-like particle (VLP)-based vaccines. Semin Immunol 2017; 34: 123-32.
        [http://dx.doi.org/10.1016/j.smim.2017.08.014] [PMID: 28887001]

[92]   https://www.pharmaceutical-technology.com/news/medicago-covid-19-vaccine/

[93]   https://clinicaltrials.gov/ct2/show/NCT04450004?term=vaccine&cond=covid-19&draw=2

[94]   BCG vaccination to protect healthcare workers against COVID-19 (BRACE). 2020. https://clinicaltrials.gov/ct2/show/NCT04327206

[95]   https://clinicaltrials.gov/ct2/show/NCT04328441

[96]   https://clinicaltrials.gov/ct2/show/NCT04387409

SUBJECT INDEX

A

www.ingramcontent.com/pod-product-compliance
Lightning Source LLC
Chambersburg PA
CBHW050819220326
41598CB00006B/255